Handbook of Neurologic Music Therapy

Handbook of Neurologic Music Therapy

Edited by

Michael H. Thaut

Volker Hoemberg

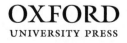

OXFORD
UNIVERSITY PRESS

OXFORD
UNIVERSITY PRESS

Great Clarendon Street, Oxford, OX2 6DP,
United Kingdom

Oxford University Press is a department of the University of Oxford.
It furthers the University's objective of excellence in research, scholarship,
and education by publishing worldwide. Oxford is a registered trade mark of
Oxford University Press in the UK and in certain other countries

© Oxford University Press 2014

The moral rights of the authors have been asserted

First published 2014
First published in paperback 2016

Published in the United States of America by Oxford University Press
198 Madison Avenue, New York, NY 10016, United States of America

British Library Cataloguing in Publication Data
Data available

Library of Congress Cataloging in Publication Data
Data available

ISBN 978-0-19-969546-1 (Hbk.)
ISBN 978-0-19-879261-1 (Pbk.)

Contents

The audio samples referred to in chapter 13 can be found at
www.oup.co.uk/companion/thaut

Contributors

Mutsumi Abiru MM MT-BC NMT Fellow
Department of Human Health Science,
Graduate School of Medicine,
Kyoto University, Kyoto, Japan

Miek de Dreu PhD
Faculty of Human Movement Science, VU
University, Amsterdam, The Netherlands

**Shannon K. de L'Etoile PhD MT-BC
NMT Fellow**
Frost School of Music, University
of Miami, Coral Gables, FL, USA

James C. Gardiner PhD
Neuropsychologist, Scovel Psychological
Counseling Services,
Rapid City, SD, USA

Volker Hoemberg MD
Head of Neurology, SRH Health Center,
Bad Wimpfen, Germany

**Sarah B. Johnson MM MT-BC NMT
Fellow**
Poudre Valley Health System, and
University of Colorado Health,
Fort Collins, CO, USA

Gert Kwakkel PhD
Department of Rehabilitation Medicine,
VU University Medical Center,
Amsterdam, The Netherlands, and
Department of Rehabilitation Medicine,
University Medical Center, Utrecht, The
Netherlands

A. Blythe LaGasse PhD MT-BC
Coordinator of Music Therapy,
Colorado State University School of
Music,
Fort Collins, CO, USA

Gerald C. McIntosh MD
Department of Neurology, University
of Colorado Health, Fort Collins,
CO, USA

Kathleen McIntosh PhD
Speech/Language Pathology,
University of Colorado Health,
Fort Collins, CO, USA

Stefan Mainka MM NMT Fellow
Department of Neurologic Music Therapy,
Hospital for Neurologic Rehabilitation
and Neurologic Special Hospital for
Movement Disorders/Parkinsonism,
Beelitz-Heilstaetten, Germany

Grit Mallien MS
Department of Speech Language
Pathology, Hospital for Neurologic
Rehabilitation and Neurologic Special
Hospital for Movement Disorders/
Parkinsonism, Beelitz-Heilstaetten,
Germany

Crystal Massie PhD OTR
UMANRRT Post-Doctoral Research
Fellow, Physical Therapy and
Rehabilitation Science Department,
University of Maryland School of
Medicine, Baltimore, MD, USA

Kathrin Mertel MM NMT Fellow
Department of Neurologic Music Therapy,
Universitätsklinikum Carl Gustav Carus,
Dresden, Germany

Audun Myskja MD PhD
Department of Geriatric Medicine,
Nord-Troendelag University College,
Steinkjer, Norway

Ruth Rice DPT
Department of Physical Therapy,
University of Colorado Health,
Fort Collins, CO, USA

Edward A. Roth PhD MT-BC
NMT Fellow
Professor of Music, Director, Brain
Research and Interdisciplinary
Neurosciences (BRAIN) Lab, School of
Music, Western Michigan University,
Kalamazoo, MI, USA

Corene P. Thaut PhD MT-BC
NMT Fellow
Program Director, Unkefer Academy
for Neurologic Music Therapy; Research
Associate, Center for Biomedical Research
in Music, Colorado State University, Fort
Collins, CO, USA

Michael H. Thaut PhD
Professor of Music, Professor of
Neuroscience, Scientific Director,
Center for Biomedical Research
in Music, Colorado State University,
Fort Collins, CO, USA

Erwin van Wegen PhD
Department of Rehabilitation
Medicine, VU University
Medical Center, Amsterdam,
Netherlands

Barbara L. Wheeler PhD
NMT Emeritus
Professor Emerita, School of Music,
Montclair State University,
Montclair, NJ, USA

Abbreviations

AAC	alternative and augmentative communication	MACT-SEL	MACT for selective attention skills
ADD	attention deficit disorder	MAL	Motor Activity Log
ADHD	attention deficit hyperactivity disorder	MD	mean difference
		MEFT	musical executive function training
ADL	activities of daily living	MEG	magnetoencephalography
AMMT	associative mood and memory training	MEM	musical echoic memory training
		MET	metabolic equivalent
AMTA	American Music Therapy Association	MIDI	musical instrument digital interface
AOS	apraxia of speech	MIT	melodic intonation therapy
APT	auditory perception training	MMIP	musical mood induction procedures
ASD	autism spectrum disorder	MMT	mood and memory training; musical mnemonics training
BATRAC	bilateral arm training with rhythmic auditory cueing	MNT	musical neglect training
BIAB	Band-in-a-Box	MPC	music in psychosocial training and counselling
bpm	beats per minute		
CBMT	Certification Board of Music Therapy	MPC-MIV	MPC mood induction and vectoring
CIMT	constraint-induced movement therapy	MPC-SCT	MPC social competence training
		MRI	magnetic resonance imaging
CIT	constraint-induced therapy	MSOT	musical sensory orientation training
COPD	chronic obstructive pulmonary disease	MUSTIM	musical speech stimulation
		NMT	neurologic music therapy
CPG	central pattern generator	OMREX	oral motor and respiratory exercises
CVA	cerebrovascular accident	PD	Parkinson's disease
DAS	developmental apraxia of speech	PECS	Picture Exchange Communication System
DMD	Duchenne muscular dystrophy		
DSLM	developmental speech and language training through music	PET	positron emission tomography
		PNF	proprioceptive neuromuscular facilitation
EBM	evidence-based medicine		
EEG	electroencephalography	PROMPT	prompts for restructuring oral muscular phonetic targets
EF	executive function		
EL	errorless learning	PRS	perceptual representation system
EMG	electromyography	PSE	patterned sensory enhancement
FFR	frequency following response	QoL	quality of life
FMA	Fugl-Meyer Assessment	QUIL	quick incidental learning
FOG	freezing of gait	RAS	rhythmic auditory stimulation
fMRI	functional magnetic resonance imaging	RCT	randomized controlled trial
		RMPFC	rostral medial prefrontal cortex
LITHAN	living in the here and now	ROM	range of motion
MACT	musical attention control training	RSC	rhythmic speech cueing

RSMM	rational scientific mediating model
SLI	specific language impairment
SLICE	step-wise limit cycle entrainment
SMD	standardized mean difference
SPT	sound production treatment
SYCOM	symbolic communication training through music
TBI	traumatic brain injury
TDM	transformational design model
TIMP	therapeutical instrumental music performance
TME	therapeutic music exercise

TMI	therapeutic music intervention
TS	therapeutic singing
TUG	Timed Up and Go (test)
UNS	*Untersuchung neurologisch bedingter Sprech- und Stimmstörungen*
UPDRS-II	Unified Parkinson's Disease Rating Scale-II
VAM	vigilance and attention maintenance
VIT	vocal intonation therapy
VMIP	Velten Mood Induction Procedure
WMFT	Wolf Motor Function Test

Chapter 1

Neurologic Music Therapy: From Social Science to Neuroscience

Michael H. Thaut, Gerald C. McIntosh, and Volker Hoemberg

1.1 Introduction

Modern music therapy, starting around the middle of the twentieth century, has traditionally been rooted mostly in social science concepts. The therapeutic value of music was considered to derive from the various emotional and social roles it plays in a person's life and a society's culture. Music has been given the age-old function of emotional expression, of creating and facilitating group association, integration, and social organization, of symbolically representing beliefs and ideas, and of supporting educational purposes.

However, the role of music in therapy has undergone some dramatic shifts since the early 1990s, driven by new insights from research into music and brain function. In particular the advent of modern research techniques in cognitive neuroscience, such as brain imaging and brain-wave recordings, has enabled us to study humans' higher cognitive brain functions *in vivo*. A highly complex picture of brain processes involved in the creation and perception of music has emerged. Brain research involving music has shown that music has a distinct influence on the brain by stimulating physiologically complex cognitive, affective, and sensorimotor processes. Furthermore, biomedical researchers have found not only that music is a highly structured auditory language involving complex perception, cognition, and motor control in the brain, but also that this sensory language can effectively be used to retrain and re-educate the injured brain.

The fascinating consequence of this research for music therapy has been a new body of neuroscientific research that shows effective uses of music with therapeutic outcomes that are considerably stronger and more specific than those produced within the general concept of "well-being." Research provides evidence that music works best in very different areas of therapeutic applications than was previously imagined or tried.

Translational biomedical research in music has led to the development of "clusters" of scientific evidence that show the effectiveness of specific music interventions. In the late 1990s, researchers and clinicians in music therapy, neurology, and the brain sciences began to classify these evidence clusters into a system of therapeutic techniques that are now known as *neurologic music therapy (NMT)*. This system has resulted in the unprecedented development of standardized clinical techniques supported by scientific evidence. Currently, the clinical core of NMT consists of 20 techniques that are defined by (1) the diagnostic treatment goal and (2) the role of the music—or mechanisms in the processes of music perception and music production—for achieving the treatment goal. This book will cover all 20 techniques from a clinician's point of view, including the technique definitions, diagnostic applications, research background, and—most importantly—examples of exercise protocols using each technique for clinical application. However, since NMT was developed out of a research database, it will continue to evolve, shaped by the emergence of new knowledge.

This transition is a very critical step in the historical understanding of music in therapy and medicine. Rather than being viewed as an ancillary and complementary discipline that can enhance other forms of "core" therapy, the therapeutic music exercises (TMEs) in NMT—applied within a neuroscientific framework—can be applied effectively in core areas of training or retraining of the injured brain, such as motor therapy, speech and language rehabilitation, and cognitive training.

By shifting one's notion of music in therapy from functioning as a carrier of sociocultural values in the therapeutic process to a stimulus that influences the neurophysiological basis of cognition and sensorimotor functions, a historical paradigm shift has emerged, driven by scientific data and insight into music and brain function. We can now postulate that music can access control processes in the brain related to control of movement, attention, speech production, learning, and memory, which can help to retrain and recover functions in the injured or diseased brain.

Six basic definitions articulate the most important principles of NMT:

1 NMT is defined as the therapeutic application of music to cognitive, affective, sensory, language, and motor dysfunctions due to disease or injury to the human nervous system.

2 NMT is based on neuroscientific models of music perception and music production and the influence of music on changes in non-musical brain and behavior function.

3 Treatment techniques are standardized in terminology and application, and are applied as TMEs which are adaptable to a patient's needs.

4 The treatment techniques are based on data from translational scientific research, and are directed towards non-musical therapeutic goals.

5 In addition to training in music and neurologic music therapy, practitioners are educated in the areas of neuroanatomy and physiology, neuropathology, medical terminology, and (re)habilitation of cognitive, motor, speech, and language functions.

6 NMT is interdisciplinary. Music therapists can meaningfully contribute to and enrich the effectiveness of treatment teams. Non-music therapists who are trained in other allied health professions can effectively adapt the principles and materials of NMT for use in their own certified practice.

1.2 **The rational scientific mediating model (RSMM)**

Music is an ancient intrinsic biological language of the human brain. Esthetically complex "modern" art works (e.g. statuettes, figurines, paintings, ornaments, functional musical instruments) appear with the advent of the modern human brain roughly 100,000 years ago—tens of thousands of years before artifacts of written language and numeracy.

Research now shows a fascinating reciprocal relationship between music and the brain. Music is a product of the human brain. However, the brain that engages in music is also changed by engaging in music. Brain changes due to music learning and performance have been well documented. However, music does not engage "music-specific" brain areas, but rather music processing engages in a highly distributed and hierarchical fashion—from spinal and various subcortical levels to cortical regions—"multimodal" brain areas that mediate general cognitive and motor control centers. There is also strong evidence that music shares processing centers with speech and language functions. One can safely say that music engages widely distributed neural networks that are shared with general "non-musical" cognitive, motor, and language function. This is an important rationale for understanding music as a "mediating" language in the therapy process. Music processing in the brain does not stop at music. Music processing can engage, train, and retrain non-musical brain and behavior function.

This is an important point for music in therapy, because it means that its theoretical models have to be based on an understanding of the processes involved in music perception first, before translational therapeutic concepts can be developed. This evolution of a path of discovery to translate music into a "mediating" language of therapy and rehabilitation is conceptualized in the rational scientific mediating model (RSMM) (Thaut, 2005).

There are suggestions in the music therapy literature that such a scientific anchoring of music therapy in psychological and physiological models of musical behavior was originally envisioned by pioneers such as Gaston (1968), Sears (1968), and Unkefer and Thaut (2002) in their thinking about the future foundations of music therapy. NMT has picked up these strands of early thinking and exploration, aiming to build them into a coherent scientific theory and clinical system.

The RSMM functions as an epistemological model—that is, a model to show ways of generating knowledge concerning the linkage between music and therapy. In the epistemological application, the RSMM helps us to know how to know, and to know how to investigate (or to learn how to learn). It does not predetermine the specific content of the mechanisms in music that produce therapeutic effects; it shows how to find them in a logical, systematic structure by linking the proper bodies of knowledge and showing what information is needed to logically support the next steps of inquiry and thus build a coherent theory.

The RSMM is based on the premise that the scientific basis of music therapy is found in the neurological, physiological, and psychological foundations of music perception and production. On this basis, the logical structure of the RSMM proceeds according to the following steps of investigation:

1 *musical response models*: investigating the neurological, physiological, and psychological foundations of musical behavior with regard to cognition and affect, speech/language, and motor control

   parallel non-musical response models: investigating overlaps and shared processes between musical and non-musical brain/behavior function in similar areas of cognition, speech/language, and motor control

   mediating models: investigating whether, where shared and overlapping processes are found, music can influence parallel non-musical brain and behavior functions

2 *clinical research models*: investigating, where mediating models are found, whether music can influence (re)learning and (re)training in therapy and rehabilitation.

1.2.1 Step 1: musical response models

In this step, the RSMM requires investigations into neurobiological and behavioral processes underlying music perception and performance in the areas of cognition, motor control, and speech/language.

Relevant questions addressed by research include, among others, the following:

◆ What processes in music learning build effective memories for music?

◆ Which processes in music shape and control musical attention?

◆ How do music perception and performance engage executive functions?

◆ What processes in music shape and influence mood and affective responses?

◆ How does music learning shape vocal control?

◆ What are the processes underlying effective musical motor control?

1.2.2 Step 2: parallel non-musical response models

In this step the RSMM requires a two-step investigative process, with each step built logically upon the other. In the first step, basic relevant concepts and mechanisms, as well as the structure and organization of non-musical processes in cognition, motor control, and speech/language function are investigated. In the second step, these findings are compared for shared processes in the parallel musical functions.

Relevant questions addressed by research include, among others, the following:

◆ Are there processes shared between non-musical and musical attention control, memory formation, executive operations, affective experiences, motor control, sensory perception, and speech/language perception and production?

◆ Are there shared processes in music that can enhance or optimize parallel non-musical functions?

If shared processes exist that may entail—at least theoretically or within the music domain—enhancing or optimizing mechanisms, the RSMM model would proceed to a third step, investigating this potential effect.

Three examples may illustrate this search for shared processes.

◆ Optimizing timing is critical for non-musical and musical motor learning. In music, motor timing is driven by the auditory rhythmic structure of the music. So can auditory rhythm as a temporal template not only facilitate motor learning on musical instruments, but also enhance neuromuscular control and motor planning in (re)training of functional non-musical upper and lower extremity movements?

◆ Music and speech, especially in singing, share multiple control processes with regard to auditory, acoustical, temporal, neuromuscular, neural, communicative, and expressive parameters. So can music—by engaging these shared parameters—enhance speech and language perception and production (e.g. by accessing alternative speech pathways, controlling timing of speech motor output, strengthening respiratory and neuromuscular speech control), enhance comprehension of communication symbols and language learning, or shape speech acoustics such as pitch, inflection, timbre, or loudness?

◆ Temporal processing (e.g. with regard to sequencing) plays an important role in cognitive functions such as attention, memory formation, and executive control. Music is an abstract auditory language that shapes attention, memory, and executive control to a large extent through its intrinsic temporal structure. So can musical structure enhance cognitive processes outside of music, such as non-musical attention and memory?

1.2.3 **Step 3: mediating models**

Investigations at this step proceed by building and studying hypotheses based on the discoveries in Step 2. The effect of music on non-musical behavior and brain function at this step may involve studies with healthy subjects or with clinical cohorts, but looking at mechanisms or short-term effects, providing evidence for the feasibility of future clinical research. For example, Step 3 research has investigated the effect of rhythmic-musical cues on motor control (gait, arms) or the effect of using musical instruments to simulate functional arm and hand movements in upper extremity rehabilitation. Studies have investigated whether speech fluency or intelligibility can be enhanced while following a rhythmic timing cue. Cognitive research has investigated whether musical mood vectoring changes the self-perceived mood state in healthy subjects or patients, and whether a song can be a mnemonic device or scaffold for remembering non-musical information ("ABC song"). If significant changes in non-musical behavior with clinical relevance due to music are found, the RSMM would proceed to Step 4.

1.2.4 **Step 4: clinical research models**

Research at this step takes the findings from Step 3 and applies them to investigations in a clinical, translational context. Step 4 research proceeds with patient populations and looks at meaningful therapeutic effects of music in (re)training brain and behavior function. Step 4 research studies the effects of interventions or intervention models on long-term learning and training. It is important to remember that NMT utilizes in most techniques the structural perceptual attributes of music to exercise therapeutic or rehabilitative functions or access alternative pathways to facilitate recovery and brain plasticity. Only the technique known as *music in psychosocial training and counseling (MPC)* also utilizes interpretative and emotionally expressive functions in musical responses for therapy. Exercises in the technique known as associative *mood and memory training (MMT)* are based on paradigms of learning and remembering through classical conditioning (Hilgard and Bower, 1975) and associative network theory mechanisms (Bower 1981) to connect mood and memory facilitation.

1.3 Summary

By following the principles of evidence-based medicine, neuroscience-guided rehabilitation, and data-driven therapy, NMT has quickly established itself within the mainstream of therapy and rehabilitation. Furthermore, NMT focuses on music as a biological language whose structural elements, sensory attributes, and expressive qualities engage the human brain comprehensively and in a complex manner. In NMT, music as a therapeutic agent does not operate as a cultural artifact, but rather it operates as core language of the human brain. In this way, the function of music as a language of learning and retraining the injured brain can be fully comprehended and appraised by clinicians, scientists, and musicians alike. NMT is advanced and evidence-based music therapy practice. However, since the basis for its techniques and the mechanisms whereby music affects the brain are based on neurobiological principles of brain and behavior, NMT allows music to be integrated into an interdisciplinary context of rehabilitation modalities.

References

Bower G H (1981). Mood and memory. *American Psychologist*, 36, 129–48.

Gaston E T (1968). *Music in Therapy*. New York: MacMillan Company.

Hilgard E L and Bower G H (1975). *Theories of Learning*. Englewood Cliffs, NJ: Prentice Hall.

Sears W W (1968). Processes in music therapy. In: E T Gaston (ed.), *Music in Therapy*. New York: Macmillan Company. pp. 30–46.

Thaut M H (2005). *Rhythm, Music, and the Brain: scientific foundations and clinical applications*. New York: Routledge.

Unkefer R F and Thaut M H (2002). *Music Therapy in the Treatment of Adults with Mental Disorders*. St Louis, MO: MMB Music.

Chapter 2

A Neurologist's View on Neurologic Music Therapy

Volker Hoemberg

All rehabilitation is aimed at improving the independence of the patient physically as well as psychologically, and at increasing their chances of engaging in activities of daily living by improving their functioning and abilities. One of the major routes for reaching the patient is language in its broadest and most comprehensive sense. In rehabilitation in particular it is very important that physicians, nurses, therapists, and caregivers speak to the patient and provide appropriate sensory stimulation. In this respect, music—conceived as a non-verbal auditory temporal language-like semantic and syntactic structure—can help to improve the patient's functioning. Therefore rehabilitative neurology is necessarily interested in exploiting music as a treatment tool.

Rhythm is a major characteristic of music. However, rhythmic oscillations also play a major role in the neurosciences. The human brain waves detected by electroencephalography (EEG) and magnetoencephalography (MEG) are very good examples of this. Higher-frequency oscillations in the gamma band (above 40 Hz) seem to provide clues to the understanding of elementary mechanisms involved in perception (Engel et al., 1999; Gold, 1999).

Central pattern generators located in the brainstem and spinal cord are essential for the control of locomotor abilities in vertebrates (Duysens and van de Crommert, 1998; Grillner and Wallen, 1985).

One of the intriguing questions arising in this context is whether a sensory stimulus such as music that has a complex spectral and temporal rhythmic–acoustic structure can shape the intrinsic rhythmic brain oscillations underlying cognitive, perceptual, and motor function (Crick and Koch, 1990).

Over the last decade, the focus of interest in the invention, design, and efficacy evaluation of motor therapies in neurorehabilitation has changed dramatically. This has involved three paradigmatic changes. First, there was a change from confession to profession (i.e. increasing use of evidence-based approaches, rather than intuitively driven procedures that followed unproven theoretical assumptions). Secondly, this development was accompanied by a change from "hands-on" treatment to "hands-off" coaching approaches, which now dominate most of the evidence procedures. This change in treatment philosophy has also had a marked impact on the self-understanding of the therapists as their relationship to the patient has changed from that of "treater" to that of teacher or coach. Thirdly, both of these developments were accompanied by a transition from intuitively marshaled individual one-to-one treatments to quality proven group treatments.

In parallel with the advances in the neurosciences and behavioral sciences during this period, a very large number of new approaches evolved to guide or refine statistical and biometric methods following the framework of evidence-based medicine (EBM). One prominent research element in EBM has been the emphasis on the design of randomized controlled trials (RCTs), which are increasingly being used to evaluate the efficacy of treatment approaches in neurorehabilitation (for a review, see Hoemberg, 2013).

- ◆ The classical physiotherapy schools such as the Bobath concept or the proprioceptive neuromuscular facilitation (PNF) concept and many more have been widely challenged on this basis. In addition, their claim to be based on sound principles of neurophysiology has received much criticism.

- ◆ In turn, the use of concepts of EBM has had an increasingly powerful influence on the selection of therapeutic procedures, especially in motor neurorehabilitation, and has influenced the drawing up of the best practice guidelines that are issued by many of the national societies for neurorehabilitation.

- ◆ The use of the evidence-based concepts has a number of advantages. In particular, it has a high biometric reliability in avoiding false-positive results (known in statistics as type I errors). Furthermore, within this framework the results from multiple RCTs can be condensed into meta-analyses, and the outcomes can help therapists and clinicians to be more critical when evaluating claims of the effectiveness of certain procedures.

However, there are also several disadvantages to relying exclusively on RCTs, which argue against the application of this rationale for decision making about treatment in neurorehabilitation. The concept of RCTs was primarily designed and is most often used for pharmacological studies, which usually involve fairly large numbers of patients. These studies are generally very expensive to conduct and are commonly sponsored by pharmaceutical companies. The EBM concept is not readily applicable to the small sample sizes and heterogeneous clinical populations that are often used in neurorehabilitation studies. A reliance on meta-analyses when making treatment decisions may introduce additional errors and sample biases. Finally, individual treatment responsivity (e.g. genetic predisposition) cannot be adequately addressed.

Therefore the question arises of the extent to which we should rely on EBM concepts when selecting treatment options. Are there other approaches that can be used to solve this dilemma for clinical practice? Certainly the results from RCTs and associated meta-analyses have to be very carefully read and interpreted in order to avoid statistical type II errors (i.e. false-negative results). Therefore we should probably place greater reliance on positive than on negative results of meta-analyses.

However, we also have to consider that there is other important scientific information available to the clinician that can be used to make evidence-based clinical decisions or to devise treatments. A wealth of scientific information is available offering insight into elementary rules and mechanisms of brain function—derived from neuroscientific and neurobehavioral studies—which we may find helpful when seeking rational forms of treatment even in the absence of evidence provided by the EBM framework. For example, as most approaches in motor rehabilitation are related to motor learning, elementary knowledge about motor learning derived from the neurosciences and behavioral sciences can offer clues to the design of new and effective therapeutic strategies.

Box 2.1 gives a list of such elementary rules which can be derived from studies of motor learning, and which may be used to design or refine therapeutic strategies in motor rehabilitation.

The single most important elementary rule in motor learning is probably repetition. A high number of repetitions are necessary to optimize movement trajectories. Elegant studies conducted in healthy subjects (Fitts and Posner, 1967) as well as in patients (Bütefisch et al., 1995; Sterr et al., 2002) have demonstrated the power of this rule.

The next important elementary rule is the use of feedback (i.e. informing the learner or patient about the progress of the quality and accuracy of their motor behavior). For this principle, too, elegant experimental studies have provided ample evidence (for a nice example, see Mulder and Hulstijn, 1985).

The presence of external cues is another important rule for guiding the patient, especially in the absence of sufficient intrinsic cues to control movement. Cues that provide information for the anticipation and planning of movement are of particular importance. Here rhythmic temporal cues can play a particularly critical role (Thaut et al., 1999a).

Furthermore, for optimal learning it is important to keep the learner at an optimal level of motivation. For this purpose, task difficulty has to be adjusted or "shaped" to balance the learner's abilities with the difficulty of the task. The teacher has to avoid both creating a boring situation (by using task elements that are too easy) and triggering frustration (by using tasks that are too difficult). In this sense it is the role of the therapist or coach to select the optimally appropriate level of task difficulty.

Box 2.1 Elementary rules for learning-oriented motor therapy

- Repetition
- Feedback (knowledge of results)
- Cueing
- Task orientation
- Active learning
- Ecological validity
- Shaping (adjusting task difficulty to the patient's abilities)
- Motivation

In addition, the selected task should be oriented to real-life situations in order to allow an effective transfer into the day-to-day behavior that the patient wants to be prepared for. This means avoiding tasks that are too "abstract" or "unrealistic", and instead selecting motor acts that have functional relevance.

The techniques and principles of neurologic music therapy (NMT) blend nicely with both the EBM approach and the new concepts of motor rehabilitation that are rooted in elementary motor learning rules. The first and most important step toward a neuro-biologically based use of music in the treatment of patients with motor problems was the scientific development of the technique of *rhythmic auditory stimulation (RAS)*.

The therapeutic principles and underlying neurophysiologic mechanisms were primarily developed at the laboratory of Michael Thaut and colleagues at Colorado State University. The basic idea behind this concept is that a repetitive rhythmic acoustic sensory signal can entrain and facilitate rhythmic movements.

It has been shown that RAS helps to improve motor function in patients with a variety of locomotor problems, such as those with Parkinson's disease (Thaut et al., 2001), Huntington's disease (Thaut et al., 1999b), and stroke (Thaut et al., 1993a, 1993b, 1997). The findings of Michael Thaut's group have been extensively replicated and extended by other groups, especially in the areas of stroke and Parkinson's disease.

Neuroimaging studies have recently shown that clearly defined parietal, frontal, and cerebellar areas are involved in the processing of rhythmicity (Thaut et al., 2009). By organizing upper extremity movements or full body coordination into patterned sequences that can be cyclically repeated, these movements can also be rhythmically cued. As an example of this approach, a study using auditory rhythmic cueing as patterned sensory enhancement (PSE) showed significant reductions in paretic arm-reaching trajectories after stroke (Thaut et al., 2002).

The mechanism underlying the facilitatory influence on movement organization and control is based on the theory of rhythmic entrainment, in which acoustical rhythms entrain neural responses in auditory and motor structures, and with regard to cueing of gait couple into central pattern generators in the brainstem and spinal cord (Duysens and van de Crommert, 1998).

Over the past decade, translational research in music and brain function has driven the broadening of the scope of neurologic music therapy to address non-motor functions as well, such as perception, cognition, linguistics, and emotion. Music provides a uniquely richly textured and temporally structured auditory environment that offers efficient stimuli to shape auditory attention, to overcome hemispatial neglect, to create basal sensory stimulation for disorders of consciousness, to offer mnemonic "scaffolds" for memory training, to access and train alternative language centers in the brain, or to challenge and exercise "creative reasoning strategies" in executive function training.

It is safe to say that the research evidence and learning and training rationales for NMT are at least as well evidenced and supported by valid rationales as they are for its sister disciplines in rehabilitation and therapy. Neurologic music therapists are not specialized in separate sub-diagnoses or specific cognitive or motor behaviors. They are specialists in technique and stimulus, which are applied to a broad range of developmental, behavioral, and neurologic disorders, and in this context they become extremely important "connecting" core members of efficient interdisciplinary patient-oriented treatment teams.

References

Bütefisch, C., Hummelsheim, H., Denzler, P., and Mauritz, K. H (1995). Repetitive training of isolated movements improves the outcome of motor rehabilitation of the centrally paretic hand. *Journal of the Neurological Sciences, 130*, 59–68.

Crick, F. and Koch, C. (1990). Towards a neurobiological theory of consciousness. *Seminars in the Neurosciences, 2*, 263–75.

Duysens, J. and van de Crommert, H. W. A. A. (1998). Neural control of locomotion; Part 1: The central pattern generator from cats to humans. *Gait and Posture, 7*, 131–41.

Engel, A. K. et al. (1999). Temporal binding, binocular rivalry, and consciousness. *Consciousness and Cognition, 8*, 128–51.

Fitts P and Posner M (1967). *Human Performance*. Belmont, CA: Brooks/Cole Publishing Co.

Gold, I. (1999). Does 40-Hz oscillation play a role in visual consciousness? *Consciousness and Cognition, 8*, 186–95.

Grillner, S. and Wallen, P. (1985). Central pattern generators for locomotion, with special reference to vertebrates. *Annual Review of Neuroscience, 8*, 233–61.

Hoemberg V. (2013). Neurorehabilitation approaches to facilitate motor recovery. In: M Barnes and D Good (eds), *Handbook of Clinical Neurology. Volume 10*. New York: Elsevier. pp. 161–74.

Mulder, T. and Hulstijn, W. (1985). Sensory feedback in the learning of a novel motor task. *Journal of Motor Behavior, 17*, 110–28.

Sterr, A., Freivogel, S., and Voss, A. (2002). Exploring a repetitive training regime for upper limb hemiparesis in an in-patient setting: a report on three case studies. *Brain Injury, 16*, 1093–107.

Thaut, M. H., McIntosh, G. C., Rice, R. R., and Prassas, S. G. (1993a). The effect of auditory rhythmic cuing on stride and EMG patterns in persons residing in the community after stroke: a placebo-controlled randomized trial. *Archives of Physical Medicine and Rehabilitation, 84*, 1486–91.

Thaut, M. H., McIntosh, G. C., Rice, R. R., and Prassas S. G. (1993b). The effect of auditory rhythmic cuing on stride and EMG patterns in hemiparetic gait of stroke patients. *Journal of Neurologic Rehabilitation, 7*, 9–16.

Thaut, M. H., McIntosh, G. C., and Rice, R. R. (1997). Rhythmic facilitation of gait training in hemiparetic stroke rehabilitation. *Journal of the Neurological Sciences, 151*, 207–12.

Thaut M H, Kenyon G, Schauer M L, and McIntosh G C (1999a). The connection between rhythmicity and brain function: implications for therapy of movement disorders. *IEEE Engineering in Medicine and Biology Magazine, 18*, 101–8.

Thaut, M. H et al. (1999b). Velocity modulation and rhythmic synchronization of gait in Huntington's disease. *Movement Disorders, 14*, 808–19.

Thaut, M. H., McIntosh, G. C., McIntosh, K. W., and Hoemberg, V (2001). Auditory rhythmicity enhances movement and speech motor control in patients with Parkinson's disease. *Functional Neurology, 16*, 163–72.

Thaut, M. H et al. (2002). Kinematic optimization of spatiotemporal patterns in paretic arm training with stroke patients. *Neuropsychologia, 40*, 1073–81.

Thaut, M. H et al. (2009). Distinct cortico-cerebellar activations in rhythmic auditory motor synchronization. *Cortex, 45*, 44–53.

Chapter 3

Music Technology for Neurologic Music Therapy

Edward A. Roth

3.1 Introduction

The sophistication, acoustic authenticity, and ease of use of electronic music technologies have improved greatly and contributed to the proliferation in their use over the last 10 to 15 years. However, as a group, music therapists have perhaps been slower to embrace these technologies in their clinical work, often favoring the use of traditional instruments. It seems that both an inclination toward and a reticence about the use of technology in music therapy exist among clinicians, fueled by a number of factors. Some have turned to technology for assistance because the requirements of therapeutic service delivery to individuals and groups of clients can exceed those that one therapist can provide. Others have utilized technology to facilitate activity and interaction among those who are most severely physically impaired, so that maximal sound is achieved through minimal action. Paradoxically, this very issue is what causes some clinicians to be disinclined to utilize one or any of the music technologies in their practice. Cost may seem prohibitive to some, in addition to concern about investing in hardware and software technologies that will quickly become obsolete or require ongoing expenses to remain current.

Wendy Magee has reported that music therapists in the UK and the USA seem to agree on a key element of music technology in healthcare, in that they generally view electronic music technology as capable of providing access to clients and therapists alike (Magee, 2006, 2011; Magee and Burland, 2008). Magee asserts that more clinicians would probably utilize the various technologies if they had a better understanding of how to select the various tools based on their capabilities, appropriate populations, applications, and intended outcomes. Although this chapter cannot be exhaustive toward that effort, due to restrictions on its length, and moreover we do not want to provide so much detail that the novice is overwhelmed (a common complaint), an overview is provided as well as introductory applications of electronic hardware (instruments), software, and hand-held devices.

3.2 Musical instrument digital interface (MIDI)

Before the available hardware and software are discussed, the device or "language" that allows the two to communicate with each other will be addressed. If you have explored the use of technology in music applications, you are likely to have used, heard of, or read about

MIDI. The *musical instrument digital interface (MIDI)* has been a major development and force driving the explosive growth in music technology in the last 15 to 20 years, allowing musicians at all levels of skill to utilize electronic instruments for performance and compositional purposes. Its onset dates back to the early 1980s, with the original goal of allowing electronic instruments from different manufacturers to connect with each other using the same electronic coding to control various note, timing, patch (instrument), and pedal events. This was originally achieved by simply cabling the instruments to each other and to a single controller, which was eventually replaced when computers became available.

3.2.1 The basics

The first—and typically most daunting—issue for first-time MIDI users is simply how to connect all of their MIDI-capable equipment, including instruments, computers, interfaces, and sound output/amplification devices. All MIDI instruments come equipped with a series of ports for sending information to and receiving it from other instruments and/or a controller, sound module, or computer. The instruments connect by cabling via MIDI IN, MIDI OUT, and MIDI THRU ports (or jacks or receptacles, if you prefer). The MIDI IN ports receive information, the MIDI OUT ports send information, and the MIDI THRU ports allow multiple instruments to be "daisy-chained" to each other. One simple rule of thumb to remember, no matter what types of MIDI instruments, interfaces, or other devices you are connecting, is that the connection between two ports is always via MIDI IN to MIDI OUT (see Figure 3.1).

One way to conceptualize it is that each port performs import or export functions—MIDI OUT exports to MIDI IN, which imports. There are exceptions, of course, and one example is connecting a computer to a single device such as a musical keyboard. In this

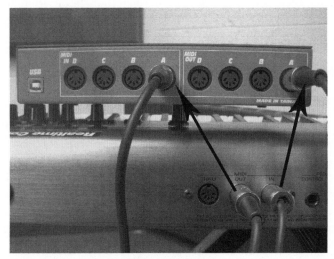

Fig. 3.1 Main connections between sound source (MIDI keyboard at bottom) and MIDI interface (at top).

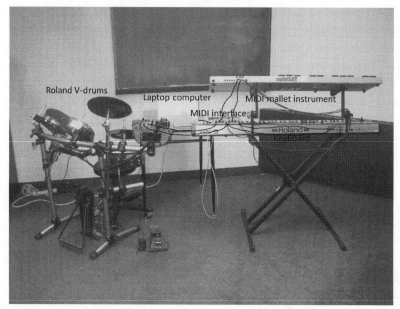

Fig. 3.2 MIDI workstation, including laptop computer, keyboard, drum set, and mallet instrument all connected through the MIDI interface.

case, you may only need to run a single cable from the USB port on your computer to the MIDI *or* USB port(s) on your keyboard. More often, however, an intermediary device known as a MIDI interface is required to connect your computer to your instruments, and in particular if you have more than one instrument, for example, a MIDI keyboard, drum set, guitar, and mallet instrument. The series of connections begins from the USB port on your computer to the USB port on the MIDI interface, and then the series of connections between the interface and various instruments (see Figure 3.2).

3.3 **Hardware**

3.3.1 **Instruments and triggers**

Virtually all MIDI-based instruments function in one form or another as a trigger. That is to say, the player of the instrument applies force by striking, strumming, or supplying air pressure to a series of sensors inside the instrument, which actuates a sound. Regardless of the shape and appearance of the instrument, it sends a similar signal to some source of sound generation, usually a keyboard or computer. It does not matter whether the instrument is an electronic keyboard, string, mallet, or wind-based device—they all function as transmitters of numerical data that represent the various note on/off signals, timbres, velocities, duration, and amplitude profiles of any given sound. These data are converted into sounds that are selected by the player or therapist. Depending on the type and quality, instruments have varying degrees of responsiveness to force, and many can be calibrated so that the amplitude of the sound playback requires greater or lesser force depending on the client's therapeutic needs. As mentioned earlier, this provides clients who have limited mobility—due to either strength or range-of-motion issues—to effect maximum sound by only lightly touching an instrument. Of course, the opposite is true as well, in that the instruments can be calibrated so that they have to be played with greater force, perhaps even more than on an acoustic version of the instrument—for example, to evoke a sound in an exercise to develop strength.

3.3.1.1 Keyboards

For most MIDI workstations, the computer and keyboard function as the two central op-erating devices. In some set-ups, the keyboard functions as either the single or central unit by which music is produced and therapeutic exercises are delivered, and there is a wide range of MIDI-capable keyboards with a spectrum of capabilities and prices. If you are simply looking for a keyboard that functions as a lightweight and portable piano, with two and a half to four octave ranges, prices at the time of writing can be found under US$ 100. On the other hand, if you require keyboards with weighted or semi-weighted keys, that have sound banks which include hundreds of sounds (including single instrument sounds, full band and orchestral accompaniment, "nature" sounds, theatrical sound effects, and so on), prices vary widely from a few hundred to several thousand dollars. Determining how you will use your keyboard will help you to decide which will best suit your needs. Will you travel from room to room within a single building? Will patients travel to you to engage in therapy in your clinic, studio, or therapy room? Do you have to use a car to travel from site to site? Will you or your clients actually play the keyboard or are you using it simply as a sound source for other MIDI instruments? If the clients are going to play the keyboard, for what purposes will they play it? Will it be for strength and dexterity exercises, such as in therapeutical instrumental music performance (TIMP), or for cognition, affect, and/or social experiences, such as in musical attention control training (MACT), musical execu-tive function training (MEFT), or music in psychosocial training and counseling (MPC)? If your clients will actually play the keyboard in order to develop strength and coordina-tion, a keyboard with weighted or semi-weighted keys is preferable as it provides resistance and a stronger finish point to each keystroke, both of which are useful in rehabilitation exercises. Alternatively, if you require greater portability or you will primarily use your keyboard as a sound bank with minimal musical input, a keyboard (or MIDI controller) without weighted keys, with a smaller number of keys, and that can be easily fitted into a small case or bag will be more useful for you. There are many brands available, and Casio, Kawai, Korg, Kurzweil, M-Audio, Roland, and Yamaha all produce multiple keyboards for you to consider.

If you work in a clinic or your use of a keyboard does not require portability, and you have an ample budget, the Yamaha Disklavier can be an enormously useful instrument in rehabilitation therapy. In one sense, it is a modern version of a player piano in that it is an acoustic instrument that can "play itself", but it has capabilities that far surpass this simple explanation. For instance, a neurologic music therapist can record a series of cueing sequences to be used for TIMP and PSE exercises with clients, and the Disklavier will provide an exact replication of the therapist's recording in real time so that the therapist can physically assist the client if necessary. Furthermore, because the information is stored digitally, it can be manipulated to adjust for individual patient needs with minimal effort and disruption to the therapy session. Its authenticity as an acoustic instrument is highly desirable, perhaps, and its ability to function as a MIDI instrument makes it a perfect match between the desire for a "real" instrument and the access that is created through its technological capabilities. A significant obstacle to using the Disklavier in therapy can be its price tag, which often is the equivalent of total annual expenses or exceeds the budget for many therapy departments and individual practitioners.

3.3.1.2 Drums and percussion

Multiple electronic and digital percussion options exist, including drum sets, drum modules, hand drums, and mallet instruments.

- *Drums.* Drum sets are produced and distributed by multiple companies. Alesis, Roland, Simmons, and Yamaha all produce multiple and useful models with prices ranging from approximately US$ 400 to US$ 3,000. Differences in capabilities include available sounds, on-board recording, number of drum and cymbal pads, quality of hardware, whether or not strike sensitivity can be calibrated, and the material used for drum "heads", which ranges from soft rubber to a flexible nylon-like material, or real drum shells and heads on the higher-end models. These drum sets are particularly useful in TIMP exercises, as they allow for spatial configuration and provide scalable angular modification for lower/upper extremity and trunk control training.

- *Hand drums.* Roland also produces a digital hand drum called the HandSonic that includes a great deal of the technology used in their V-drums drum sets. It includes 15 separate pads that can trigger up to 15 different sounds simultaneously, so it can be used in both individual and small group therapy (15 people cannot fit around the instrument to play it at the same time). The HandSonic 15 includes over 300 percussion sounds, including typical band and orchestral instruments as well as traditional instruments from around the world. The authenticity of the sound is rather remarkable, and when played in conjunction with other percussion instruments, depending on the quality of the amplification system, it is difficult to tell the difference between the acoustic instruments and their reproduced counterparts on the HandSonic. Similar to the V-drums (and other similar digital drum sets), the pads are touch-sensitive so they allow greater expressivity and can be calibrated for use in TIMP exercises based on the client's rehabilitation needs. (*For individuals who are experiencing extreme weakness, the HandSonic and other MIDI percussion instruments present a potential latency issue, where the sound occurs with a delayed onset in relation to the patient's touch.*) The HandSonic includes MIDI IN/OUT jacks, so it can be used to record patient performance for playback and analysis as well as to receive a MIDI signal from a computer or other device. At the time of writing its retail price is approximately US$ 1,200.

◆ *Mallet instruments.* The MalletKat is a MIDI-based mallet instrument that has the appearance of an acoustic vibraphone. It differs from an acoustic xylophone and marimba in that the row of chromatic "black keys" (as they relate to a piano) is not vertically raised above the main row of keys. It comes with three octaves as standard, and expansion models can be purchased that extend its range to four or five octaves. The pads are made of a soft foam-like material, and are intended to be played with marimba or vibraphone mallets. This instrument has been useful in motor exercises such as those involving range of motion at the shoulder, elbow, and wrist. Like other MIDI triggers, it can produce any sound available from the sound source, providing a great deal of flexibility depending on the purpose of the therapeutic exercise.

3.3.1.3 Wind instruments

MIDI-based wind controllers work in a similar way to their percussion counterparts in that they serve as a source of data—created by playing the instrument—that are sent to a sound source (often a keyboard or computer, although sound modules now appear on most models) for audio output. The main difference, of course, is that passing air over a pressure-sensitive sensor and bite plate rather than striking a key or pad produces the sound. Use of these instruments in TIMP (for finger dexterity, strength, and coordination) and OMREX (for oral motor and respiratory exercises) can be useful. Most models allow for various fingering configurations that are customizable for individual client needs. Like other MIDI triggers, "performance" data can be collected, analyzed, and expressed to demonstrate the client's recovery in quantifiable terminology. However, the data are expressed in digital music parameters, not clinical language, so translating the musical data (e.g. velocity and duration of exhalation) into clinically relevant outcomes is a process required of the therapist. Akai and Yamaha produce several models, with prices ranging from US$ 300 to US$ 700 at the time of writing.

3.3.2 Movement sensors

3.3.2.1 Soundbeam

Soundbeam is a motion-sensor-based system that converts physical movement through space into sound. Where other systems utilize video-based sonification systems (Lem and Paine, 2011), the Soundbeam tracks the perturbation of a signal (or beam) generated by the device and sends it back to the sensor for sonification, via either MIDI or an available sound module. Like other MIDI trigger devices, it sends data back to its own sound module or to a computer for conversion into audio output. Similar to other MIDI instruments, the sound that is produced is based on the available sounds on the module, keyboard, or computer to which it is connected. As a person moves their whole body, individual body part, or even an instrument such as a drum stick or mallet through space, the sensor(s) track the movement and send spatial data back to the sound source for conversion and sound production. This takes place at a speed that provides the experience of simultaneous movement to sound reproduction. The distance and amount of movement required to access the full spectrum of sound available can be calibrated so that clients who have limited mobility, as well as those who can move freely through space, are able to access the entire multi-octave spectrum, whether it be through a few centimeters or several meters of movement. Soundbeam may be a useful tool in recovery through interventions that include musical sensory orientation training (MSOT), TIMP, PSE, and MPC.

In the later stages of recovery of consciousness through an MSOT experience, the patient can reconnect their physical behavior to the outside world with the auditory feedback provided as a result of their movement. Because the sound is electronically produced, volume levels can be adjusted to clinically appropriate levels, and harmonic structures can be electronically calibrated to include only desirable pitch combinations or sequences.

Soundbeam can be an effective tool in TIMP exercises in that it allows the sensor to be aimed at an instrument selected by the therapist and/or client, calibrated so that it is triggered by movement similar in space to its acoustic counterpart, and maximum sound can be created with minimal movement through volume control. This is an important clinical consideration that should be monitored closely by the therapist so that the client experiences success afforded by the device, but is continually challenged toward improvement by not using Soundbeam to overcompensate for deficits in movement.

The applications of Soundbeam to PSE expand beyond the following description, but have been primarily useful in the creation of the auditory cueing sequences used in PSE experiences. If connected to a computer, a therapist can record a movement sequence to later be practiced by the client, such as sit-to-stand exercises, and the spatial and temporal characteristics of the movement are captured by the Soundbeam sensors, which can later be used to produce the optimal auditory cueing sequences. An important missing feature is the ability of Soundbeam to capture and reproduce force characteristics of a given movement sequence. This will have to be done via software manipulation so that the cueing of muscle contraction and release sequences is appropriately conveyed through dynamic expressions in the sound.

The use of Soundbeam in MPC is valuable as it allows clients who have very limited mobility to actively engage in improvisational experiences purposefully, "equally", and in a manner that is esthetically pleasing.

3.3.3 Digital hand-held devices

Hand-held music devices are arguably the most widely utilized music technology in the general population and, as such, perhaps the most familiar to people as they begin therapy (Nagler, 2011).

3.3.3.1 iPod/iPad

Just as it is difficult to adequately describe all the features and applications of the various electronic instruments and software identified in this chapter, it is impossible to do so for the iPad and iPod manufactured by Apple Inc. Both have the tremendous advantage of being portable playback devices that are useful in the delivery of several therapeutic music interventions (TMIs), including but not limited to RAS, TIMP, and MPC-MIV. The iPod has been a useful tool in the delivery of ambulation training exercises, in that the songs used for auditory–motor cueing can be saved in a playlist at multiple frequencies (e.g. 60 bpm, 63 bpm, 66 bpm) and presented based on the client's current state of functioning and rehabilitative progress. Headphones can be used when ecologically required, and a headphone splitter can be utilized so that the client and therapist both hear the music simultaneously. This is particularly helpful when a patient requires hands-on assistance for mobility, making it impossible for the neurologic music therapist to provide a live cue.

There are also many music-based software applications (apps) that have been created for the iPad and iPod, and which turn these devices into electronic sequencers, loop generators/recorders, composition aids, and touch-sensitive instruments. Some apps provide all three (and other) capabilities, so that the client can create a chord progression, add preloaded or acoustically recorded loops, and improvise by tapping instrument images that then reproduce the appropriate related timbres. In addition to the facilitation of domain-specific goal attainment (e.g. motor, speech, cognition), these devices can be successfully utilized to reduce the social isolation and withdrawal that are so commonly observed during hospitalization and long-term treatment.

3.3.3.2 Kaossilator

The Kaossilator, produced by Korg, functions by creating sound in response to manipulation of a touch pad on the face of the device. It provides the capability to create musical and rhythm-only phrases by converting the manner in which a "player" touches the touch pad and produces sound sequences through bass, realistic instrument sounds, electronic instrument sounds, and percussion sequences or drum beats. As well as being a touch-activated synthesizer, it functions as a loop recorder in that multiple tracks that are 1, 2, 4, 8, or 16 beats long can be input and stacked on top of each other to produce a rich arrangement of grooves, beats, and effects. When functioning in this way it can be a useful tool in the compositional application of MEFT to aid the development of decision-making and organizational skills. In a similar way to the Soundbeam, the Kaossilator can be a useful instrument in an MSOT exercise in that clients with extremely limited mobility, dexterity, and strength can manipulate the sound in satisfying ways with small finger movements across the touch pad. Because of its motivational qualities for some patients, the Kaossilator may be an effective tool in compositional exercises aimed at mood modification within an MPC format. Prices at the time of writing are in the range US$ 120–350.

3.4 Software

3.4.1 GarageBand

GarageBand is Mac-specific software produced by Apple Inc. as part of the iLife suite that has multiple applications for the use of music in rehabilitation therapy. Although it has many functions with several creative applications, at its core GarageBand is music-sequencing software that includes hundreds of digital and pre-recorded audio loops, as well as serving as an on-board mixer and recording studio for live acoustic instruments. By utilizing the loops that come with the basic software and those available for secondary purchase, therapists and clients can create compositions in a series of "tracks"—for instance, in an MEFT intervention. The client can be given or asked to provide a relevant theme or scenario on which to build their composition. Directions to select appropriate musical representations of some aspect of their chosen theme or scene from the available loops (which also include a series of sound effects) require the client to exercise both abstract thinking and decision-making behavior. Layering the different tracks and timbres on top of each other allows the practicing of sequencing and organizational skills, as the client is encouraged to consider and select those compositional features that best fit each other to represent their chosen compositional theme. Live recordings of acoustic instruments and voice can be directly added as tracks into the composition. This is just one simple example, and the software provides for a wide range of complex features in a simple-to-learn format for recording, performance, and improvisational purposes.

3.4.2 **Band-in-a-Box**

Band-in-a-Box (BIAB) is music composition software, produced by PG Music, which utilizes a lead-sheet visual interface for song composition in both Windows and Mac formats. The user simply inputs their chords as they would on a jazz/pop/rock lead sheet (e.g. C, F7, Dm, G13b9), selects from the hundreds of available style presets, and BIAB creates a stylistically congruent arrangement that typically includes piano, bass, drums, guitar, and strings or horns. The quality of the arrangements has improved dramatically over the years, and the software now includes digitally recorded samples, which increases the quality of the audio output as well. With simple technical manipulations, compositions can be tailored for specific use in clinical applications, such as the ability to "trade 4's" during improvisation, change the tempo in real time, and follow a compositional map through a series of repeats that are also individually customizable. This is useful in performance and improvisational experiences. The software can utilize the on-board sounds of a computer, and is MIDI-compatible, so it can access and utilize the sounds of the user's MIDI keyboard. One useful feature is the ability to save songs in MIDI (.mid) format and export them to another application (e.g. GarageBand) for further editing, conversion to.mp3 or AAC formats, and export to a portable music device.

3.4.3 **Ableton Live**

Ableton Live is a powerful software application that, among many other compositional and improvisational functions, allows the user to import and manipulate pre-recorded music. For example, when you need to create music for a client to use during ambulation training (RAS), and you want to utilize the client's preferred music without the esthetically diluting effects of creating MIDI-based or even live versions of the piece, Ableton Live allows you to manipulate the original recording so that it becomes clinically useful. After assessing the client's musical preferences and determining which songs most closely match his or her current resonant frequency, you can import them into Ableton Live and manipulate the tempo without impairing the presentation of tonality (e.g. decrease the tempo without lowering the pitch, increase the tempo without increasing the pitch). This functionality is available in multiple applications. However, Ableton Live is particularly useful in that it allows you to embed a metronomic click on the strong beats to cue heel strikes using a timbre of your choice (e.g. clave, woodblock, cowbell, etc.), and it also gives you the capability to create amplitude modulation patterns so that the strong beats in the music are accented. This is a scalable feature, so you can create music that is esthetically compatible with the client without sacrificing the necessary cueing for optimal motor synchronization.

3.5 Brain–computer music interfacing and music video games in rehabilitation

Attempts have been made over the last few years to improve the process by which brain activity, which is typically detected and analyzed by electroencephalography (EEG), is used to create music. In a gross simplification for the purposes of brevity, the most common approach involves the conversion of EEG signals into musical sequences based on the translation of mathematical representations of brain activity into some pre-determined musical analog as a form of auditory biofeedback. The notion is that as the patient gains the ability to control some function or behavior (e.g. eye-gaze, level of arousal, state of attention), they are essentially gaining control over their brain activity and resultant musical output. Miranda et al. (2011) have reported in a proof-of-concept paper the successful use of such a system with an adult patient who had experienced a stroke. The patient was able to quickly understand and utilize the procedures toward the intended behavioral and musical outcomes. Miranda and colleagues suggest that for patients who have acquired severe physical limitations as a result of damage to the central nervous system, this type of brain–music interface system could be employed to provide them with the ability to exercise control over their environment while engaging in active music-making experiences for cognitive and emotional rehabilitation. These researchers argue for the application of the system with the goal of increased socialization through simultaneous use of multiple units in a group format.

People who have experienced neurological damage or disease commonly show loss of emotional stability and sense of self. Benveniste et al. (2012) argue for the use of music in a video-game format for patients who have Alzheimer's disease and are struggling with issues related to the obvious—cognitive atrophy—as well as with social isolation, emotional withdrawal, and related self-esteem issues. They report the use of the Nintendo Wii platform for the delivery of music improvisation and performance experiences for people with mild to moderate Alzheimer's disease. In both modalities, the patient—with assistance from a therapist—points the Wiimote (hand-held remote) at a television or video screen which controls a white dot that appears over a sequence of 8 or 12 preselected notes. When the patient clicks the Wiimote, it causes whichever note they are aiming at to sound. The authors readily acknowledge the high level of assistance required by the participants, and actually highlight feedback from the participants indicating that the human interaction required during the music-making experiences was highly pleasurable and rewarding. Parameters of the task, audio output, and on-screen images allowed the participants to experience musical success, resulting in vivid and comprehensive recollections, which the participants experienced as motivating and socially connecting. The authors designed what they refer to as "failure-free gameplay", and they emphasize the musical interaction aspect that the game requires and facilitates.

As great progress has been made toward the useful adaptation and application of music technology in clinical scenarios, further refinement is required to avoid the need to compromise clinical logic or esthetic quality in the delivery of therapeutic music interventions. Ramsey (2011) has identified several salient issues in the development of music hardware and software to be used specifically in rehabilitation medicine. These issues are reflected in the description of instrument and software applications that differ from available MIDI and other electronic resources in that they are being developed for the specific purpose of motor rehabilitation therapy. They appear to be in prototype stages of development, but a cursory review indicates the potential for promising results. Until such software and instruments are available commercially, music therapists will probably need to continue to modify and translate both MIDI hardware and software applications for purposeful use in the delivery of music therapy services.

While simultaneous enthusiasm and counter-indications exist for the use of music technology in therapy and medicine (Whitehead-Pleaux et al., 2011), maintaining a focus on the clinical application of technology is an important feature of the delivery of clinically relevant experiences that conform to good therapeutic logic. As others have cautioned (Magee et al., 2011), keeping the therapeutic process at the forefront when designing technology-assisted experiences should help the neurologic music therapist to avoid the allure of technology-centered approaches and be well positioned to utilize the existing technologies to develop exciting therapeutic goal-centered care.

References

Benveniste, S., Jouvelot, P., Pin, B., and Péquignot, R. (2012). The MINWii project: renarcissization of patients suffering from Alzheimer's disease through video game-based music therapy. *Entertainment Computing*, 3, 111–20.

Lem, A. and Paine, G. (2011). Dynamic sonification as a free music improvisation tool for physically disabled adults. *Music and Medicine*, 3, 182–8.

Magee, W. L. (2006). Electronic technologies in clinical music therapy: a survey of practice and attitudes. *Technology and Disability*, 18, 139–46.

Magee, W. L. (2011). Music technology for health and well-being: the bridge between the arts and science. *Music and Medicine*, 3, 131–3.

Magee, W. L. and Burland, K. (2008). An exploratory study of the use of electronic music technologies in clinical music therapy. *Nordic Journal of Music Therapy*, 17, 124–41.

Magee W L et al. (2011). Using music technology in music therapy with populations across the life span in medical and educational programs. *Music and Medicine*, 3, 146–53.

Miranda E R et al. (2011). Brain–computer music interfacing (BCMI): from basic research to the real world of special needs. *Music and Medicine*, 3, 134–40.

Nagler J C (2011). Music therapy methods with hand-held music devices in contemporary clinical practice: a commentary. *Music and Medicine*, *3*, 196–9.

Ramsey D W (2011). Designing musically assisted rehabilitation systems. *Music and Medicine*, *3*, 141–5.

Whitehead-Pleaux, A. M., Clark, S. L., and Spall, L. E. (2011). Indications and counterindications for electronic music technologies in a pediatric medical setting. *Music and Medicine*, *3*, 154–62.

Useful websites

Ableton Live. www.ableton.com/live

Alternate Mode MalletKAT. www.alternatemode.com/malletkat.shtml

Apple Inc. www.apple.com

Korg Kaossilator. www.korg.com/KAOSSILATOR

PG Music Band-in-a-Box. www.pgmusic.com

Roland. www.roland.com

Soundbeam. www.soundbeam.co.uk

Chapter 4

Clinical Improvisation in Neurologic Music Therapy

Edward A. Roth

4.1 Introduction

Improvisation is a method commonly employed by music therapists across a broad spectrum of clinical populations and toward a diverse breadth of therapeutic outcomes. The application of improvisation is widely acknowledged within the discipline as beneficial in the assessment, treatment, and reassessment or evaluation of patients with a variety of neurological, psychological, and physiological disorders. It is commonly reported in the extant literature as being effective within individual and group formats toward the development of cognitive, affective, sensorimotor, and communicative behaviors. In particular, improvisation is often utilized as a medium for self-expression and toward the development or rehabilitation of appropriate socio-emotional functioning (Davis and Magee, 2001; Gooding, 2011; Hilliard, 2007; McFerran, 2010; Silverman, 2007; Wigram, 2004). The literature base abounds with theories, examples, and arguments for the use of improvisation in therapy and medicine, but Hiller (2009) points out that although improvisation is widely used by clinicians, instruction at the undergraduate/equivalency level is both inconsistent and limited across academic training programs in the USA. It is not possible within the parameters of one chapter to provide a comprehensive review of clinical improvisation. However, clinical improvisation has an important place in neurologic music therapy (NMT), and is utilized as one of several therapeutic experiences across the various therapeutic music interventions (TMIs).

This chapter is primarily intended to provide the musical materials and a few basic examples of clinical improvisation within NMT. The provision of a basic structure around which to discuss the use of music for clinical purposes seems useful, and one definition may read as follows:

> The use of improvisation through instrumental, vocal, or other media, and movement modalities, is a process by which the therapist and client, or groups of clients, engage each other for purposes of assessment, therapeutic experience, or evaluation. Improvisational exercises typically are implemented within rule-governed parameters along a continuum of definition based on the needs of the client(s) and aims of the experiences. Among the primary functions of improvisation used for clinical purposes is to provide clients with an apparatus in which to experience and practice non-musical functioning and behaviors.

With reference to the *transformational design model (TDM)* (Thaut, 2008), the identification of functional non-musical behaviors and exercises (following an assessment and identification of goals and objectives) is an important step in the process of creating clinical improvisation experiences. Once those issues have been addressed, it is then possible to move forward to Step 4 of the TDM—that is, the transference of functional non-musical stimuli and experiences into functional therapeutic music stimuli and exercises. During this translation, the selection of appropriate musical analogs for the various features of non-musical behavior can have a direct impact on the effectiveness and efficiency of treatment. These characteristics will vary widely, of course, depending on the diagnosis, presentation of symptoms, delivery format, goals and objectives, age, and other characteristics of the client(s), and should be considered carefully when designing clinical improvisation exercises. For example, when translating social interaction experiences into clinical musical exercises, the form of the interaction(s) to be practiced should be considered while designing an appropriate parallel improvisation experience. Additional considerations include what non-musical roles the client will play within the improvisation, and how the various tonal, timbrel, dynamic, and temporal features of music can be utilized to facilitate a musical exercise that promotes the desired non-musical behavior and/or experience. The isomorphic conformity of the musical exercise to the non-musical experience and behavior that is being practiced is an important consideration. That is, the degree to which the improvisational experience resembles the non-musical behavior in structure and function can determine its efficacy and translation to post-therapy generalization to the client's daily life.

4.2 **Musical concepts and materials**

4.2.1 **Temporal constructs**

The primary temporal aspects of improvisation include pulse, tempo, meter, and rhythm. All of these elemental features are ways in which we define and organize time in music. They contribute to our overall perception of music, including syntactical structure (phrasing), emotional quality, energy, and movement parameters, and thus essentially communicate much of what an improvisation may musically "mean" to a group or an individual client.

4.2.1.1 **Pulse**

The core—or better put perhaps, the foundation—of temporal organization in music is referred to as the pulse, and is often described as the "basic beat." Some have distinguished between the terms "pulse" and "beat" by describing a beat as a single acoustic event which, when it occurs at repetitive and temporally equal intervals, creates a sense of "pulse" that is "felt" rather than heard. This most basic structure of time is based on felt patterns of stable periodically recurring amplitude modulations. The pulse provides predictability via the temporal distance between each acoustic event, rather than simply the perception of the events (i.e. beats) themselves. The individual beats that comprise a felt sense of pulse provide consistent reference points in time, but the sense of stability, predictability, and comfort in some scenarios is probably derived from the perception of equidistant intervals between each beat.

4.2.1.2 Meter

Depending on the placement of amplitude modulations (or other types of accents), one large-scale subdivision of the pulse created by short cyclical repetitions is described as "meter." A sense of meter is created when sound is organized in groupings of twos (duple meter) and threes (triple meter) through the predictable and repetitive use of amplitude modulation within the basic beat. Accents are used (usually on the first beat of a grouping) to create a felt sense of repetitive two-beat, four-beat, and three-beat sequences. This is truer in western than in non-western music, where pulse organization can consist primarily of long rhythmic phrases. Multiple combinations and sequences exist and form a secondary layer of temporal organization within the pulse in which to frame rhythmic patterns.

4.2.1.3 Rhythm

Rhythms, or rhythmic patterns, are smaller subdivisions within the metrical structure of a given song or improvisation. They are created by fluctuating durations of each event or note, intervals between each note, and the placement of accents within a particular sequence. The complexity (or simplicity) of rhythms exists along a continuum, from minor subdivisions of the pulse to highly complex sequences of varying levels of subdivision of the meter, as well as those whose accent patterns and numerical structures fall outside of the metrical structure of the pulse. More than pulse and meter perhaps, rhythms create the "feel" or "groove" of an improvisation and contribute to the perception of phrases within the meter. They can contribute to the communication of multiple streams of information, from motor cues to cultural identity (consider rhythms such as those linked to Latin American cultures, e.g. bossa nova, mambo, merengue, rumba) (see Figure 4.1).

4.2.1.4 Tempo

Tempo is almost universally understood as the "speed" or "velocity" of music, and is determined by the frequency rate of repetition of beats within a given time frame. This is typically expressed as beats per minute (bpm), and is generally in the range 40–200 bpm. Tempo variably influences a multitude of responses, from motor activity to perception of emotion in music, to arousal and motivation. Elevated tempi tend to require and induce increased muscle contractions, whereas slower tempi tend to be associated with muscle relaxation. Tempo also affects perception of mood in music. However, the effect may be mediated by the influence of tempo on arousal, more than a straight-line effect on mood. Whereas tempo seems to function as an amplifier of sorts, influencing in part the extent to which we experience mood states, mood seems to be influenced to a greater degree by tonal aspects of music, specifically by mode or scale.

(a)

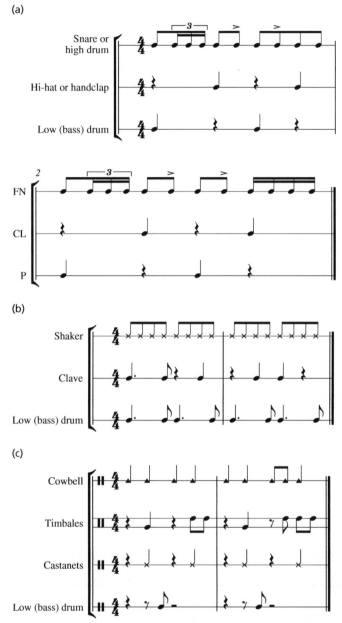

Fig. 4.1 Latin rhythms. (a) Bolero (ballroom rumba). (b) Bossa nova (Brazil). (c) Cha-cha (Afro-Cuban). (d) Mambo (Afro-Cuban). (e) Merengue (Dominican Republic). (f) New Orleans 2nd line. (g) Reggae, one drop (Jamaica). (h) Samba (Brazil). (i) Samba II (Brazil).

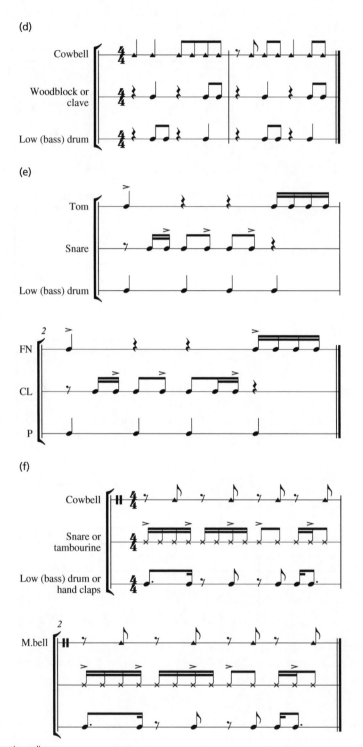

Fig. 4.1 (continued)

(g)

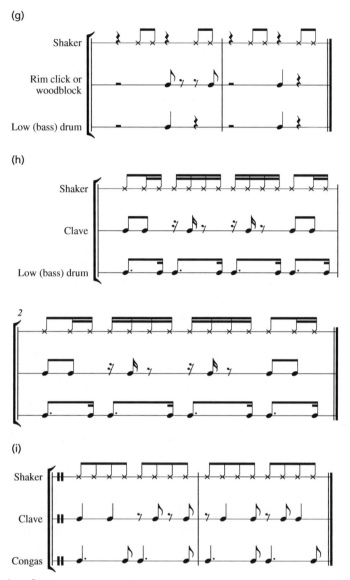

(h)

(i)

Fig. 4.1 (continued)

4.2.2 Tonal constructs

The organization of pitches, both vertically (played simultaneously) and horizontally (played sequentially), creates the tonal characteristics used in improvisation that are commonly referred to as melody, harmony, modality, and tonality.

4.2.2.1 Modes

Modal scales and modal polyphony offer several opportunities and advantages when structuring the tonal characteristics of a clinical improvisation experience. Although attempts have been unsuccessfully made throughout history to impose consistent referential meaning and inferences on music (Berlyne, 1971; Meyer, 1956), and in particular the various musical modes, some observable patterns in perception may have developed across listeners native to western musical structures. Relatedly, Brown and Jordania (2011) provide a list and description of musical universals that identifies a probabilistic set of putative characteristics found cross-culturally in musical behavior. Despite the existence of idiosyncratic differences and the acknowledgement that music does not intrinsically communicate extra-musical meaning, it appears that some similarities could perhaps exist in perception and reaction to the various modal organizations of pitch, at least among trained musicians. The data in Table 4.1 were collected, over a period of eight academic semesters from 2009 to 2012, from undergraduate and equivalency music therapy students who were enrolled in the author's clinical improvisation course. The students were instructed to complete improvisational exercises at the piano individually and in pairs and to simply write down any thoughts, feelings, or images that arose as a result of their improvisations. Although not originally intended for research or publication purposes, the information would seem to be relevant to the content of this chapter.

Gardstrom (2007) has presented a useful table with represented modes and scales all beginning on D. She logically indicates that presenting the modes/scales in D tonality is inclusive of the various ranges of pitches available on most chromatic percussion instruments. A revised representation of that table appears below, in C tonality, as Orff xylophones and metallophones typically come standard with C as the lowest or first tone, and extra bars can be purchased to create the various scales and modes (see Table 4.2 and Figure. 4.2).

Perhaps the most obvious advantage to utilizing any of the various modes for improvisational purposes is the absence or diminution of notes and note combinations that are perceived as dissonant or "wrong" by clients. This is, of course, no guarantee that clients will respond positively to the musical qualities of an improvisation experience, but the use of modal frameworks provides tonal structure in which to organize, guide, develop, and interpret the client's musical expressions within a readily accessible tonal format. Because there are no chordal implications, patients can extemporaneously create music together heterophonically, which can be esthetically pleasing as well as clinically useful. Pentatonic modes can be particularly useful as the note ranges are limited to five tones, perhaps creating a more accessible apparatus for patients who require less complexity. To increase the complexity of an improvisation while maintaining the esthetic appeal and simplicity of improvising within a pentatonic mode, the therapist may consider utilizing the authentic and plagal configurations of each mode. The terms "authentic" and "plagal" refer to the range or ambitus of the melody in relation to the modal scale and tonic. In an authentic configuration, the scale ranges from tonic to tonic (the way that we typically conceptualize scales). In the plagal configuration, the range goes from dominant to dominant (see Table 4.3). The simultaneous combination of authentic and plagal formats can allow richer textures and potentially more interesting note combinations, leading toward better arousal, attention, and overall cognitive stimulation.

Pentachordic modes are also five-note scalar segments taken from the diatonic scale: C-D-E-F-G, D-E-F-G-A, E-F-G-A-B, F-G-A-B-C, (G-A-B-C-D), (A-B-C-D-E), B-C-D-E-F.

Table 4.1 Comparison of mode characteristics

Dorian	Phrygian	Lydian	Mixolydian	Aeolian	Locrian	Ionian
Minor scale, ominous, earthy, depressing, urgent, feels like more minor-scale sound	Regal, imposing, intimidating, dark, angry, resolves, drive, powerful, morbid, mysterious, foreboding, angst	Happy, alive, slower, thoughtful, hopeless, loneliness, contemplative, bright	On a journey (turning point), looking forward, positive	Empty, intensity, dark, journey	Flat, centerless, without resolution, void of substance, no foundation	Train moving through hills, wheelbarrows, rolling fields, sunrise, long winding roads, dandelions blowing in the wind
Slower, thoughtful, hopeless, loneliness, contemplative, dream-like, sad	Powerful, like being pushed forward, morbid, sharp, stinging, piercing, mysterious	Sweet, mellow, light, positive, uplifting, touch of melancholy	Insistent, walking fast, light, dancing, unfazed, single-minded, in motion, neutral	Arabian nights, on a chase, dark Christmas carols, traveling	Ethereal, sad, unsettled, even emptier	Church, Bach, calmness, empty, walking, spaciousness
Somber, deliberate, determined, troubled, feels like minor scale, ominous	Morbid, marching to gallows, chant from church, cold, ice, pain, heartache, alone, homeless, despair	Happy, alive, freedom, purpose, journey, hard times in between	Forgiving, new beginning, fresh, fixing screw ups, hope not manifested but insistent, unfazed, in motion	Empty feeling, alone in an unknown place	Tranquil, (uncomfortably) warm, calm, melancholy, bittersweet	Light-hearted, chipper, skipping, having fun, bells in a church, meeting of lovers, light-hearted
Ominous, intensify, darkness with moments of light, night, ice, driven, seriousness	Unsettled, unresolved, melancholy, wistful, nostalgic, someone alone, moments of uplift	More bright sound, sounds like a little child jumping all around	Ireland, warm, light, carefree, on a path, hopeful	Not happy but not depressing either, mature, independent, but still sad, resolved pain, tolerable pain	Creepy and haunting, horror film, very uncomfortable but no desire to quit	Happy, warm, and calm; pictured a park that was very green and had balloons
Mixed major/minor feelings, moments of excitement and energy, mellow feeling, uncertainty/wonder	Agitation, aggression, annoyance, at some points passive aggressive, feelings of war	Pretty, ballet-like, folk song	Taking a trip, dreamlike, bubbly, walking (skipping) through a field	Serious, hard to breathe, sad, empty	Chaotic, anxiety and it sounds very intense, like it's building toward something. Reminds me of a scary movie soundtrack	Peaceful and calming, sounds like reminiscent music; religious

Table 4.1 (continued)

Dorian	Phrygian	Lydian	Mixolydian	Aeolian	Locrian	Ionian
Escaping, running away, time pressure, passion, earthy, dirt, blue, moody, relaxed, depressed, stuck, closed, brown, melancholy	Jewels, mysterious, energy, dark and beautiful, foreboding, demands attention, dark eroticism	Space, ungrounded, high-school band, floating, aiming	Hiking or biking somewhere in the middle of a trip, looking forward to the "next step"	When rhythmic drive was faster: determined, grandiose, epic, important	Dark, menacing, creepy, intense with a hint of anger and aggression	Religious
Depressing, urgent, sense of change, dragging, shift of content to discontent or vice versa	Angst, black, tired, frustration, abandonment/ alone, cry for help, inner conflict—OK to be angry	Gray, empty, apathetic, numb, aimless, floating, soulless, no foundation, playful, fun, enlightening, liberating		When rhythmic drive was slower: sad, tragic, melancholy, depressed, mournful	Ominous, sneaky, abrasive, curious, unresolved, at times evil, haunting, frightening	Cheerful, majestic, at times playful or child-like, happy, content, centered, predictable
Depressing at slow tempo, more thoughtful, steady bass line, rainy-day imagery, reliable, steady, hopeless, deep loneliness, methodical	Morbid, dark, foreboding, intense, driven, resolves, melodic motive	Interest, change in routine, uncomfortable at times, uncertainty, positive, movement overall, open, fun, running in field, peaceful, spacious				Sounded like a song or something familiar, I think that had to do with the use of chords
Unfinished, contemplative with underlying optimism, ethereal, striving toward rhythmic consistency	Angry, resolved, letting emotions out, aggressive energy, driving	Debussy-esque, peaceful, hopeful, whimsical, spacious peaceful feeling, jazzy				

Table 4.2 Scales and modes in C tonality

	C	C#/Db	D	D#/Eb	E	F	F#/Gb	G	G#/Ab	A	A#/Bb	B	(C)
Chromatic	C	C#/Db	D	D#/Eb	E	F	F#/Gb	G	G#/Ab	A	A#/Bb	B	(C)
Ionian	C		D		E	F		G		A		B	(C)
Dorian	C		D	Eb		F		G		A	Bb		(C)
Phrygian	C	Db		Eb		F		G	Ab		Bb		(C)
Lydian	C		D		E		F#	G		A		B	(C)
Mixolydian	C		D		E	F		G		A	Bb		(C)
Aeolian	C		D	Eb		F		G	Ab		Bb		(C)
Locrian	C	Db		Eb		F	Gb		Ab		Bb		(C)
Arabic/gypsy	C	Db			E	F		G	Ab			B	(C)
Egyptian	C		D	Eb			F#	G	Ab			B	(C)
Pentatonic 1 Chinese pentatonic (1) (major pentatonic)	C		D		E			G		A			(C)
Pentatonic 2	C		D			F		G			Bb		(C)
Pentatonic 3	C			Eb		F			Ab		Bb		(C)
Pentatonic 4 Chinese pentatonic (2)	C		D			F		G		A			(C)
Pentatonic 5 (minor pentatonic)	C			Eb		F		G			Bb		(C)
Japanese pentatonic	C	Db				F		G	Ab				(C)
Spanish scale	C	Db			E	F		G	Ab		Bb		(C)
Blues (minor)	C			Eb		F	F#	G			Bb		(C)
Blues (major)	C		D	Eb	E			G		A			(C)
Whole tone	C		D		E		F#		G#		A#		(C)

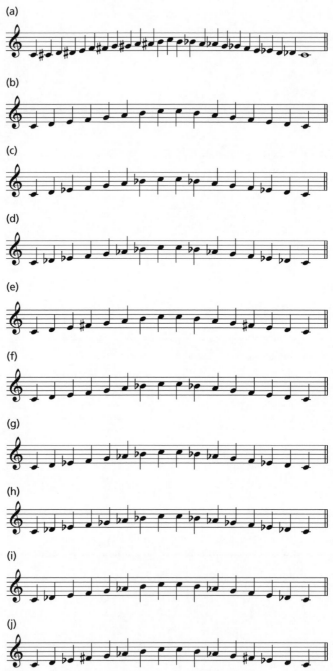

Fig. 4.2 Modes and scales. (a) Chromatic. (b) Ionian. (c) Dorian. (d) Phrygian. (e) Lydian. (f) Mixolydian. (g) Aeolian. (h) Locrian. (i) Arabic gypsy. (j) Egyptian. (k) Chinese pentatonic. (l) Chinese pentatonic II. (m) Japanese pentatonic. (n) Spanish. (o) Blues (minor). (p) Blues (major). (q) Whole tone.

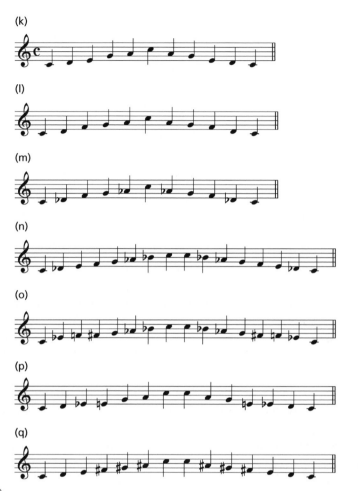

Fig. 4.2 (continued).

Table 4.3 Pentatonic scales in their authentic and plagal configurations

Mode	Tonic	Configuration							Configuration						
1	C	Authentic	C	D	E	G	A	C	Plagal	G	A	C	D	E	G
2	D	Authentic	D	E	G	A	C	D	Plagal	A	C	D	E	G	A
3	E	Authentic	E	G	A	C	D	E	None						
4	G	Authentic	G	A	C	D	E	G	Plagal	D	E	G	A	C	D
5	A	Authentic	A	C	D	E	G	A	Plagal	E	G	A	C	D	E

Table 4.4 Pentachordic modes

C	D	E	F	G
D	E	F	G	A
E	F	G	A	B
F	G	A	B	C
G	A	B	C	D
A	B	C	D	E
B	C	D	E	F

There are only five unique pentachordic scales, as the two groups in parentheses have identical intervals to the first two groups (see Table 4.4). Similar in use to authentic and plagal combinations of pentatonic scales, pentachordic modes add complexity and interest and can be utilized in a way that maintains a five-note range, but excludes the leaps that exist in the five pentatonic scales identified in this chapter. This could be useful when improvising on an instrument with fixed keys (e.g. piano, keyboard, some tuned percussion instruments) and the patient's range of motion or other limitations allow for no more than single-key movement.

4.2.3 Form

Arguably the most logical musical analog to social and interpersonal behavior is the complex concept of musical form. As in social paradigms where certain processes take place over expected periods of time, musical form in improvisation can also be utilized over varying degrees of time. One might consider the form of improvisation as it relates to a single experience and the similarities to and differences from the process of ongoing therapy. Wigram (2004) discusses sonata form, as it possesses similarities in the structure and ongoing processes related to a single improvisation, making friends, a therapeutic relationship, and the overall process of therapy. Consider, for instance, the symbolic similarities within a single improvisation and sonata form. Early-stage exploration of sound can be seen as akin to the *introduction*, where the clients explore the various sonorous capabilities of their voice or instrument. The *exposition* stage provides for the expression of early-stage musical ideas between therapist and client(s) and among clients. Those musical ideas are further expanded in the *development* stage using parts of the original motives while exploring new directions, taking note of what individuals in the group find pleasant, meaningful, or rewarding in some way. *Recapitulation* brings the improvisers back to the original musical notions, and the *coda* is utilized to carry the improvisation to an esthetically pleasing end.

Often described as having a "shaken sense of self", which includes a modified sense of personal identity, people who require neurological rehabilitation can subsequently experience difficulties socially. As described above, the use of musical form, in particular as it relates to social interaction, is a crucial consideration when constructing clinical improvisation experiences. One useful structure for practicing various aspects of social functioning within the safety of a predictable sequence of events is *rondo* form (ABACA-DAEAF etc.). "A" represents group improvising, and the subsequent sequence of letters represents emphasis on individuals within a group. Rondo form is often utilized to give clients the opportunity to individually explore their post-event capabilities within a socio-emotionally supportive structure that continually retreats to the safety of simultaneous group music making.

4.2.4 Timbre

Another important consideration when designing clinical improvisation experiences is the use of timbre and its effects on motor, cognitive, affective, and social responses. For instance, variation in timbre from gentle to harsh can be utilized to facilitate different states of muscle contraction during improvisation exercises designed to aid motor development or rehabilitation.

Another example is the use of timbre to help to establish auditory figure–ground relationships that are used to simulate and practice selective attending behavior, such as might be implemented in MACT for selective attention skills (MACT-SEL). One or more clients provide an underlying stable structure or ground—for instance, via a large drum or low-pitched tone bar played quietly with a soft mallet—while one or more other client(s) function as the figure or featured component. In this scenario, an instrument with a contrasting timbre (e.g. triangle, soprano Orff xylophone, kalimba, agogo bells) utilizes, in part, the difference in timbre to create distinction from the ground, and provides the auditory material to be selected and responded to by other members of the group.

4.2.5 Dynamics

Dynamics in music generally refer to changes in the intensity or amplitude of the sound, often spoken of in terms of "loudness" and "softness." As many improvisation experiences are conducted utilizing percussion instruments, including piano, dynamic ranges are created by fluctuations in the use of force applied to these instruments. The more force you apply, or the harder you strike the drum, Orff xylophone, or triangle, the greater the amplitude, and vice versa. Dynamics can be modified over extended periods of time, as observed in multi-measure crescendos and decrescendos, but can also include instantaneous changes from one note to the next. Dynamics can be utilized to elicit desired responses in multiple domains, including muscle activation (e.g. the greater the amplitude, the greater the muscle contraction) and emotional responses (e.g. gradual decrescendos may elicit a decreasing sense of the emotions experienced while the music was improvised at a greater volume.)

One interesting way to structure an improvisation, in particular for patients who cannot maintain a steady pulse, is to do so by utilizing primarily dynamic elements. Through the use of structured soundscapes created by combinations and variations of timbres, tempi, registers, rhythmic flourishes, glissandos, and entry and exit points, multiple players can improvise in a way that maintains temporal organization without the requirement to "keep the beat." An example is provided in Section 4.3 in the context of a musical executive function training experience.

4.3 **Musical executive function training (MEFT)**

The use of improvisation in MEFT can be successfully employed in both individual and group formats to practice executive function skills, including abstract thinking, organization, reasoning, planning, use of working memory to connect past experience to present task, and problem solving. Other related behaviors include the initiation of appropriate actions and inhibition of those considered to be inappropriate, error detection and mid-course correction, use of novel responses rather than automatic reactions, and other behaviors that require the overcoming of a habituated response.

These behaviors and areas of functioning can be practiced, as stated earlier, within the context of dynamically varying soundscapes. One application in a group format involves a patient being given the role of director, and, using the available instruments and group members, then being asked to create an auditory analog of some particular scene or environment that changes over time. For instance, in the case of a beach scene, some clients may be directed to utilize an ocean drum to resemble the sounds of the waves, while others use wind chimes or rub their hands together to resemble the sound of wind, and yet other group members play glissandos on an Orff xylophone to help to further create the mood of the scene. As the scenario develops over time, another client may be directed to play on a thunder sheet or deep drum to represent thunder, while another client uses a rain stick to create the sound of gentle rain as a storm moves into the beach scenario. Through the use of directing or physical gestures, the group, and individual members within the group, can be cued to change the dynamics of their playing to represent changes in the oncoming and outgoing durations of the storm. Eye contact and a head nod, perhaps along with physical movement resembling that which is required to play an instrument, may be used to initiate playing, while a hand in a stop position would cue the client(s) to stop playing. Moving the hands with the palms up in an upward and outward motion can be used to indicate a desired increase in volume and intensity, while moving the hands downward and inward with the palms down can be used to indicate a decrease in dynamic volume. In this way the group improvises dynamically within a temporal structure that changes in broad structure (similar to musical form, perhaps), avoiding the requirement to improvise within any rhythmic or tonal framework.

Conversely, another way to organize an improvisation experience is to build it in successive layers using the musical materials described earlier in this chapter. The score in Figure 4.3 can be utilized as a framework to begin an improvisation, and is written with multiple parts for rhythmic and tonal improvisers, with tonal parts comprising the top five staves (moving from less to more complex from bottom to top) and rhythmic parts comprising the bottom seven staves (also generally moving from less to more complex from bottom to top). One way to use the score is to assign clients with more limitations the lower rhythmic and tonal parts of the score, and clients who require greater challenge can be assigned successively more complex parts of the score. Clients can be directed to start and stop playing via physical cues, and parts can be conveyed via demonstration. The score is intended only as a starting point, and therapists will need to modify the procedure as necessary to determine their available instrumentarium, how much extemporaneous playing should take place, and which timbres, rhythms, melodies, and dynamic changes (not included) are most appropriate for their clients.

4.4 Music in psychosocial training and counseling (MPC)

Using improvisation experiences within the context of MPC interventions, music is utilized to assist mood stabilization, expression of emotion, clarity of thought, and appropriate social functioning. It should be noted that these experiences are to be provided with careful planning and consideration of the needs and vulnerabilities of individual clients and client groups. Indeed, music has been known throughout history to have a powerful influence on the mood of individuals, and in recognition of the influence that one individual could have in the manipulation of another's mood, Aristotle considered music to be a rather ignoble profession. Understanding the dynamic nature of clinical improvisation and its mechanistic principles should aid the clinician in the careful planning and implementation of improvisation experiences. Although many musicians and music therapists use improvisation to express thoughts, concepts, and feeling states, very little is understood about the underlying neural mechanisms of extemporaneously produced music.

In their study of professional jazz pianists, Limb and Braun (2008) described patterns of neural activity involved in improvisation that differed from those involved in the performance of over-learned music. Using functional magnetic resonance imaging (fMRI), they found a significant dissociated pattern of activity whereby improvisation resulted in activation of the medial prefrontal cortex and deactivation of the dorso-lateral prefrontal and lateral orbital cortices. Connected to behavioral output, Limb described the process as activation of brain regions thought to be involved in self-expression, including the generation of autobiographical information, and deactivation of areas involved in self-monitoring or inhibition. Like others (Patel, 2010), Limb and Braun also identified activation of the left posterior inferior frontal gyrus when two musicians were improvising together in a back-and-forth manner commonly utilized by jazz musicians, known as "trading 4's." This would seem to suggest that these participants were engaged in a socially communicative experience, as this region, also referred to as Broca's area, is most commonly associated with speech production.

4.4.1 MPC social competence training (MPC-SCT)

MPC-SCT gives clients the opportunity to utilize music as a method of aiding the development of skills necessary for appropriate and useful social interaction (Gooding, 2011). Rather than serving as a metaphor for psychosocial functioning, through its elements, music is used to allow the client to directly practice the various non-musical behaviors used while interacting with other people, as follows:

(a)

Arab

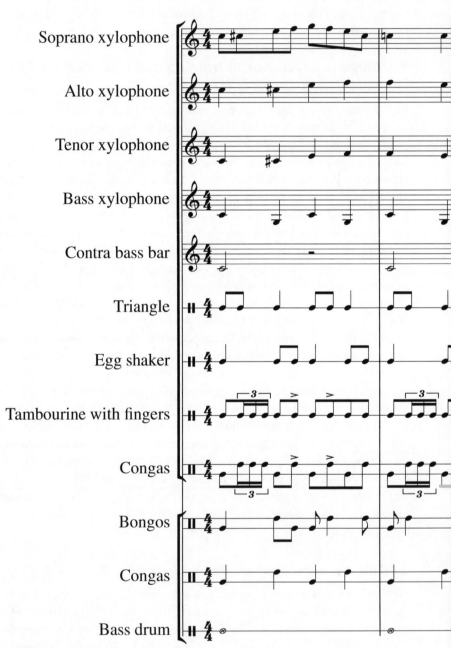

Fig. 4.3 Arabic mode with bolero rhythm framework.

lode with Bolero Rhythm

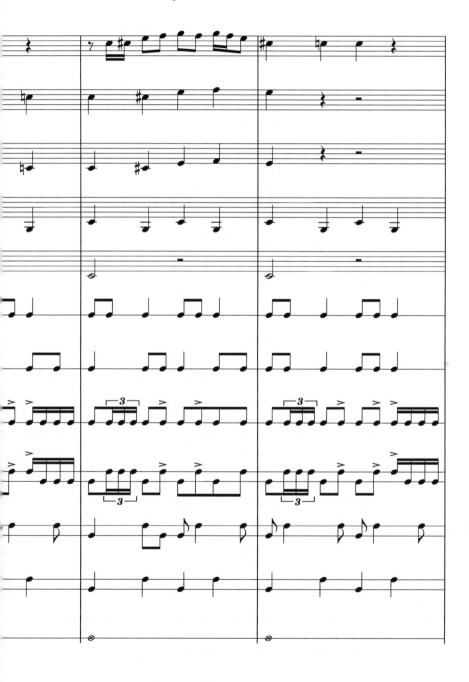

(b)

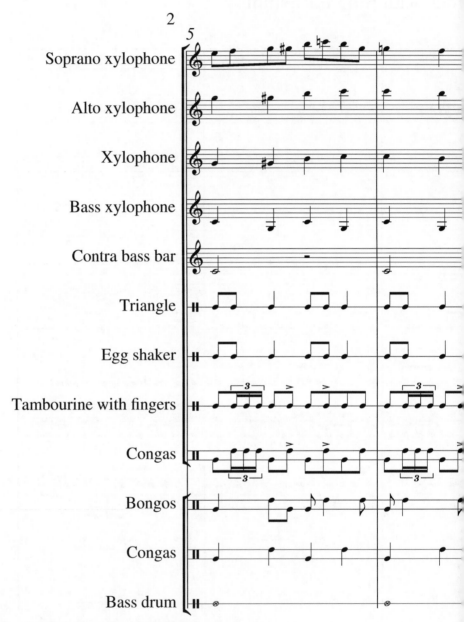

Fig. 4.3 (continued) Arabic mode with bolero rhythm framework.

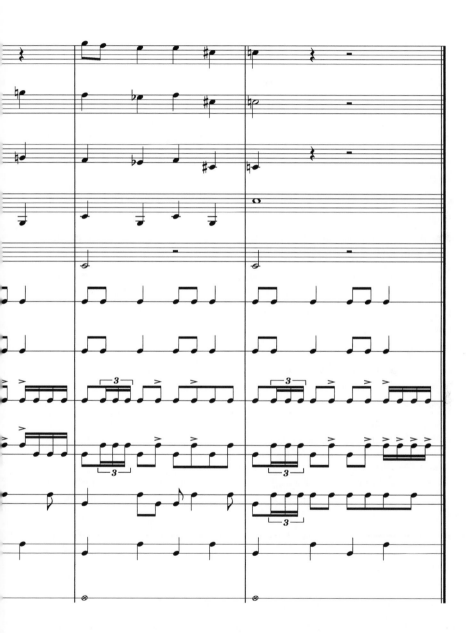

General goal area: Social

Specific skill: Initiation and reciprocation

Outcome behavior: Each member will be able to appropriately initiate and reciprocate interaction with another individual

Materials/equipment: Percussion instruments, including drums (djembe, tubano, doumbek, etc.) and Orff xylophones/metallophones

Setting: Group (2 to 10 people)

Procedure:

1 Clients are asked to consider the characteristics of a greeting to which they are most likely to be responsive. If necessary, they can be further prompted to consider various specific aspects (e.g. loudness, use of speech inflection, length, speed, choppy or smooth phrases, etc.).

2 Musical parallels or "analogs" are then identified (e.g. volume, pitch/notes, duration, tempo, rhythm).

3 The same process is repeated for the identification of pleasant or satisfying responsive phrases and the related musical analogs.

4 Using the identified non-musical characteristics and related musical elements considered to be pleasing for greetings and responses, each member of the group plays a brief musical excerpt to which the group responds musically. This continues until each member has had at least one turn initiating a musical interaction.

5 Using clinical logic to determine a good stopping point, the group can be asked to identify the musical characteristics they heard that contributed most to eliciting a response. A secondary question may be asked regarding the nature and characteristics of the responses that felt most satisfying.

6 After the musical characteristics of the most effective greetings and satisfactory responses have been identified, a second round of improvisation should be initiated.

7 If it is deemed appropriate to verbally process after the experience, clients can be guided to relate the musical experience to their immediate objectives within the context of non-musical interaction. Facilitation of the connection between the therapeutic music experience and non-musical behavior can be further explored by helping the participants to connect the clinical improvisation experience to their long-term goals and post-session real-life scenarios.

4.4.2 MPC mood induction and vectoring (MPC-MIV)

The extra-musical associations presented in Table 4.1 may be of some use when creating clinical improvisation exercises used to aid the development of social and emotional functioning, such as mood modification, interpersonal communication, and expression of emotion. That information is included with the intention of it being used, metaphorically speaking, more as an analog compass that provides general guidance, rather than as a digital global positioning system that communicates precise direction.

The following is one such example:

General goal area:	Emotion/affect
Specific skill:	Mood modification
Outcome behavior:	Each member will be able to experience, identify, and express feelings related to a state of relaxation
Materials/equipment:	A variety of percussion instruments, including drums, Orff xylophones, metallophones, auxiliary effect instruments (e.g. ocean drum, rainstick, wind chimes, thunder sheet, temple blocks)
Setting:	Group (2 to 10 people)

Procedure:

1 Tonal percussion instruments are presented to clients in one of two prearranged sequences, in either Phrygian or Mixolydian mode. Non-pitched instruments are used to further facilitate mood induction and expression.

2 Clients who chose or were assigned instruments prearranged in Phrygian mode are instructed to explore the individual sounds and combination of sounds that can be produced within that sequence of pitches. This can be done within a prescribed rhythm context, one that emerges as the improvisation develops, or outside of rhythmic organization altogether. All of the group members are asked to consider and take note of any thoughts, emotions, and/or images that may arise while they are improvising or listening.

3 Once established, those participants who chose or were assigned instruments prearranged in Mixolydian mode are instructed to begin quietly improvising and exploring the sonorous capabilities of that sequence of pitches, eventually increasing their volume to match that of those improvising in Phrygian mode.

4 After both modes are established in the improvisation, participants improvising in Phrygian mode are asked to search for the tones on their instrument that are coincident, or sound pleasant, with those on the instruments in Mixolydian mode, and begin to utilize those tones to a greater degree.

4.5 **Conclusion**

As mentioned at the outset, the purpose of this chapter was to provide the musical materials and a few brief examples of clinical improvisation as utilized in NMT. Good clinical logic and isomorphic conformity of improvisation exercises to non-musical behavior should guide the clinician in the planning and implementation of therapeutic experiences.

References

Berlyne, D. E. (1971). Perception. In: *Aesthetics and Psychobiology*. New York: Meredith Corporation. pp. 96–114.

Brown, S. and Jordania, J. (2011). Universals in the world's musics. *Psychology of Music, 41*, 229–48.

Davis, G. and Magee, W. L. (2001). Clinical improvisation within neurological disease: exploring the effect of structured clinical improvisation on the expressive and interactive responses of a patient with Huntington's disease. *British Journal of Music Therapy, 18*, 78–9.

Gardstrom, S. C. (2007). *Music Therapy Improvisation for Groups: essential leadership competencies*. Barcelona: Gilsum (NH).

Gooding, L. F. (2011). The effect of a music therapy social skills training program on improving social competence in children and adolescents with social skills deficits. *Journal of Music Therapy, 48*, 440–62.

Hiller, J. (2009). Use of and instruction in clinical improvisation. *Music Therapy Perspectives, 27*, 25–32.

Hilliard, R. (2007). The effects of Orff-based music therapy and social work groups on childhood grief symptoms and behaviors. *Journal of Music Therapy, 44*, 123–38.

Limb, C. J. and Braun, A. R. (2008). Neural substrates of spontaneous musical performance: an fMRI study of jazz improvisation. *PLoS One, 3*, e1679.

McFerran, K. (2010). *Adolescents, Music and Music Therapy: methods and techniques for clinicians, educators and students*. London: Jessica Kingsley Publishers.

Meyer, L. (1956). *Emotion and Meaning in Music*. Chicago: University of Chicago Press.

Patel, A. (2010). *Music, Language, and the Brain*. New York: Oxford University

Silverman, M. J. (2007). Evaluating current trends in psychiatric music therapy: a descriptive analysis. *Journal of Music Therapy, 44*, 388–414.

Thaut, M. H. (2008). *Rhythm, Music, and the Brain: scientific foundations and clinical applications*. New York: Routledge.

Wigram, T. (2004). *Improvisation: methods and techniques for music therapy clinicians, educators, and students*. London: Jessica Kingsley Publishers.

Chapter 5

Patterned Sensory Enhancement and Constraint-Induced Therapy: A Perspective from Occupational Therapy to Interdisciplinary Upper Extremity Rehabilitation

Crystal Massie

5.1 Introduction

Research demonstrating the ability of the brain to change and reorganize following injury or insult (i.e. neuroplasticity) has established conceptual shifts in neurorehabilitation approaches over the past couple of decades. Facilitating neuroplasticity requires a sufficient behavioral mechanism to promote use-dependent plasticity—the avenue for which upper-extremity interventions have a fundamental role in recovery from stroke. Neurorehabilitation efforts to improve upper-extremity function following a stroke often require structured and intensive interventions incorporating motor learning, motor control, and neurophysiologic principles. The structure of interventions and tasks should be a consideration for clinicians and rehabilitation scientists, as this may influence outcomes. For example, constraint-induced therapy (CIT) is one extensively studied approach that is based on forced-used paradigms and incorporates many functional based tasks, whereas concepts for neurologic music therapy (NMT) rely heavily on the beneficial properties of auditory–motor entrainment and repetition. A detailed account of considerations for clinicians is presented in this chapter, including interventions and single-session studies that highlight movement strategy differences in survivors of stroke when reaching cyclically and with rhythmic auditory cues.

5.2 Constraint-induced therapy (CIT)

Current perspectives in stroke rehabilitation are focused on intense, structured interventions designed to facilitate use-dependent plasticity. Although the intensity and structure of interventions can take many forms, CIT is one extensively researched intervention (Wolf et al., 1989, 2006). CIT was based on the behavioral neuroscience work of Taub and colleagues, who demonstrated that learned non-use was a conditioned suppression of movement, a powerful behavioral phenomenon (Taub and Uswatte, 2003). However, this suppression of movement could be remediated by protocols of forced use of the affected extremity. A similar learned non-use behavior was observed in survivors of stroke, and led to the development of CIT. The standard CIT protocol was implemented as 6 hours of therapy a day for 10 consecutive weekdays, although many variations exist (Page et al., 2008; Wu et al., 2007a). A number of motor learning principles are incorporated in CIT, and the main principles can be summarized as follows:

1 *Restraint.* The less affected side is restrained, typically in a padded mitt to discourage use. Many protocols suggest that the less affected side should be restrained for up to 90% of waking hours, with removal of the mitt when warranted for safety (e.g. when using a walker or cane).

2 *Task practice.* Patients complete individual functional tasks, for 15- to 20-minute blocks of time, that require repetitive practice.

3 *Shaping.* This requires a progressive increase in the difficulty of training tasks as performance improves (Uswatte et al., 2006a).

4 *Massed practice.* This involves engaging in more practice than rest. Because rest breaks are only indicated for fatigue as needed, patients are encouraged to be engaged in massed practice.

These elements are combined throughout the course of the training period, yet the specific therapeutic tasks are highly dependent on the goals and functional ability of each patient. An example of a typical CIT training day is shown in Table 5.1. The amounts of task practice and shaping varied for each patient, but each training day typically consisted of a combination of both. One of the challenges for task practice in CIT is to use tasks that are unilateral, as the less affected side is restrained in a padded safety mitt. If the task cannot be completed unilaterally, alternatives are often considered, such as additional equipment (e.g. card holder), or the therapist-trainer assists as the second hand. In our experience, we attempted to have patients complete tasks that were as functional as possible, depending on the specific impairments of each patient. Although all of the patients had at least 10–20 degrees of extension in the wrist and fingers, the degree of fine motor impairment can certainly have an impact on the types of training tasks that are possible. We used a mix of activities that incorporated gross motor movements, fine motor elements, and combinations of both. The use of shaping within CIT training tasks is a fundamental component, such that tasks are made progressively more difficult as function improves. This requires a focused effort by the clinician to formulate tasks that can be made more difficult over time, and to provide appropriate feedback to promote functional return of movement. For example, if the goal was to put canned goods in a cupboard, the activity could be shaped by starting with moving small cans to a raised platform on a table. The vertical distance could then be increased as the first goal was achieved. As the patient continued to progress, larger and/or heavier cans could be used. The clinician must provide a challenge that is "just right", such that the patient is challenged, but not to the point of frustration or inability to succeed. The complexity of CIT as an intervention should not be underestimated.

Table 5.1. Example of daily activities for a typical CIT training day: patients would work on a one-to-one basis with a trainer to complete these activities using the principles of CIT. Each activity is completed in blocks of about 15–20 minutes to ensure high rates of repetition of each task within an activity.

Time	Activity
9:00–9:15 a.m.	Review home diary and mitt compliance
9:15–9:30 a.m.	Bouncing/stretching with a therapy ball
9:30–10:00 a.m.	Work on fine motor skills with dominoes
10:00–10:20 a.m.	Removing and putting canned goods in cupboard
10:20–10:30 a.m.	Break
10:30–11:00 a.m.	Gardening, using hand tools
11:00–11:20 a.m.	Using a Rolodex
11:20–11:40 a.m.	Rolling out Play-Doh™ with hand/fingers
11:40 a.m.–12:00 p.m.	Lunch preparation
12:00–12:30 p.m.	Lunch
12:30–1:00 p.m.	Clean up and wipe counters
1:00–1:20 p.m.	Shaping activity with marbles, small wooden pieces for in-hand manipulation
1:20–1:50 p.m.	Playing Bocce ball
1:50–2:00 p.m.	Break
2:00–2:30 p.m.	Card game
2:30–2:50 p.m.	Hanging up hangers and clothes
2:50–3:00 p.m.	Wrap-up

The clinician is responsible for determining the precise intensity and structure required to facilitate improved functional ability in survivors of stroke.

5.3 **Constraint-induced therapy and motor control**

CIT was developed as an intervention to overcome learned non-use. Indeed, research has demonstrated that CIT is efficacious in improving the amount of hemiparetic arm use, with sustained improvements being observed over a year (Wolf et al., 2006). Less research attention has been focused on determining the impact of CIT on movement strategies and movement quality. The recovery versus compensation debate has subsequently been regarded as an important aspect of evaluating neurorehabilitation interventions (Levin et al., 2009). Kinematic motion analysis is one technology available for precisely quantifying changes in reaching strategies for survivors of stroke completing intensive interventions. This technology can quantify movement strategies that may not be observable to the clinician. The number of studies using kinematic motion analysis before and after interventions has increased over the past few years (Malcolm et al., 2009; Massie et al., 2009; Michaelsen et al., 2006; Woodbury et al., 2009; Wu et al., 2007b).

We used kinematic motion analysis to determine the impact of CIT on movement strategies (Massie et al., 2009). We were specifically interested in characterizing compensatory movement strategies before and after CIT. We asked subjects to complete a continuous reaching task between two targets in a parasagittal plane while cameras recorded their movement. The movements were then digitized to quantify the degree of compensatory trunk movement that was used to accomplish the reaching task, how much shoulder flexion and elbow extension were used, and the movement time and reaching velocity. We demonstrated that CIT did not improve compensatory trunk movement, and that the amount of shoulder abduction increased following CIT. The degree of shoulder flexion used to accomplish a forward-reaching task significantly increased following CIT, but there was no change in the degree of elbow extension. The changes in the amount of trunk, elbow, and shoulder movement from pre- to post-CIT are illustrated in Figure 5.1. In addition to the kinematic motion analysis, we used commonly implemented assessments, including the Motor Activity Log (MAL) (Uswatte et al., 2006b) and the Wolf Motor Function Test

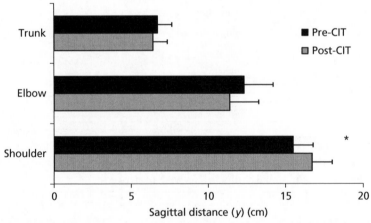

Fig. 5.1 Trunk rotation is represented in the upper set of bars and depicts the amount of forward trunk movement. There was no difference between the amount of compensatory trunk displacement before (black bar) or after (gray bar) CIT. The middle set of bars depicts the amount of forward reach that was covered by the elbow extending. This value was calculated by taking the ratio of elbow extension to shoulder flexion and applying that to the distance between the targets after the amount of trunk displacement was removed. There was a slight decrease in the amount of movement generated by elbow extension following CIT (gray bar), but this was not statistically significant. The bottom set of bars depicts the amount of movement generated by shoulder flexion. Clearly visible is the significant increase (indicated by the asterisk) in the amount of movement generated by shoulder flexion following CIT.

Data from Massie C, Malcolm M P, Greene D, and Thaut M (2009). The effects of constraint-induced therapy on kinematic outcomes and compensatory movement patterns: an exploratory study. *Archives of Physical Medicine and Rehabilitation*, 90, 571–9.

(WMFT) (Wolf et al., 2001), for measures of real-world upper-extremity use and functional motor capacity, respectively. The MAL is a subject-reported assessment of how well a patient perceives use of their stroke-affected side in activities of daily living. The WMFT provides a measure of functional motor capacity, and consists of a number of different subtasks ranging from placing the hand on the table, to picking up a pencil, to folding a towel. The findings of our study were consistent with other studies demonstrating an improvement in the amount of use and functional capacity of movement, and was one of the first studies to demonstrate that CIT did not improve compensatory movements. These were not necessarily surprising findings, because CIT was developed to improve the amount of use rather than the quality of use; limited attention is given to how the patients complete the task but are encouraged about the amount of use. CIT improved the quantity of movement but not necessarily the quality of movement, and these conclusions led us to consider alternative and/or complementary interventions that may have an impact on both areas. Although the question of whether movement quality limits functional return or has negative long-term consequences remains debatable, we felt that the quality of movement following stroke was still an important aspect to consider. This perspective was certainly congruent with reviews calling for more in-depth analyses of interventions (Levin et al., 2009).

5.4 Patterned sensory enhancement and quality of movement

As a result of some of our work with CIT, we wanted to study an intervention that could facilitate better movement quality. We directed our research endeavors toward incorporating elements of neurologic music therapy (NMT) for upper-extremity neurorehabilitation for survivors of stroke. NMT techniques such as rhythmic auditory stimulation (RAS) improve the quality of post-stroke gait, such as stride symmetry and stride length (Thaut et al., 1997). This technique capitalizes on the rhythmic/cyclic nature of gait. In comparison, reaching can be considered more complex because of the variety of movements required during activities of daily living (i.e. reaching is not entirely cyclic). Certainly many activities of daily living involve reaching movements that have some cyclic/reciprocal patterns. For example, wiping a table, brushing one's teeth, and stirring a pot all require some degree of cyclic motion. The concepts of patterned sensory enhancement (PSE) are better applied to upper-extremity interventions because of the complexity of upper-extremity movements. PSE provides an ideal opportunity for relearning upper-extremity movements because of the repetition inherent in PSE training and the feedback elements involved.

While developing the incorporation of PSE into an intervention for survivors of stroke, we have conducted a couple of studies that highlight the beneficial effects of a rhythmic auditory cue and the unique reaching strategies incorporated during cyclic reaching compared with discrete reaching. One of our research projects demonstrated that reaching kinematics in survivors of stroke immediately improved when a rhythmic auditory cue was provided that was set to the same self-selected pace as the condition with no cue

(Thaut et al., 2002). A total of 21 participants completed kinematic motion analysis testing during a single session of reaching continuously and as steadily as possible between two targets in a sagittal plane for 30 seconds. Some of the key outcome measures included trajectory variability and elbow range of motion. The variability in the wrist trajectories was significantly reduced when participants reached in time with a metronome cue. The participants also used significantly more elbow extension when they were reaching with the auditory cue. These profound results provided evidence that survivors of stroke could entrain upper-extremity reaching movements to an auditory cue to improve their reaching characteristics. These effects were essentially instantaneous. We felt that PSE could be expanded as a reaching intervention for survivors of stroke based on these findings. More recently we have studied how survivors of stroke performed discrete versus cyclic reaching to determine whether the basic structure of a reaching task alters how the movements are generated (Massie et al., 2012). We asked 17 survivors of stroke to perform two forward-reaching tasks—five reaching cycles in a cyclic task without any rhythmic auditory cues, and five discrete reaches. We instructed the participants to reach as quickly and as accurately as possible between two targets in a parasagittal plane 35 cm apart. One of the interesting findings from this project was the greater amount of trunk rotation used when reaching cyclically compared with discrete reaches. This represents a movement strategy for cyclic reaching with the stroke-affected side, yet this is not likely to be a negative compensation, because the degree of rotation did not different greatly from that when the participants reached with the less affected side. Another interesting finding from this study was that the participants did not show differences in the accuracy at target contact when reaching cyclically. This suggests that the motor performance was not affected by having to generate cyclic reaching that is continuous during the five trials and requires real-time afferent feedback and efferent motor output. Taken together, these studies highlight the distinct motor control strategies that are involved when survivors of stroke are asked to reach cyclically, and the added benefits of reaching in synchronization with a rhythmic auditory cue.

Based on our initial study of rhythmic cued reaching compared with non-cued reaching, we developed a PSE training program for reaching in survivors of stroke. This program was a combination of supervised therapy and a home training program. Patients completed 1 hour of supervised training in the research clinic 3 days per week. The first day of therapy was used to provide patients with an overview of the program and familiarize them with the training protocol. At subsequent visits, patients completed 1 hour of PSE exercises under the guidance of a therapy trainer. Patients were asked to complete a further 2 hours of practice the same day, and then 3 hours on the subsequent day (Tuesday/Thursday). A therapist trainer phoned the subjects at home on their "days off" to check on their progress and to make modifications to the home program if necessary. No practice schedules were given for the weekends, and patients completed 2 weeks of therapy for a total of 30 hours of training.

A target matrix (see Figure 5.2) was used for this study, and participants were given a matrix to take home with them. A total of 28 consecutively numbered targets were

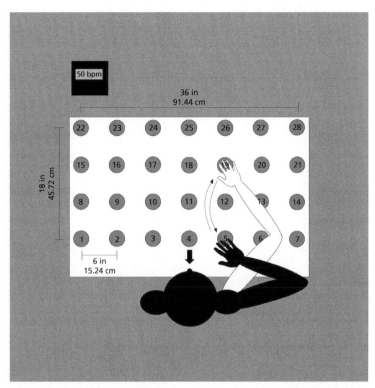

Fig. 5.2. A schematic diagram of the training template used in PSE. The therapist trainer would determine pairs of targets individually for each patient to work on specific movements that were challenging. The frequency at which movements were made was also set by the therapist, as illustrated in Table 5.2.

organized in a 36-inch by 18-inch grid with 6 inches between targets. An arrow centered on the matrix indicated where the patient was to center his or her body in front of the matrix. The matrix was secured on to a standard-height table, and patients were instructed to use a standard table at home and to center their chair in front of the arrow. A metronome was used to determine the reaching frequency, and patients were instructed to reach in time with the metronome beat. The initial frequency was set to match the self-selected timing which was observed during a practice trial with no metronome beat.

During the hour of supervised training, patients completed five to ten 30-second trials for a given target array. This allowed for many repetitions of each movement, a critical component of relearning. To ensure massed practice, 15–20 seconds of rest were allowed between trials (i.e. patients completed more training than rest). One to two minutes of rest were allowed between blocks of trials. A block of trials consisted of a set of target arrays, and the metronome beat could be changed. Table 5.2 shows an example of progression through a therapy session. One of the unique aspects of this training program was the ability to alter the reaching tasks spatially and temporally. Sets of targets were determined to

Table 5.2. Example of the progression through a PSE protocol: patients are required to move between pairs of targets at a specified metronome frequency, with increases in distance or frequency increased as the patient progresses through the therapy protocol

Training day	Trial set	Number of trials	Number of trials completed	Metronome frequency (bpm)	Target pairs
1	1	5	XXXXX	45	3,10
	2	10		40	2,11
	3	10		40	4,10
	4	10		50	2,9
	5	–			
2	1	10		50	3,10
	2	5		40	2,11
	3	5		40	2,18
	4	5		45	4,10
	5	5		50	4,10
	6	–			

elicit reaching movements in different directions. For example, a set of targets could be in the sagittal plane, frontal plane, or diagonal planes. Because of this, we could target movements that were more difficult to generate or that required specific retraining. In addition to changing the direction of the reach, the distance could also be modified to include shorter or longer reaching movements. Reaching could be changed temporally by making the metronome beat faster or slower. Many of these parameters were manipulated for individual patients depending on the specific movement impairments, but our goal was to progress each patient through the protocol to improve the distances and speed at which the trials could be completed.

Patients underwent assessments prior to starting the training program and immediately after the training program. We measured impairment by using the Fugl-Meyer Assessment (FMA), which is a sensory–motor assessment that quantifies reflexes, movements within and outside of synergies, fine motor function, and coordination (Fugl-Meyer et al., 1975). We found that participants generally showed increased FMA scores, indicating a decrease in the level of impairment. Functional capacity was measured using the WMFT, which quantifies how quickly an individual can generate movements in the upper extremity. We found that participants were able to complete the tasks faster following the training period.

We also measured the participants' ability to reach by quantifying movement with kinematic motion analysis techniques (see Figure 5.3). We asked them to complete a continuous, cyclic reaching task between two targets in a parasagittal plane without any rhythmic auditory cues. The outcome measures included how much compensatory trunk movement

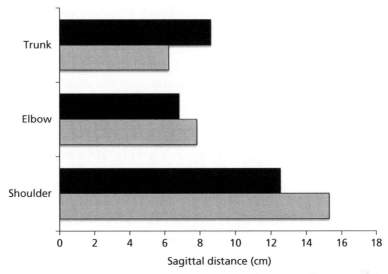

Fig. 5.3. The degree of linear distance that was generated by the degree of anterior trunk displacement, elbow extension, and shoulder flexion, similar to the data presented in Figure 5.2. The top bars represent the amount by which the trunk flexed forward while reaching between the proximal and distal targets before (black) and after (gray) PSE training. Clearly visible is the significant decrease in compensatory trunk displacement following the training. This finding paralleled a significant increase in the amount of movement generated by shoulder flexion following the training, represented in the bottom set of bars. A slight but statistically non-significant increase in the degree of elbow extension was also observed. The improvement in compensatory trunk movement was counterbalanced by the improvement in shoulder flexion.

Data from Malcolm M P, Massie C, and Thaut M (2009). Rhythmic auditory-motor entrainment improves hemiparetic arm kinematics during reaching movements: a pilot study. *Topics in Stroke Rehabilitation*, 16, 69–79.

was used to accomplish the reaching task, how much shoulder flexion and elbow extension were used, and the movement time and reaching velocity. We found that, following PSE, the participants used significantly less compensatory trunk movement. This was accomplished by using significantly more shoulder flexion. We also found that they were able to reach faster after the training period. Combining these findings with the experimental data from the single session of cyclic reaching suggests that cyclic reaching is distinct from discrete reaching, and that practicing cyclic reaching tasks with PSE can improve movement strategies, generalizes to reaching without PSE, and promotes better functional ability.

Our study demonstrated that PSE has the potential to reduce compensatory trunk movements in addition to improving the functional capacity to use the stroke-affected arm and hand (Malcolm et al., 2009). This was an important finding for the study because we did not include a fine motor element in the training. Although our study is just one example of the potential to incorporate PSE as an intervention, a number of other studies have implemented cyclic upper-extremity movement tasks with a metronome cue (Beckelhimer et al., 2011; Richards et al., 2008; Senesac et al., 2010; Whitall et al., 2000). The pilot study by Whitall et al. (2000) included 14 chronic survivors of stroke in a 6-week intervention using the repetitive bilateral arm training with rhythmic auditory cueing (BATRAC) protocol. This protocol was utilized for 20 minutes three times a week, and required the participant to slide handles of the BATRAC apparatus in time with a metronome cue that was set at his or her preferred movement speed. Improvements in functional ability were noted during the follow-up period. Subsequently, Richards et al. (2008) performed a study using the BATRAC apparatus with slightly different training parameters, and the improvements were not as dramatic as those in the initial study. Senesac et al. (2010) reported the kinematics for an intervention study with 14 survivors of stroke in the chronic phase of recovery using the BATRAC apparatus. This training protocol consisted of 2.25-hour sessions four times a week for 2 weeks. When kinematic motion analysis was used to determine outcome measures, improvements were found in the peak velocity and the smoothness of the reaching movement, and the path of the hand was straighter when reaching (Senesac et al., 2010). These authors suggest that although the BATRAC device trains movements in a limited range of forward reaching, this training may develop the building blocks of movements required for more complex movements for those survivors of stroke who are just regaining the capacity to move. This group of studies using the BATRAC system is one example of how rhythmic auditory cues can be used in upper-extremity movements that are constrained to the track's gliding surface. There has also been an application of a commercially available product as a treatment modality with two survivors of stroke, but very few details of the protocol were provided (Beckelhimer et al., 2011). All of these studies feature the use of a rhythmic auditory cue combined with cyclic reaching, and implementation of these types of interventions is likely to expand.

5.5 Clinical applications of PSE

One benefit of PSE is the ability to grade and modify the training based on the individual needs of the patient. For example, this training could be beneficial as a precursor to interventions requiring more dexterous use of the hand if a patient has some gross motor movement but not much fine motor ability. The PSE protocol that we implemented was well suited for this, as we could focus on improving more proximal gross motor movements. The benefits from training the proximal control should subsequently benefit distal training by reducing the amount of training required for proximal control. Greater movement potential in the shoulder and elbow should facilitate a greater working area for which fine motor components could be trained.

The potential also exists for PSE to promote better quality of movement for survivors of stroke who have learned compensatory movements. These can be clinically difficult to remediate, but PSE may facilitate better movement quality by entraining movement patterns with an auditory cue coupled with therapist expertise to select movements that will prevent or limit compensatory movements. This can be accomplished by selecting a set of target arrays that will prevent the compensatory movement, and by limiting the travel distance until sufficient movement is possible without having to compensate with the trunk or shoulder abduction. For example, selecting a target array in a diagonal pattern across the body will facilitate elbow extension, shoulder horizontal adduction, and shoulder flexion. Care should be taken to start with a distance that does not elicit trunk flexion. The distance can then be graded as greater movement is possible without eliciting compensatory movements. The advantage of PSE is that the focus of movements is on the synchronization with the metronome cue, and not necessarily on how the movements are generated. This is an interesting area for clinicians, because the focus of attention during a task can alter reaching kinematics. Fasoli et al. (2002) demonstrated that asking survivors of stroke to attend to their arm or to how the movement was generated was detrimental to the overall motor performance compared with attending to an external focus. This concept is likely to extend to the benefits of PSE, such that patients are attending to the task rather than to how the movements are generated, and the rhythmic auditory cue provides a subliminal stimulus by which the motor system can entrain movements.

Grading of movements within a PSE context is essentially unlimited as the patient progresses and their function improves. For example, it is possible to include more planes of movement. This can be accomplished by using targets in a vertical plane or by having more complex target arrays (i.e. more than two targets). Although all of our targets were located on a transverse/horizontal plane, the use of targets in a vertical plane would not be difficult. We also graded the reaching tasks by asking patients to complete movements to more than two targets such that they would make a continuous triangular or rectangular motion. Elements of fine motor control could also be incorporated into a PSE training program. Without requiring any additional equipment, we encouraged greater fine motor control by asking patients to try to make contact with the targets with their fingers extended. We graded this by encouraging extension of different fingers on repetitions, or by opening and closing the hand on successive contacts. The expansion of PSE concepts is feasible, and the option of grading movements is one of the benefits of implementing this type of training for survivors of stroke.

5.6 PSE and CIT in joint application

PSE can be expanded to include more complex upper-extremity tasks. In this way, concepts from PSE and CIT could be integrated. A rhythmic auditory cue could be easily integrated into a task that is cyclic in nature, such as wiping a counter or stirring a pot. Another example is to use a metronome cue while rolling dough back and forth. There also are a number of opportunities in which movements that are typically performed discretely can be modified to incorporate cyclic movements. For example, an activity such as playing cards or dominoes that is often a discrete movement can be modified to incorporate cyclic elements by asking the patient to move the playing pieces to specified locations (targets) with an auditory cue. Another example is to have a rhythmic auditory cue playing while moving cans into a cupboard. The patient could be instructed to grasp, transport, and release cans in synchronization with a metronome beat. This would probably require a slower frequency to allow for a grasping component, depending on the functional level of the patient. A task such as replacing hangers on a rod could be accomplished in synchronization with a metronome cue. Completing these types of tasks with an auditory cue would use the feed-forward temporal planning advantages of PSE while incorporating the principles of task practice and shaping that are used within interventions such as CIT.

There is a growing evidence base for incorporating PSE as a clinical approach for upper-extremity interventions for survivors of stroke, and this is supported by both basic/translational data and intervention studies. Our data suggest that survivors of stroke use a distinct motor control strategy when reaching cyclically, and that these movements can be enhanced when reaching to a patterned sensory cue (Thaut et al., 2002). Extending these benefits to interventions is also supported by our intervention data (Malcolm et al., 2009) and research studies by others. PSE represents a protocol that can be easily adapted and implemented in the clinic and used as a structured home program. The only requirement is a metronome (low cost) or other device to play an auditory rhythmic cue at variable frequencies—this represents one of the major benefits of PSE, because these interventions do not require large expensive items of sophisticated equipment. Although targets are not necessarily required, they can be easily created and/or adapted. We used a printed target template for participants, but any target could be used. For example, two targets could be made from colored paper or plastic, placed on a surface, and then moved or altered for the next set of trials. The advantage of this type of flexibility is that movements are not constrained, but rather they are built on repetitions and improvements in motor performance—that is, motor learning variables that are important to attend to in rehabilitation contexts. The PSE techniques incorporating motor–auditory entrainment are easy to implement clinically with survivors of stroke either as structured home programs or as a combination of home and in-clinic training.

References

Beckelhimer, S. C. et al. (2011). Computer-based rhythm and timing training in severe, stroke-induced arm hemiparesis. *American Journal of Occupational Therapy, 65*, 96–100.

Fasoli, S. E., Trombly, C. A., Tickle-Degnen, L., and Verfaellie, M. H. (2002). Effect of instructions on functional reach in persons with and without cerebrovascular accident. *American Journal of Occupational Therapy, 56*, 380–90.

Fugl-Meyer, A. R. et al. (1975). Post-stroke hemiplegic patient.1. Method for evaluation of physical performance. *Scandinavian Journal of Rehabilitation Medicine, 7*, 13–31.

Levin, M. F., Kleim, J. A., and Wolf, S. L. (2009). What do motor "recovery" and "compensation" mean in patients following stroke? *Neurorehabilitation and Neural Repair, 23*, 313–19.

Malcolm, M. P., Massie, C., and Thaut, M. (2009). Rhythmic auditory–motor entrainment improves hemiparetic arm kinematics during reaching movements: a pilot study. *Topics in Stroke Rehabilitation, 16*, 69–79.

Massie, C., Malcolm, M. P., Greene, D., and Thaut, M. (2009). The effects of constraint-induced therapy on kinematic outcomes and compensatory movement patterns: an exploratory study. *Archives of Physical Medicine and Rehabilitation, 90*, 571–9.

Massie, C., Malcolm, M. P., Greene, D. P., and Browning, R. C. (2012). Kinematic motion analysis and muscle activation patterns of continuous reaching in survivors of stroke. *Journal of Motor Behavior, 44*, 213–22.

Michaelsen, S. M., Dannenbaum, R., and Levin, M. F. (2006). Task-specific training with trunk restraint on arm recovery in stroke: randomized control trial. *Stroke, 37,* 186–92.

Page, S. J. et al. (2008). Modified constraint-induced therapy in chronic stroke: results of a single-blinded randomized controlled trial. *Physical Therapy, 88,* 333–40.

Richards, L. G. et al. (2008). Bilateral arm training with rhythmic auditory cueing in chronic stroke: not always efficacious. *Neurorehabilitation and Neural Repair, 22,* 180–84.

Senesac, C. R., Davis, S., and Richards, L. (2010). Generalization of a modified form of repetitive rhythmic bilateral training in stroke. *Human Movement Science, 29,* 137–48.

Taub, E. and Uswatte, G. (2003). Constraint-induced movement therapy: bridging from the primate laboratory to the stroke rehabilitation laboratory. *Journal of Rehabilitation Medicine, 35,* 34–40.

Thaut, M. H., McIntosh, G. C., and Rice, R. R. (1997). Rhythmic facilitation of gait training in hemiparetic stroke rehabilitation. *Journal of Neurological Sciences, 151,* 207–12.

Thaut, M. H. et al. (2002). Kinematic optimization of spatiotemporal patterns in paretic arm training with stroke patients. *Neuropsychologia, 40,* 1073–81.

Uswatte, G. et al. (2006a). Contribution of the shaping and restraint components of Constraint-Induced Movement therapy to treatment outcome. *Neurorehabilitation, 21,* 147–56.

Uswatte, G. et al. (2006b). The Motor Activity Log-28: assessing daily use of the hemiparetic arm after stroke. *Neurology, 67,* 1189–94.

Whitall, J., McCombe Waller, S., Silver, K. H., and Macko, R. F. (2000). Repetitive bilateral arm training with rhythmic auditory cueing improves motor function in chronic hemiparetic stroke. *Stroke, 31,* 2390–95.

Wolf S L, Lecraw D E, Barton L A, and Jann B B (1989). Forced use of hemiplegic upper extremities to reserve the effect of learned nonuse among chronic stroke and head-injured patients. *Experimental Neurology, 104,* 125–32.

Wolf, S. L. et al. (2001). Assessing Wolf motor function test as outcome measure for research in patients after stroke. *Stroke, 32,* 1635–9.

Wolf, S. L. et al. (2006). Effect of constraint-induced movement therapy on upper extremity function 3 to 9 months after stroke: the EXCITE randomized clinical trial. *Journal of the American Medical Association, 296,* 2095–104.

Woodbury, M. L. et al. (2009). Effects of trunk restraint combined with intensive task practice on poststroke upper extremity reach and function: a pilot study. *Neurorehabilitation and Neural Repair, 23,* 78–91.

Wu, C. Y. et al. (2007a). A randomized controlled trial of modified constraint-induced movement therapy for elderly stroke survivors: changes in motor impairment, daily functioning, and quality of life. *Archives of Physical Medicine and Rehabilitation, 88,* 273–8.

Wu, C. Y. et al. (2007b). Effects of modified constraint-induced movement therapy on movement kinematics and daily function in patients with stroke: a kinematic study of motor control mechanisms. *Neurorehabilitation and Neural Repair, 21,* 460–66.

Chapter 6

Assessment and the Transformational Design Model (TDM)

Michael H. Thaut

6.1 Principles of assessment

Assessment is a critical element in evidence-based therapy. Assessments give the therapist the framework and basis on which to select the optimal care options and track treatment progress based on the patient's level of functioning. Assessment is therefore the basis for treatment that follows best-practice standards. These standards involve a process of treatment selection based on available research evidence, or at least preliminary evidence of effectiveness for best treatment outcome. In this context, it is important to distinguish between two types of assessment, namely *diagnostic assessment* and *clinical assessment*.

Diagnostic assessment usually involves complex medical or psychological procedures and tests to determine diagnoses, carried out by professionals who have specialized knowledge of the diagnostic and etiologic aspects of disorders.

Clinical assessment serves two different functions. The first function is to track the level of functioning of the patient during the therapy process, starting with intake assessments and continuing with regular assessment updates throughout the duration of therapy until discharge. This function should be the basis for determining the progress of therapy as objectively as possible, and establishing a framework of data-driven therapy to ensure an optimal treatment outcome for the patient. The second function of clinical assessment is concerned with optimal treatment selection. It addresses the question of what is the most promising treatment option, based on the assessment of functioning of the patient and the available research data. For example, several research studies (Pilon et al., 1998; Thaut et al., 2001) have shown that rhythmic speech cueing (RSC) is more effective in more severe speech dysarthria (intelligibility rates of 60% or lower) than in moderate or mild forms of the condition. Thus intelligibility assessment would allow one to decide—based on clinical research data—whether RSC is the most promising treatment technique for a patient with speech dysarthria.

In summary, clinical assessment enables (1) optimal treatment selection and (2) the monitoring of patient progress throughout the therapy process. Most therapists are involved in clinical assessment in their daily work. Therefore this chapter will focus on the principles of and resources for clinical assessment.

In order to apply assessment outcomes meaningfully to clinical practice, two criteria for the therapeutic approach must be met. First, the therapeutic applications (i.e. the clinical techniques) must be defined and standardized according to some form of consistent treatment protocol, and secondly, there must be research data about the effectiveness of their clinical application. Fortunately, because the techniques of neurologic music therapy (NMT) evolved as the clinical translation of research data, NMT fulfills both conditions, and successful assessment can be incorporated within and applied to the daily routines of NMT work.

Effective assessments should provide meaningful information about a patient's status and progress when recovering from impairments, and when learning new or relearning former functional skills and behaviors. Therefore clinical assessment tools should be standardized, and their validity and reliability tested, so that they provide information about the patient's general level of functioning in relation to certain standards of health and ability, rather than just indicating how successful the patient is in performing the therapeutic exercises. In other words, assessments should give us benchmarks about the patient's status. Based on these requirements, assessments in most NMT techniques are conducted separately from the therapeutic music exercises. In rhythmic auditory stimulation (RAS), gait assessments are built into the clinical exercise protocol, and functional performance data can be extracted from the exercise performance. However, RAS is the exception among the 20 NMT techniques currently in use. In the other techniques, separate assessments are necessary to benchmark the patient's performance. Yet even in RAS one may want to assess beyond the treatment protocol—for example, one may wish to test general lower-extremity function and gait adaptations in order to gain a more comprehensive picture of the patient's functional mobility.

Fortunately, over the past 20 years there has been much progress in the development of reliable and valid clinical assessment tools that are relatively easy to apply and have normative scores for comparative benchmarking. It is important for the music therapist to bear in mind that most of them are not music based. However, this allows the music therapist to conduct generalizable assessments about the patient's functional status. One music-based test that is actually used in neurologic assessments is the rhythm test of the Seashore Tests of Musical Ability, which tests for non-verbal auditory perception, auditory acuity, temporal (rhythmic) pattern discrimination, and sustained auditory attention (Reitan and Wolfson, 2004). Contrary to previous notions, research has shown that this Seashore test does not discriminate between patients with right and left temporal lobe damage (Boone and Rausch, 1989). The Seashore rhythm test is used in the Halstead–Reitan Neuropsychological Battery.

It is important to note that most assessment tools are not "owned" by professional disciplines, but can be administered by a wide range of healthcare professionals with the appropriate education, test training, and clinical background, and if used with appropriate clinical populations. In the USA, assessment falls within the official scope of practice of the Certification Board of Music Therapy (CBMT) and the standards of practice of the American Music Therapy Association (AMTA). With appropriate knowledge, music therapists can and should implement clinical assessments or collaborate with other disciplines in patient assessment in their respective areas of clinical practice, such as motor, speech/language, and cognitive rehabilitation. Becoming familiar with clinical assessment tools for the practitioner is therefore an essential component of NMT education, both in academic training and in professional continuing education. Assessments of musical preference, familiarity, or musical background and skills in patients can be very useful for appropriate selection of musical stimuli for effective therapeutic music exercises. However, these assessments do not offer data for monitoring therapy progress or selecting optimal treatment.

6.2 **Assessment in the transformational design model (TDM)**

Assessment plays a critical role in two steps of the *transformational design model (TDM)* for NMT practice. The TDM was developed to help the clinician to translate research findings from the *rational scientific mediating model (RSMM)* into functional music therapy practice (Thaut, 2005). The RSMM provides a model of how to translate basic music research from the neurosciences and behavioral sciences into applied clinical music research. The TDM guides music therapists through the basic mechanisms of designing functional therapeutic music applications whose validity is based on the RSMM. It also averts two traditional potential weaknesses of therapeutic music interventions: first, an activity-based approach in which therapeutic goals are retroactively incorporated into generic music activities, and secondly, the use of therapeutic music techniques that address therapeutic goals very broadly and generally, and are only weakly related to functional therapeutic outcomes. The five steps in the original TDM (Thaut, 2005) are here expanded into six basic steps:

1 diagnostic and functional/clinical assessment of the patient

2 development of therapeutic goals/objectives

3 design of functional, non-musical therapeutic exercise structures and stimuli

4 translation of Step 3 into functional therapeutic music exercises

5 outcome reassessment

6 transfer of therapeutic learning to functional applications for "activities of daily living" (ADL).

Steps 1 to 3 and Steps 5 and 6 in the TDM are basic processes common to all therapy disciplines. Step 1 entails understanding the diagnostic and etiological assessment of the client and applying clinical assessments for optimal treatment selection and monitoring of the patient's progress. Step 2 consists of the development of appropriate and measurable therapy goals and objectives. Step 3 consists of the design of therapeutic exercises, structures, or therapeutic stimuli to accomplish the clinical goals and objectives.

This design process is based upon functional behaviors of the patient and does not yet include musical considerations. The planning of these therapeutic experiences is similar to, or at times even based on, therapeutic plans that are utilized across rehabilitation disciplines. This approach also ensures patient-centered rather than discipline-centered therapy programs. In patient-centered approaches, all disciplines work together to support the same therapeutic goals from different angles, using as many collaborative and interdisciplinary techniques as possible. In discipline-centered therapy, patients move from one therapy session to the next through their daily schedule, being treated for different aspects of rehabilitation with little consideration given to collaborative planning and treatment.

The crucial clinical process for neurologic music therapists occurs in Step 4. Here their unique professional role emerges—that of translating functional and therapeutic exercises, elements, and stimuli into functional therapeutic music exercises and stimuli that are "structure equivalent" (i.e. have all functional exercise elements translated into musical elements) to the non-musical exercise plan.

For example, social interaction exercises are translated into musical role plays expressed in group improvisation structures that simulate the content of the specifically intended interaction and communication exercises. Emotional communication exercises are translated into musical, possibly non-verbal, group dynamic improvisation exercises to express emotions. Access to positive cognitive networks in psychotherapy and counseling is facilitated by mood vectoring through guided music listening, putting the client into the desired mood state to be able to access positive cognitive networks.

Speech pacing in dysarthria rehabilitation may be accomplished through rhythmic cues in musical stimuli. For divided attention training in a small group improvisation, two different instruments give two different "action" cues simultaneously to the third player, who thus trains his or her divided attention capability (e.g. xylophone signals to the "target" client play or do not play, high or low drum signals play high register or low register).

Memory training may be facilitated by music-based mnemonic devices (e.g. songs, chants, rhymes). Exercises to improve the range of motion and limb coordination are translated into structures of therapeutic instrument-playing exercises. Functional reaching and grasping exercises are regulated by cues in rhythmically structured beat sequences or strongly accentuated rhythms in music. Gait-training exercises are facilitated by rhythmic entrainment and audio-spinal stimulation. It is important to remember that it is not the goals or objectives that are translated into music applications, but the structure, process, and elements of functional non-musical exercises and stimuli.

The translational or transformational process is guided by three principles:

1 *Scientific validity*: the translation process must be congruent with the scientific information developed in the RSMM. For example, appropriately connected research models in musical and non-musical memory formation allow for the development of valid techniques using music as a mnemonic device for cognitive retraining. If music is used for memory training without considering the basic and clinical research knowledge about musical memory and its parallels to non-musical memory processes, non-functional and only spuriously effective techniques are likely to evolve.

2 *Musical logic*: the musical experience in therapy has to conform, even at the most basic level, to the esthetic and artistic principles of good musical forms. In other words, the

musical experience has to be esthetically well composed and performed, whether active or receptive music techniques are applied (e.g. listening exercises, improvisation, rehearsed performance, movement to music). The beneficial influence of music on structuring, organizing, and enhancing perception, learning, and training in the therapeutic process can unfold only within optimal musical patterns, regardless of the level of complexity. However, we must remember that the application of a certain musical technique, such as improvisation, does not in itself create a theoretical model of music therapy practice.

3 *Structural equivalence*: the therapeutic music exercise has to be isomorphic in therapeutic structure and function to the non-musical functional design. For example, the group dynamic structure of a psychotherapy exercise has to be captured and simulated in the structure of the musical experience in order to truly facilitate and enhance the intended therapeutic process (e.g. exercises designed to improve the range of arm motion by playing musical instruments must entail the functional motions of the non-musical therapy goals in order to accomplish useful training for the patient). Thus a well-trained music therapist needs to learn how to create appropriate musical analogs for non-musical behavior and stimuli. Here the logic and creativity of functional musicianship and translational "non-musical to musical" thinking and reasoning form a necessary third prerequisite for isomorphically molding functional therapy into functional music therapy.

In Step 5 the music therapist should reassess the patient's progress using the same clinical assessment tools from Step 1 to be able to compare and benchmark the effectiveness of treatment. Step 5 assessment may occur after each session, intermittently during the treatment process, or only at the end of treatment and at follow-ups. The schedule of assessment administration depends on the clinical setting, patient needs, and the assessment tool. Some assessments are very sensitive to capturing small changes, possibly over just one session or over short periods of time. Other tests only capture larger changes or confound the assessment by creating a "test learning" effect in the patient.

Step 6 deals with transfer exercises from treatment training to activities of daily living. One of the most important considerations in transfer is to prepare the patient to continue exercising and using functions. One of the main underlying principles in therapeutic training to recover functions or learn new functions is based on neuroplasticity—that is, the ability of the brain to reorganize or "rewire" itself to build new neural connections. However, brain plasticity is experience driven, following the "use it or lose it" principle. Effective transfer preparation of the patient may also involve the preparation of materials such as electronic audio devices, learning materials, music instruments, and so on.

The TDM in neurologic music therapy is a practical guide to enable the therapist to compose goal-oriented therapeutic music experiences based on a functional reasoning process that links assessments, goals, and learning and training experiences. The TDM is the clinical complement or practical extension of the scientific theory model, the RSMM. The validity of the isomorphic transformation of a therapeutic experience into a therapeutic music experience is measured against the scientific evidence in Step 4 of the RSMM. For example, the musical and transformational logic of a certain therapeutic music exercise may be fulfilled (e.g. a well-structured, musically creative, and motivating exercise using the reading and play-ing of musical notation in order to help the reading of letters), but the scientific logic is missing because no evidence for the therapeutic value of music exists in a certain area of application (reading musical symbols does not transfer to enhanced reading of letters). Thus the RSMM functions as a check on the validity of NMT techniques developed within the TDM system. On the other hand, the use of the TDM allows the music therapist to examine the research evidence relating to the RSMM for applicable information to optimize treatment variables. The use of the RSMM may also help to identify weak areas in bodies of knowledge, and may stimulate the ongoing and dynamic development of new research agendas in NMT. Through this exchange, the clinician shares in the three basic principles of data-based therapies, namely skepticism, determinism, and empiricism. The available scientific evidence relating to the RSMM allows us to understand why Step 4—the translation of functional therapy into functional music therapy—is not an unnecessary detour of the treatment process rather than a facilitating and optimizing process to provide "best-practice" interventions.

6.3 **Assessment instruments**

In this section a selection of common clinical assessment instruments will be listed by treatment domain. In addition, some major assessment databases will be listed, excluding any commercial ones which may be selected by the consumer in follow-up purchase. The development of assessment tools is a very dynamic and fast-changing area, so continuous personal updating through web searches and professional networking is recommended. The following list of resources is not exhaustive, but rather is intended as an introduction to finding resources. Assessment tools can be found directly in databases or via web searches. Some are referenced and can be found in published papers. Others require purchase from vendors. Handbooks containing assessment scales are also available.

6.3.1 **Quality-of-life scales**

For a review, see McDowell and Newell (1996).

6.3.2 **Neurologic rating scales**

For a review, see Herndon (2006).

6.3.3 **General use scales**

- Ashworth Scale and Modified Ashworth Scale for spasticity (motor)
- Walking While Talking (dual task, attention/motor)
- Timed Up and Go (motor)

- Mini Mental State Examination (cognition)
- Barthel Index of Activities of Daily Living (activities of daily living)
- Rivermead Activities of Daily Living (ADL) Scales (activities of daily living)
- Functional Activity Scale (FAS) (activities of daily living)
- Functional Independence Measure (FIM) (motor/cognition)
- Clock Drawing Test (cognition)

6.3.4 Pediatric developmental scales

- Peabody Picture Vocabulary Test
- Pediatric Evaluation of Disability Inventory (PEDI)
- Bruininks–Oseretsky Test of Motor Proficiency
- Wide Range Assessment of Memory and Learning
- Gross Motor Function Measure (recommended for cerebral palsy)
- Purdue Perceptual–Motor Survey
- Psychoeducational Profile (PEP) (autism and communicative disabilities)

6.3.5 Motor scales

- Fugl-Meyer Assessment of Motor Recovery after Stroke
- Wolf Motor Function Test (WMFT)
- Action Research Arm Test (ARAT)
- Rivermead Motor Assessment (RMA)
- Rivermead Mobility Index (RMI)
- Berg Balance Scale (BBS)
- Nine Hole Peg Test (recommended for Parkinson's disease and multiple sclerosis)
- Box and Block Test (BBT)
- 10-Meter Walk Test
- Motor Activity Log (MAL)
- Jebson–Taylor Hand Function Test

6.3.6 Cognition scales

- Rey Auditory Verbal Learning Test (for mood and memory training)
- Trail Making Test (TMT) Parts A and B (for musical executive function training)
- Digit Span Test (Forward and Backward) (for mood and memory training)
- Seashore Rhythm Test (for musical attentional control training, and aptitude testing)

- Paced Auditory Serial Addition Test (PASAT) (for musical attentional control training)
- Albert's Line Crossing Test (for musical neglect training)
- Star Cancelation Test (for musical neglect training)
- Line Bisection Test (for musical neglect training)
- Montreal Cognitive Assessment (MoCA) (for musical attention control training, associative mood and memory training, and musical executive function training)
- Geriatric Depression Scale (GDS) (for music in psychosocial training and counselling)
- Recognition Memory Test (for mood and memory training)
- Multiple Affect Adjective Check List (MAACL) (for music in psychosocial training and counselling)
- State–Trait Anxiety Inventory (STAI) (for music in psychosocial training and counselling)

6.3.7 **Speech/language scales**

- Stuttering Severity Instrument (for rhythmic speech cueing)
- Test of Childhood Stuttering (for rhythmic speech cueing)
- Peabody Picture Vocabulary Test (for developmental speech and language training through music (DSLM))
- Correct Information Unit (CIU) analysis (for melodic intonation therapy, musical speech stimulation (MUSTIM))
- Boston Diagnostic Aphasia Examination

6.3.8 **Websites with multiple assessment tools**

A list of such websites is given at the end of this chapter.

References

Boone K B and Rausch R (1989). Seashore Rhythm Test performance in patients with unilateral temporal lobe damage. *Journal of Clinical Psychology*, 45, 614–18.

Herndon R M (ed.) (2006). *Handbook of Neurologic Rating Scales*. New York: Demos Medical Publishing.

McDowell I and Newell C (eds) (1996). *Measuring Health*. New York: Oxford University Press.

Pilon M A, McIntosh K H, and Thaut M H (1998). Auditory versus visual speech timing cues as external rate control to enhance verbal intelligibility in mixed spastic-ataxic dysarthric speakers: a pilot study. *Brain Injury*, 12, 793–803.

Reitan R M and Wolfson D (2004). Theoretical, methodological, and validational bases for the Halstead–Reitan Neuropsychological Test Battery. In: G Goldstein and S Beers (eds) *Comprehensive Handbook of Psychological Assessment. Volume 1. Intellectual and Neuropsychological Assessment*. Hoboken, NJ: John Wiley & Sons. pp. 105–8.

Thaut M H (2005). *Rhythm, Music, and the Brain: scientific foundations and clinical applications*. New York: Routledge.

Thaut M H, McIntosh G C, McIntosh K H, and Hoemberg V (2001). Auditory rhythmicity enhances movement and speech motor control in patients with Parkinson's disease. *Functional Neurology*, 16, 163–72.

Websites with multiple assessment tools

StrokEngine-Assess. http://strokengine.ca/assess

The Internet Stroke Center. www.strokecenter.org/professionals/stroke-assessment-scales

Iowa Geriatric Education Center (geriatric assessment tools). www.healthcare.uiowa.edu/igec/tools

Society of Hospital Medicine (quality initiatives, clinical tools, and geriatric care).
www.hospitalmedicine.org

Chapter 7

Rhythmic Auditory Stimulation (RAS) in Gait Rehabilitation for Patients with Parkinson's Disease: A Research Perspective

Miek de Dreu, Gert Kwakkel, and Erwin van Wegen

7.1 Introduction

What are the effects of rhythmic auditory stimulation (RAS) provided by a metronome or music in patients with Parkinson's disease (PD)? People with PD typically walk slowly, with short shuffling steps, and often fall, due to a decreased balance, festination, and freezing of gait (FOG). Since walking is essential for many activities of daily living (ADL), these problems can have a detrimental effect on independence and quality of life (QoL).

RAS, provided by a metronome, can be described as a relatively simple technique for improving gait of patients with PD. RAS can also include rhythmic cues embedded in music, which can additionally provide a cultural and motivational context.

Cross-sectional studies are summarized to explain the immediate effects of RAS on gait and insight in the optimal application. A meta-analysis of randomized controlled trials (RCTs) investigating RAS provided by a metronome provides strong evidence for an increase in gait speed and stride length. A second meta-analysis, which included studies of full body movement and dance, revealed improvements in balance, stride length, Six-Minute Walk Test (6MWT), dual-task walking speed, Timed Up and Go (TUG) test, and the Unified Parkinson's Disease Rating Scale-II (UPDRS-II). Even though the evidence is promising, further research should continue to broaden the applications of RAS, fine-tune study designs, and elucidate the underlying working mechanism of RAS.

7.2 Background

Facilitation of gait in patients with PD with sensory cues was reported for the first time in 1942 (Von Wilzenben, 1942). A detailed analysis of the effect of external (visual) cueing on gait was provided by Martin (1963). A few years later a "Dr. Trombly noticed that a patient who would severely 'freeze' while walking did not freeze while dancing. He envisioned the possibility of causing the patient to function continuously by feeding sound into his ears" (Ball, 1967). Auditory cues have been applied in the form of music as well as a metronome in combination with other physiotherapeutic techniques within a functional rehabilitation program with a long-term (1-year) follow-up (Gauthier et al., 1987). The first systematic investigation of auditory rhythmic cues in gait training for PD was carried out by Thaut et al. (1996) and Miller et al. (1996), who studied the effect of a 3-week daily home-based rhythmic training program compared with self-paced gait exercise and no specific gait training. Pre- and post-tests were assessed without rhythmic training cues. Subsequently, Thaut et al. (1996) introduced the term *rhythmic auditory stimulation (RAS)*. In the 1990s and the beginning of the twenty-first century, the scientific focus on auditory cueing continued, resulting in studies specifically directed at the evaluation of auditory cueing (e.g. Cubo et al., 2004; Ebersbach et al., 1999; Enzensberger et al., 1997; Freedland et al., 2002; Howe et al., 2003; McIntosh et al., 1997). However, the majority of these studies were of relatively low methodological quality (Lim et al., 2005). Based on this evidence, the use of RAS provided as a rhythmic beat was recommended as part of physical therapy interventions in guidelines to improve gait and gait-related activities for patients with PD (Keus et al., 2007). However, at that time it was still unknown whether the improvements during walking with RAS would transfer to uncued walking and activities of daily life.

7.3 **RAS definitions**

RAS can be defined as the application of rhythmical (temporal) auditory stimuli associated with the initiation and ongoing facilitation of gait and gait-related activities (Thaut et al., 1996; Keus et al., 2007; Lim et al., 2005), by providing a reference for the timing of movements. Clinically, RAS has been implicated as a relatively simple technique for improving the walking performance of patients with PD.

RAS may consist of a rhythmic beat, often provided by a metronome (Lim et al., 2005), or a more complex musical structure (de Bruin et al., 2010), or a combination of both (i.e. music with an enhanced beat) (Thaut et al., 1996, 1997), to which the user is asked to synchronize their movements or steps. Unfortunately, studies quantifying the adjustment of gait to the beat are scarce, despite their potential for improving the efficacy of RAS in clinical gait rehabilitation. RAS is one of several types of rhythmic external cueing. Other types of cueing are somatosensory cues (pulses of vibration on the wrist) or visual cueing (light flashes from specially designed glasses). When the participants were allowed to choose between these different cueing modalities, the majority ($n = 103$) of the included PD patients preferred RAS, and 51 patients preferred somatosensory cues. None of the participants preferred visual cues in the form of light flashes, even though this modality was shown to be feasible in a laboratory setting (Nieuwboer et al., 2007; van Wegen et al., 2006b). The preference for RAS may be related to a number of factors, including its effectiveness, its ease of use (for the patient as well for the specialist), and the fact that the patient can use it discretely, without attracting attention from bystanders. In contrast, patients with, for example, hearing deficits could benefit more from somatosensory cues than from auditory cues (van Wegen et al., 2006a).

RAS is directed at influencing cadence. However, it may indirectly affect other gait parameters, such as stride length and walking speed, as well (Lim et al., 2005). Recently it has been successfully combined with an instruction directed at influencing step length ("As you walk, try to take big steps") (Baker et al., 2007). Transverse stripes on the floor directly and effectively influence step length (Martin, 1963; Morris et al., 1996). However, whereas RAS can be used in virtually any environment, the use of visual cues is confined to areas in which these cues are available or have been applied deliberately.

7.4 Understanding RAS

The underlying working mechanism of RAS in PD is unknown. However, it has been proposed that it may function as an external timekeeper that supports the diminished function of the defective basal ganglia (McIntosh et al., 1997; Rubinstein et al., 2002), possibly through the involvement of compensatory networks in the brain (Thaut, 2005). This is an appealing explanation because it is specifically the timing and/or scaling of movements that seems to be impaired in patients with PD (McIntosh et al., 1997; Morris et al., 1994). Neuroimaging studies may substantiate this theory, as they suggest that alternative brain routes are activated during movement supported by RAS or other forms of external cueing. For example, Debaere et al. (2003) compared cyclical hand movements when a person had their eyes closed (internally generated coordination) with the same movements when the person received augmented visual feedback (externally guided coordination) on a computer screen. During the internally generated movements, among others, the basal ganglia, the supplementary motor area, and the cingulate motor cortex showed higher levels of involvement. When the movement was externally generated, other areas, such as the superior parietal cortex and the premotor cortex, showed higher activation levels (Debaere et al., 2003). A study by Cunnington et al. (2002) indicated that the basal ganglia were only involved in internally paced finger movements, and not during externally paced finger movements. A study investigating internally paced and externally paced lower limb movements (simulating walking) presented similar findings (Toyomura et al., 2012). Furthermore, differences in cerebral blood flow that were apparent in internally generated coordination tasks between patients with PD and age-matched controls decreased when external cues were provided (Jahanshahi et al., 1995).

The reported retention of up to 3 weeks after 3 weeks of training with RAS (McIntosh et al., 1998; Rochester et al., 2010a) implies a learning effect that is possibly due to plasticity of the brain with regard to the internal time-keeping and rhythm formation processes (known as *entrainment mechanisms*) (Thaut, 2005). Therefore RAS may be useful not only as a compensatory technique, but also as a training stimulus to improve non-cued performance during activities of daily living (Lim et al., 2010; Nieuwboer et al., 2007).

7.5 Effects of RAS on gait and gait-related activities

7.5.1 Overview of cross-sectional studies

The gait of people with PD is characterized by "constant" features, such as a stooped posture, slow speed, short shuffling steps, narrow step width, reduced counter-rotation of the trunk, and decreased arm swing (bradykinesia). In addition, patients experience episodal features, such as festination, FOG, and postural instability (Morris, 2006; Nieuwboer et al., 2008). FOG can be defined as an episodic inability to generate effective stepping (Giladi and Nieuwboer, 2008). When experiencing FOG, patients are unable to start or continue walking, and they feel as if their feet are glued to the ground. Although FOG is rather unpredictable, it can be triggered by navigating through small passages and/or turning (Nieuwboer and Giladi, 2008).

As mentioned earlier, RAS and/or visual cues have been suggested to be a powerful tool for improving gait performance in patients with PD (Lim et al., 2005; Rubinstein et al., 2002). The immediate effect of RAS on gait and gait-related tasks has been extensively studied during cross-sectional studies in laboratory situations (Lim et al., 2005). Table 7.1 provides an overview of the cross-sectional studies that have been reported since the most recent systematic review (Lim et al., 2005). In most of the studies a personalized mean step frequency was determined during uncued gait at comfortable speed, and was referred to as the baseline frequency of the metronome, to account for individual differences in step frequencies (Arias and Cudeiro, 2010; Baker et al., 2007; Hausdorff et al., 2007; Lee et al., 2012; Lohnes and Earhart, 2011; Nieuwboer et al., 2009; Rochester et al., 2009; Willems et al., 2006, 2007). Different frequencies provided by the metronome were determined as a percentage of the baseline frequency (Howe et al., 2003; Lohnes and Earhart, 2011; Willems et al., 2006). Cadence typically varied with the frequency of the metronome (Howe et al., 2003; Lohnes and Earhart, 2011; Willems et al., 2006), and therefore the short shuffling steps that are characteristic of gait in PD can be influenced by RAS with regard to step frequency. However, this finding does not guarantee a precise match of the steps with the RAS (Freeman et al., 1993). Gait speed generally increased compared with baseline, specifically with higher stimulation frequencies (Howe et al., 2003; Willems et al., 2007). Gait variability, represented as the coefficient of variation of either stride, step, or swing time (CV strideT, CV stepT, or swingT) decreased with RAS when provided at baseline frequency or 10% higher (Arias and Cudeiro, 2008; Hausdorff et al., 2007; Willems et al., 2007).

RAS did not appear to affect stride length consistently. Participants who experienced FOG as a symptom generally increased their step length with lower frequencies, whereas those who did not suffer from FOG increased their step length with higher frequencies (Lee et al., 2012; Willems et al., 2006). Therefore, in a more heterogeneous group of patients, the effects of RAS on stride length may have been diminished (Arias and Cudeiro, 2010; Howe et al., 2003; Suteerawattananon et al., 2004; Westheimer, 2008).

7.5.2 Effects of RAS on freezing of gait (FOG)

FOG is an episodic gait disorder characterized by an inability to generate effective forward-stepping movements (Giladi and Nieuwboer, 2008). It is difficult to investigate due to its unpredictable occurrence. With the exception of stride length (as described earlier), RAS affected gait in patients with FOG in a similar way to that in patients without FOG (Lee et al., 2012; Willems et al., 2006) (see Table 7.1).

RAS appeared to have a substantial effect on the number of freezing episodes and the duration of freezing when the medication was not functioning properly (i.e. during "off" periods or at the end of the dose) (Arias and Cudeiro, 2010; Lee et al., 2012). This is an

Table 7.1 Overview of cross-sectional trials

Reference	Comparison	Subject characteristics				Results	Main conclusion
		Subjects (n)	Age (years) M ± SD	H&Y stage M ± SD	On or off period		
Forward walking							
Hausdorff et al. 2007	Walking with RAS (100% PC) compared with non-cued preferred walking	PD = 29	PD = 67,2 ± 9.1	PD = 2.4 ± 0.4	n.r.	GS↑(+) SL↑(+) StrT SwiT↑(+) CV StrT CV SwiT	RAS at 110% reduced variability of walking, and these effects persisted 2 and 15 minutes later in uncued trials
	Walking with RAS (110% PC) compared with non-cued walking	PD = 29	PD = 67,2 ± 9.1	PD = 2.4 ± 0.4	n.r.	GS↑(+) SL↑(+) StrT↓(+) SwiT↑ CV StrT↓(+) CV SwiT↓(+)	
Arias et al. 2008	RAS, visual cues (light in glasses) and a combination compared with PW in SPD	SPD = 9	SPD = 71.33 ± 3.20	SPD = 3.11 ± 0.33	On	GS StepL (A↑) (C↑) (+) Ca (A↓) (V↓) (C↓) CV StrT (A↓) (C↓) (+) CV (StepL)	Auditory cues seemed to improve gait more effectively than visual cues in PD
	RAS at a range of frequencies from 70% to 110% of personal FW step frequency	SPD = 9	SPD = 71.33 ± 3.20	SPD = 3.11 ± 0.33	On	GS (90–110↑) (+) StepL (80–110↑) (+) Ca (70–90↓, 100–110↑) CV StrT (90 and 100↑) (–) CV(StepL)	Higher frequencies (90–110% FW) seemed to best improve gait in SPD patients
Freezing							
Willems et al. 2006	Cueing frequencies –20%, –10%, baseline, +10%, +20% of personal PW	PD+F = 10	PD+F = 68.4 ± 6.9	PD+F = 2.8 ± 0.6	On	GS (↑–10) (↑B) (↑+20) (+) SL (↑+10) (+) Ca (↑all)DST	Recommended RAS frequency for PD+F = RAS (90%), for PD–F = RAS (100%) or RAS (110%)
	Cueing frequencies –20%, –10%, baseline, +10%, +20% compared with the lower frequency	PD–F = 10	PD–F = 60.6 ± 6.2	PD–F = 2.7 ± 0.6	On	GS (–10↑) (B↑) (+10↑) (+) SL (–10↑) (B↑) (+) Ca (all↑) DST (–10↓) (+)	

Table 7.1 (continued)

Reference	Comparison	Subject characteristics				Results	Main conclusion
		Subjects (n)	Age (years) M ± SD	H&Y stage M ± SD	On or off period		
Forward walking							
Arias et al. 2010	PD+F who performed a walking trial with RAS compared with baseline	PD+F = 9	PD+F = 68.2 ±8.03	PD+F = n.r.	End of dose	GS↑ StepL Ca↑ Turning time↓ N of FOG↓ MD of FOG↓	RAS +10% prevents freezing at end of dose in combination with environmental challenges
Nieuwboer et al. 2009	Visual, auditory, and somatosensory cueing when patients were asked to pick up a tray, turn and walk back	PD-F = 65	PD-F = 66 ±8.1	PD-F = 2.5 ±0.6	On	N of FOG Turn time (A↓) (S↓)	Rhythmical cueing yielded faster performance of a functional turn in both freezers and non-freezers. RAS was more effective than visual cueing
		PD+F = 68	PD+F = 67,3 ±6.9	PD+F = 2.7 ±0.7	On	N of FOG Turn time (V↓) (A↓) (S↓)	
Lee et al. 2012	Visual cue (stripes on the floor) and auditory cue compared with baseline walking	PD+F = 15	PD+F = 69.1 ±8.1	PD+F = 2.3 ±0.5	Off	GS (V↑) SL (V↑) (A↑) Ca (V↓) (A↓) DST SST Tstep (V↓) (A↓) Ttime (V↓) (A↓) N FOG (V↓) (A↑) Pelvic tilt (V↑) HF KF(V↑) AD (V↑) (A↑)	RAS and visual cueing can positively affect gait in patients with PD+F; only RAS (not visual cueing) is advised in patients with PD-F
		PD-F = 10	PD-F = 63.2 ±7.6	PD-F = 1.60 ±0.52	Off	GS (V↓) SL Ca (V↓) (A↓) DST SST Tstep Ttime (V↑) Pelvic tilt (V↑) HF KF (V↑?) AD (V↑) (A↑)	
Dual tasks							
Baker et al. 2007	Effect of cues on a single task in PD compared with baseline	PD = 14	PD = 69.3 ± 3.4	PD = 2.7 ± 0.4	On	GS (At↑) (AAt↑) CV StepT (AAt↓) CV DLS (At↓) (AAt↓)	RAS (specifically in combination with an instruction: "As you walk try to take big steps") decreases gait variability and therefore possibly the attentional cost of walking
	Effect of cues on a dual task in PD compared with baseline	PD = 14	PD = 69.3 ± 3.4	PD = 2.7 ± 0.4	On	GS (At↑) (AAt↑) CV StepT (AAt↓) CV DLS	
Lohnes et al. 2011	Walking with an attentional cue (At), auditory (+10%), auditory (−10%), combination (+10%) and combination (−10%) compared with ...	PD = 11	PD = 70.3 ± 6.8	PD = 2.2 ± 0.3	On	Single task: GS (At↑) (C−10↑) (C+10↑) SL (At↑) (C−10↑) (C+10↑) Ca Dual task: GS SL Ca	Attentional strategy is most effective in single task; no cue strategy had an effect on gait with the current dual task

Table 7.1 (continued)

Reference	Comparison	Subject characteristics				Results	Main conclusion
		Subjects (n)	Age (years) M ± SD	H&Y stage M ± SD	On or off period		
Forward walking							
Turning							
Willems et al. 2007	Auditory cueing compared with no cueing	PD = 19	PD+F = 68.1 ± 7.3PD–F = 60.6 ± 6.2	PD+F = 2.8 ± 0.7PD–F = 2.6 ± 0.7	On	Turn StepL StepW StepD CV–StepD↓	The reduction of CV step in the cued trial may relate to a decrease in risk of falling and freezing
Cognitive impairment							
Rochester et al. 2009	Auditory cue with spatiotemporal instruction compared with auditory cue with a temporal instruction and no cue	PDCI = 9	PDCI = 74.9 ± 6.45	PDCI = 2.9 ± 0.5	On	GS↑ SL↑ Ca CV StepT CV DLS	Participants complied with testing and instructions. RAS with the instruction "Take a big step" significantly improved single- and dual-task walking

PD, Parkinson's disease; n, number of subjects; SD, standard deviation; RAS, rhythmic auditory stimulation; GS, gait speed; SL, stride length; Ca, cadence; StriT, stride time; SwiT, swing time; AMC, age-matched controls; n.r., not reported; n.a., not applicable; CV, coefficient of variation; StepL, step length; StepW, step width; StepD, step duration; StepT, step time; DST, double support time; SST, single support time; SPD, severe Parkinson's disease; FW, fast walking; PD+F, patients with Parkinson's disease who experience freezing; PD–F, patients with Parkinson's disease who do not experience freezing; B, baseline; FOG, freezing of gait; Tstep, total numbers of steps, Ttime, total time; A, auditory cues; S, somatosensory cues; V, visual cues; At, attentional cue; AAt, auditory combined with attentional cue; HF, hip flexion; KF, knee flexion; AD, ankle dorsiflexion; Turn, turn (steps, time, length, height, width, length).

↑, significantly increased; ↓, significantly decreased; +, an improvement in status despite a decrease in outcome; –, decreased gait parameters.

important finding, as FOG and postural instability are thought to be related, in view of the high incidence of falls among patients with PD (Bloem et al., 2004). Bloem and colleagues found that 50% of elderly individuals with PD had recurrent fall episodes within a year (Bloem et al., 2004), whereas only 25% of community-dwelling elderly are defined as recurrent fallers (Milat et al., 2011; Pluijm et al., 2006). When patients have experienced falls in the past, they tend to develop fear of falling during movement in general, and may consequently avoid physical activity. As gait is an integral component of activities of daily living, these impairments can have a major impact on the functioning, independence (Covinsky et al., 2006), and quality of life of the patient (Ellis et al., 2011; Rahman et al., 2011). However, when drug treatment works properly, freezing is not as prevalent, and testing the effects of RAS has been cumbersome (Nieuwboer et al., 2009; Nieuwboer and Giladi, 2008).

Currently there are differing opinions about the optimal stimulation frequency for preventing FOG. A marked decrease in stride length and a simultaneous increase in gait variability occur just before FOG (Giladi and Nieuwboer, 2008). Only stride length was found to increase with a stimulation frequency of 90% (Willems et al., 2006), whereas gait variability decreased with a stimulation frequency of 110% (Hausdorff et al., 2007). At the end of the dose, patients experienced significantly fewer freezing episodes when RAS was provided at 110% of baseline during performance of walking tasks that are known to provoke FOG (Arias and Cudeiro, 2010). Even though a stimulation frequency of 90% of uncued gait was tested on participants while they were off medication as well, this did not lead to clear results with regard to FOG (Lee et al., 2012).

Future research needs to focus on the interplay between attention and cueing in order to understand how the motor control deficits inherent in freezing are optimally influenced by external stimuli (Nieuwboer and Giladi, 2008). Assessing the precise auditory–motor synchronization as a measure of motor performance in order to determine, for example, the optimum frequency may well be essential in this regard.

7.5.3 Effect of RAS on normalizing gait

The results of the recent cross-sectional studies suggest that frequencies equal to step frequency during uncued comfortable walking, or 10% higher, may partially normalize the walking characteristics of patients with PD, specifically with regard to walking speed, cadence, and FOG. These results are in line with the systematic review by Lim et al. (2005). Furthermore, specifically with regard to FOG, these studies add to the current body of knowledge. At the time of the review by Lim et al. (2005), only two high-quality RCTs (Ellis et al., 2005; Thaut et al., 1996) were available, of which only one (Thaut et al., 1996) was specifically targeted at the evaluation of RAS, and most of the studies were conducted in laboratory settings. Therefore there were not enough high-quality RCTs to investigate whether RAS would be useful as an intervention to induce longer-term improvements in walking in everyday situations and environments. Since that time, rigorous research has been performed, specifically evaluating the effects of RAS, that was mainly directed at the longer-term effects of RAS outside laboratory environments (see Table 7.2) (Elston et al.,

Table 7.2 Overview of randomized controlled trials

Reference	Study characteristics	Intervention	Subject characteristics				Outcomes	Quality (PEDro score)
			Intensity (w/h/m)	Subjects (n)	Age (years) M ± SD	H&Y M ± SD		
Thaut et al. 1996	RCT Concealed allocation: no Baseline comparability: no Blind assessors: no Adequate follow-up: yes Intention-to-treat analysis: no	Home-based walking program with RAS with normal/quick/fast RAS compared with a similar self-paced walking program and no intervention	3/7/30	37 E = 15 NT = 11 SPT = 11	E = 69 ±8 C = 71 ± 8 C = 74 ± 3	2.3 ± 0.7	1. Gait velocity↑ 2. Inclined gait velocity↑ 3. Cadence↑ 4. Stride length↑ 5. EMG (variability/symmetry/ timing/onset and termination)	4/10
Marchese et al. 2000	RCT Concealed allocation: no Baseline comparability: yes Blind assessors: yes Ade quate follow-up: no Intention-to-treat analysis: no	Physical therapy program with the use of RAS compared with a similar program without RAS	6/3/60	20 E = 10 C = 10	E = 65.0 ± 5.8[1] C = 66.9 ± 6.3[1]	E = 2.35 ± 0.58[1] C = 2.3 ± 0.48[1]	1. UPDRS-II 2. UPDRS-III	5/10
Ellis et al. 2005	RCT (cross-over) Concealed allocation: yes Baseline comparability: yes Blind assessors: yes Adequate follow-up: yes Intention-to-treat analysis: no	A combination of medical therapy and physical therapy, containing 15 minutes of gait training with RAS compared with medical therapy alone	6/3/1.5	68 Ea = 35 La = 33	64 ± 8.4 Ea = 64 ± 8.4 La = 63 ± 8.8	2.5 ± 0.5 Ea = 2.5 ± 0.5 La = 2.4 ± 0.5	1. SIP-68 (total /mobility) (+) 2. UPDRS-I 3. UPDRS-II↓(+) 4. UPDRS-III 5. Walking speed ↑	7/10

Table 7.2 (continued)

Reference	Study characteristics	Intervention	Intensity (w/h/m)	Subjects (n)	Age (years) M ± SD	H&Y M ± SD	Outcomes	Quality (PEDro score)
Nieuwboer et al. 2007	RCT (cross-over) Concealed allocation: yes Baseline comparability: yes Blind assessors: yes Adequate follow-up: yes Intention-to-treat analysis: no	Practice of different aspects of gait with the preferred type of cue (67% choose RAS, 33% choose somatosensory cueing) compared with no intervention	3/3/30	153 Ea = 76 La = 77	Ea = 67.5[2] ± 7.8 La = 69[2] ± 7.8	Ea = 2.6[2] ± 0.7 La = 2.7[2] ± 0.7	1. PG-score↓(+) 6. FOGQ 2. 10MWT 7. NEADL (GS↑/SL↑/Ca↑) 8. FES↑ 3. FR 9. PDQ-39 4. TSLS and 10. CSI TTS↓(+) 5. TUG	7/10
Morris et al. 2009	RCT Concealed allocation: yes Baseline comparability: yes Blind assessors: yes Adequate follow-up: yes Intention-to-treat analysis: yes	Walking, turning, standing up from a chair, and obstacle negotiation with cognitive strategies and external cues compared with conventional exercise that aimed to improve general fitness and function	(2/max 16/max 45)[3] M number of sessions: E = 14 C = 13	28 E = 14 C = 14	E = 68 ± n.r. C = 66 ± n.r. Range for all patients: 52 –79 years	n.r.	1. UPDRS-II 2. UPDRS-III 3. 10MWT 4. TUG 5. Two-Minute Walk Test 6. Shoulder "tug" test↑ 7. PDQ-39	8/10
Lim et al. 2010	RCT (cross-over) Concealed allocation: yes Baseline comparability: yes Blind assessors: yes Adequate follow-up: yes Intention-to-treat analysis: no	Practice of different aspects of gait with the preferred type of cue (67% choose RAS, 33% choose somatosensory cueing) compared with no intervention	3/3/30	153 Ea = 76 La = 77	Ea = 67.5[2] ± 7.8 La = 69[2] ± 7.8	Ea = 2.6[2] ± 0.7 La = 2.7[2] ± 0.7	Percentage of time spent on: 1. dynamic activity ↑[4] 2. static activity ↓[4] 3. sitting[4] 4. standing[4] 5. walking ↑[4] 6. N walking >5 s/hour ↑[4] 7. N walking > 10 s/hour↑[4]	7/10

Table 7.2 (continued)

Reference	Study characteristics	Intervention	Subject characteristics				Outcomes	Quality (PEDro score)
			Intensity (w/h/m)	Subjects (n)	Age (years) M ± SD	H&Y M ± SD		
Rochester et al. 2010a	RCT (cross-over) Concealed allocation: yes Baseline comparability: yes Blind assessors: yes Adequate follow-up: yes Intention-to-treat analysis: no	Practice of different aspects of gait with the preferred type of cue (67% choose RAS, 33% choose somatosensory cueing) compared with no intervention	3/3/30	153 Ea = 76 La = 77	Ea = $67.5^2 \pm 7.8$ La = $69^2 \pm 7.8$	Ea = $2.6^2 \pm 0.7$ La = $2.7^2 \pm 0.7$	1. Single task no cue SL/Ca↑ 2. Single task V/A/S GS/SL↑ 3. Dual task no cue GS/SL↑ 4. Dual task V/A/S GS/SL↑	7/10
Elston et al. 2010	RCT (cross-over) Concealed allocation: yes Baseline comparability: no Blind assessors: no Adequate follow-up: no Intention-to-treat analysis: no	Use of a metronome with a frequency set for comfortable walking without further therapy	4/n.a./n.a.	42 Ea = 21 La = 20	Ea = 71.5 ± 11.3 La = 70.4 ± 8.7	Ea = 2.1 ± 0.3 La = 2.3 ± 0.5	1. PDQ-39 2. SF-36 3. Falls Diary 4. 10MWT	4/10

w, weeks; h, hours; m, minutes; n, number; M, mean; SD, standard deviation; H&Y, Hoehn and Yahr; RCT, randomised controlled trial; RAS, rhythmical auditory stimulation; E, experimental group; NT, no training; SPT, self-paced training; C, control group; EMG, electromyography; UPDRS-II, Unified Parkinson's Disease Rating Scale-ADL section; UPDRS-III, Unified Parkinson's Disease Rating Scale-motor subsection; Ea, early group; La, late group; SIP, Sickness Impact Profile; PG score, posture and gait score; 10MWT, 10-Meter Walking Test; FR, Functional Reach test; TSLS and TTS, combined timed single leg stance and timed tandem leg stance; TUG, Timed Up and Go test; FOGQ, Freezing of Gait Questionnaire; NEADL, Nottingham Extended Activities of Daily Living Scale; FES, Falls Efficacy Scale; PDQ-39, Parkinson's Disease Questionnaire-39; CSI, Carer Strain Index; n.r., not reported; max, maximum; n.a., not applicable; s, seconds; SL, stride length; Ca, cadence; GS, gait speed; SF-36, Short Form-36.

1. It is not stated whether this is an SD or standard error of the mean (SEM).

2. A median value is presented instead of the mean.

3. The frequency and duration of the therapy can vary depending on the need of the patient. This is decided by the therapist.

4. Only within-group results have been presented: ↑, significant increase; ↓, significant decrease; (+), an improvement in status despite a decrease in outcome.

2010; Lim et al., 2010; Morris et al., 2009; Nieuwboer et al., 2007; Rochester et al., 2010a). In Section 7.6 we summarize the outcomes of the RCTs that investigated the effects of RAS on gait and gait-related activities, by pooling them in a meta-analysis.

7.6 Systematic review of the literature on the effects of RAS on Parkinsonian gait

7.6.1 Effects of RAS training on (uncued) gait characteristics, activities of daily life (ADL) and quality of life (QoL) in people with Parkinson's disease

7.6.1.1 Literature search

PubMed was searched with the following MeSH terms: Parkinson disease, Cues, Music, Music Therapy, Gait, Gait Disorders, Neurologic, Walking, Mobility Limitation, Locomotion, Physical Therapy Modalities, Exercise, Exercise Therapy, Exercise Movement Techniques. It was also searched with the following search terms: Parkin*, cueing, auditory, sensory, external, rhythmic, stimulus, stimulation, stimuli. These results were limited to studies published in English and Dutch after 2004 (the year of the search of the most recent systematic review, by Lim et al., 2005). This search (conducted in March 2012) resulted in a total of 117 citations (the results are available from the corresponding author on request). Of these citations, 81 studies were excluded based on title, 20 were excluded based on abstract, and 10 were excluded based on full text. Therefore a total of six studies remained for analysis (Elston et al., 2010; Lim et al., 2010; Morris et al., 2009; Nieuwboer et al., 2007; Rochester et al., 2010a; Thaut et al., 1996), of which three were describing separate outcomes from one intervention (Lim et al., 2010; Nieuwboer et al., 2007; Rochester et al., 2010a). These three reports are displayed separately in Table 7.2. However, they are regarded as one study in the meta-analysis. Reference tracking resulted in the identification of one other study (Marchese et al., 2000). From studies with a crossover design (Lim et al., 2010; Nieuwboer et al., 2007; Rochester et al., 2010a) we only assessed the effects of the early intervention, in order to avoid problems with carryover and learning effects. In total, eight studies were analysed, involving a total of 348 patients.

7.6.1.2 Methodological quality

Table 7.2 shows the PEDro scores of the 8 included studies, which ranged from 4 to 8 points. As shown in Table 7.2, 6 out of 8 studies concealed the allocation of the participants (Ellis et al., 2005; Elston et al., 2010; Lim et al., 2010; Morris et al., 2009; Nieuwboer et al., 2007; Rochester et al., 2010a), 6 out of 8 studies presented baseline comparability (Ellis et al., 2005; Lim et al., 2010; Marchese et al., 2000; Morris et al., 2009; Nieuwboer et al., 2007; Rochester et al., 2010a), 6 out of 8 studies blinded the assessors (Ellis et al., 2005; Lim et al., 2010; Marchese et al., 2000; Morris et al., 2009; Nieuwboer et al., 2007; Rochester et al., 2010a), and 6 out of 8 studies presented adequate follow-up data (Ellis et al., 2005; Lim et al., 2010; Morris et al., 2009; Nieuwboer et al., 2007; Rochester et al., 2010a; Thaut et al., 1996). Subsequently, the studies were of relatively high methodological quality. However, most of them failed to perform an intention-to-treat analysis (Ellis et al., 2005; Elston et al., 2010; Lim et al., 2010; Nieuwboer et al., 2007; Rochester et al., 2010a; Thaut et al., 1996), with the exception of one study (Morris et al., 2009).

7.6.1.3 Quantitative analyses

Significant mean differences (MD) in favor of RAS were found for gait speed [MD (random): 0.114, 95% CI, 0.028–0.200; $Z = 2.591$; $P < 0.01$; $I^2 = 57\%$] and stride length [MD (fixed): 0.085, 95% CI, 0.022–0.148; $Z = 2.654$; $P < 0.01$; $I^2 = 47\%$] (see Figure 7.1 for forest plots). These results were consistent in a sensitivity analysis based on type of therapy, with the exception of one study, for which only a small part of the therapy consisted of RAS (Ellis et al., 2005)). A sensitivity analysis based on type of therapy (excluding the study by Ellis et al., 2005) resulted in a significant MD for quality of life [MD (fixed): 3.400, 95% CI, 0.215–6.586; $Z = 2.092$; $P = 0.04$; $I^2 = 40\%$] (not shown). Cadence, Timed Up and Go (TUG) test, and balance were not significantly affected by an intervention with RAS. The differences between studies with regard to cadence may be explained by differences in the stimulation frequencies that were provided. Thaut et al. (1996) provided training with a graded increase in stimulation frequency, whereas Nieuwboer et al. (2007) did not specify an increase in stimulation frequency. Analysis was not possible for UPDRS-II and UPDRS-III.

7.6.1.4 Interpretation

Even though the intervention periods were relatively short (mostly 3 or 4 weeks), therapy with RAS seemed to affect gait speed as well as stride length during subsequent uncued walking. The effects of RAS on gait speed have important implications, as gait speed is an important predictor of performance of activities of daily living (gait-related activities as well as non-gait-related ones, such as bathing and dressing) (Verghese et al., 2011), community walking (Elbers et al., 2013), quality of life (Ellis et al., 2011), and overall health and survival (Studenski et al., 2011). These effects may by mediated by fitness, cognition, mood (Verghese et al., 2011), and the energy cost of walking (Studenski et al., 2011). This may in turn be related to the increased percentage of time that patients with PD spend performing dynamic physical activity (mainly walking) after home-based cueing training (Lim et al., 2010).

The increase in stride length is quite consistent across intervention studies, whereas this is not the case in cross-sectional studies (see Table 7.1 and Table 7.2). Possibly patients were better able to increase their stride length after prolonged training with RAS. Alternatively, perhaps RAS was combined with unreported specific instructions regarding step length. As cadence in people with PD is often reported to be higher than that in healthy controls, an increased stride length and gait speed with a constant cadence would correspond to a normalization of the walking pattern (Morris et al., 1994; Willems et al., 2007).

The current meta-analysis showed a positive trend towards significance on quality of life. However, caution is needed when interpreting this, because only one study (Nieuwboer et al., 2007) seems to be responsible for the effect (see Figure 7.1), even though the

Study name	Outcome	Difference in means	Standard error	Variance	Lower limit	Upper limit	Z-Value	p-Value
Thaut et al. 1996 (1)	gait speed (m/s)	0.400	0.115	0.013	0.175	0.625	3.484	0.000
Thaut et al. 1996 (2)	gait speed (m/s)	0.100	0.102	0.010	-0.099	0.299	0.985	0.325
Ellis et al. 2005	gait speed (m/s)	0.100	0.052	0.003	-0.002	0.202	1.915	0.055
Nieuwboer et al. 2007	gait speed (m/s)	0.110	0.035	0.001	0.042	0.178	3.164	0.002
Morris et al. 2009	gait speed (m/s)	0.000	0.064	0.004	-0.126	0.126	0.000	1.000
		0.114	0.044	0.002	0.028	0.200	2.591	0.010
Thaut et al. 1996 (1)	stride length (m)	0.300	0.125	0.016	0.055	0.545	2.404	0.016
Thaut et al. 1996 (2)	stride length (m)	0.000	0.095	0.009	-0.186	0.186	0.000	1.000
Nieuwboer et al. 2007	stride length (m)	0.080	0.036	0.001	0.010	0.150	2.249	0.025
		0.085	0.032	0.001	0.022	0.148	2.654	0.008
Thaut et al. 1996 (1)	cadance (steps/min)	9.100	4.844	23.462	-0.394	18.594	1.879	0.060
Thaut et al. 1996 (2)	cadance (steps/min)	13.500	4.680	21.902	4.327	22.673	2.885	0.004
Nieuwboer et al. 2007	cadance (steps/min)	-0.500	2.216	4.911	-4.843	3.843	-0.226	0.821
		6.640	4.752	22.580	-2.673	15.954	1.397	0.162
Nieuwboer et al. 2007	TUG (s)	0.400	0.528	0.279	-0.635	1.435	0.758	0.449
Morris et al. 2009	TUG (s)	0.500	1.023	1.046	-1.505	2.505	0.489	0.625
		0.421	0.469	0.220	-0.498	1.340	0.898	0.369
Ellis et al. 2005	SIP-86	-0.123	0.243	0.059	-0.599	0.353	-0.506	0.613
Nieuwboer et al. 2007	PDQ-39	0.448	0.164	0.027	0.127	0.769	2.739	0.006
Morris et al. 2009	PDQ-39	-0.012	0.378	0.143	-0.752	0.729	-0.031	0.975
Elston et al. 2010	PDQ-39	-0.009	0.345	0.119	-0.686	0.668	-0.025	0.980
		0.208	0.120	0.014	-0.027	0.443	1.737	0.082

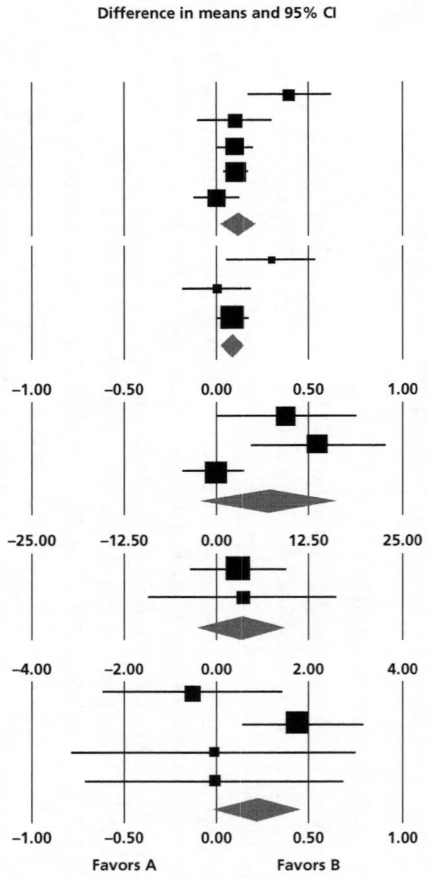

Fig. 7.1 Forest plots for RAS.

original study does not report a significant increase in quality of life (Nieuwboer et al., 2007). This is possible, because we only used the effects of the early intervention in our analysis. Furthermore, the method for calculating mean differences which is standard for a meta-analysis (no regard for pre-intervention values) may also have contributed to the observed effect (see Figure 7.1).

The fact that cadence per se (in uncued conditions) is not affected may be explained by the stimulation frequency that was provided, which is usually either near the preferred frequency of uncued walking (Elston et al., 2010; Nieuwboer et al., 2007) or not specified (Ellis et al., 2005; Marchese et al., 2000; Morris et al., 2009). However, one study gradually and systematically increased the stimulation frequency during the training sessions, and subsequently reported an increase in cadence (Thaut et al., 1996).

Specifically, automaticity of movements seems to be impaired in patients with PD, as patients normally use more brain activity when they perform automatic tasks, and tend to shift from automatic to executive control (Mentis et al., 2003). Patients are capable of taking big steps during walking when they specifically focus their attention on that aspect of gait (Baker et al., 2007). During activities of daily living, attention often needs to be divided between several tasks (e.g. talking while walking). This is an important issue for people with PD, as gait impairments are exacerbated when they are required to perform a concurrent task (O'Shea et al., 2002).

A combination of an attentional strategy and RAS ("Take big steps to the beat") may decrease the attentional cost of the strategy (Baker et al., 2008). This view was supported by a decrease in the interference of dual tasks during gait with RAS (Rochester et al., 2010b). These effects in performance may relate to more automaticity and therefore less attentional demand of movements during RAS-guided gait (Rochester et al., 2010a).

Most individual studies report no or little generalization to domains other than walking, such as activities of daily living and balance (Elston et al., 2010; Nieuwboer et al., 2007). As an exception, Marchese et al. (2000) reported improvements in activities of daily living. These effects may relate to the duration of the therapy and the frequency (6 weeks instead of 3 weeks, and 3 hours of therapy per week instead of 1.5 hours), and/or to the content of the therapy, which next to gait training contained postural control and limb mobilization in different positions. Irrespective of the content of the intervention, the intensity, duration, frequency. and dosage are essential for the desired effect (Lopopolo et al., 2006). The dosage of investigated interventions (expressed as the duration of therapy per week) varied from 1.5 to 3.5 hours per week. Only high-dosage therapy (defined as 3 hours or more of therapy per week) effectively improved habitual gait speed in healthy older adults (Lopopolo et al., 2006). Although some of the studies included in the present review (Ellis et al., 2005; Marchese et al., 2000; Thaut et al., 1996) can be regarded as high dosage according to the definition by Lopopolo et al. (2006), they account for less than 50% of the participants included in the meta-analysis (91 out of 216 patients). It is important to mention that one study (Nieuwboer et al., 2007) did report significant results despite having the lowest intensity of therapy (1.5 hours per week). The intensity of the therapy was low enough to be possibly around the intensity of normal walking (2.2–3.0 MET, depending on the speed) (Ainsworth et al., 2000). However, this was not assessed during the studies included in this review, so requires further investigation.

RAS appears to be useful as a (home-based) therapy to improve gait and gait-related activities (Nieuwboer et al., 2007; Thaut et al., 1996). It can be used as a compensatory technique, as demonstrated by the immediate improvements with respect to gait speed, cadence, and FOG during the cross-sectional studies. However, if RAS was used during a period of training it increased stride length and walking speed, and transferred to uncued gait and the effects attained during a relatively long follow-up period (up to 3 weeks after a short training program) (Nieuwboer et al., 2007; Thaut et al., 1996), although gained improvements may deteriorate after a follow-up of 6 weeks (Nieuwboer et al., 2007).

Reported effects are small, and it remains unclear what the optimal dose and content of cueing training should be. Thus dose–response studies with varying intensity of therapy are desirable. Furthermore, the ability of participants to synchronize their movements with RAS, and its role in therapeutic efficacy, have not been investigated sufficiently. The results of these studies could optimize the application of RAS.

7.7 **New applications of RAS**

7.7.1 **Music**

Recently, rhythmic music has been applied as a form of RAS in combination with gait training (de Bruin et al., 2010; Thaut et al., 1996). Through the beat, music provides basically the same rhythmic temporal structure as a metronome. A beat can be described as a perceived pulse that marks equally spaced points in time (Large and Palmer, 2002). A metronome indicates the beat with simple single regular tones. However, in music, besides the regular time interval, multiple aspects (e.g. loudness, pitch, timbre, harmony, duration of the tone) indicate the beat within a complex structure (Grahn, 2009; Krumhansl, 2000). Recent evidence indicates that the basal ganglia are necessary for beat perception (Grahn and Brett, 2009; Teki et al., 2011). However, this may not be the case for music because the beat is emphasized by the multiple aspects that were described previously (Grahn, 2009). Therefore the complex structure of music may also aid the patient in synchronization compared with a single beat.

This was exemplified by Thaut et al. (1997), as RAS embedded in a musical structure was found to significantly decrease the variability of finger tapping compared with an isochronous metronome beat. This is consistent with general functional perspectives of rhythmic music enabling and facilitating entrainment and precise synchronization of movements (McIntosh et al., 1997; Madison et al., 2011). People may subconsciously time their motor actions to an auditory rhythmic stimulus when they pay no attention to the music (Molinari et al., 2003). The attraction of making rhythmic movements to a rhythm is further exemplified by the finding that people find it more difficult to tap in between the beats than on the beat (Krumhansl, 2000). However, they may also have difficulty hearing the beat and therefore have problems synchronizing their movement to it (e.g. while dancing). Listening to music may therefore demand some additional attentional resources and could potentially adversely affect gait performance (Brown et al., 2009, 2010). The effectiveness of music as a form of RAS may depend on the distinctiveness of the musical structure for enhancing rhythm perception.

Within music, the pitch and the rhythm combined provide a melodic pattern (Krumhansl, 2000), whereas a metronome only provides a rhythm. The melody is normally a short string of tones, which is repeated in various forms throughout a musical piece (Krumhansl, 2000). Laukka (2006) found that, within an elderly population, most people (88%) felt emotions when they heard music during 33% or more of the listening time. The emotion in music is best interpreted when it is familiar and culturally embedded (Fritz et al., 2009). However, at least some of the main emotions expressed through music have been recognized cross-culturally (Fritz et al., 2009). Intensely pleasurable music seemed to elicit physiological pleasure sensations related to reward and emotions (Blood and Zatorre, 2001; Boso et al., 2006). These sensations may relate to activation of several specific brain areas, such as the insular and cingulate cortex, hypothalamus, hippocampus, amygdala, and prefrontal cortex, while listening to music (Boso et al., 2006). Moreover, several biochemical mediators, such as endorphins, endocannabinoids, dopamine, and nitric oxide, may play a role in the musical experience (Boso et al., 2006). Therefore music may alter mood, which could be a benefit in view of the incidence of depression in PD (Chaudhuri et al., 2006), and might increase therapy compliance for long-term interventions. Furthermore, music may distract from sensations such as fatigue (Hayakawa et al., 2000; Lim et al., 2011).

Patients with PD who exercised daily while listening to music with an overlaid RAS beat showed significant and more lasting improvements in gait compared with patients who received the same exercise program without RAS (Thaut et al., 1996). The effective element of RAS/gait training may actually be the RAS, rather than the gait training per se, as a study by Ito et al. (2000) showed that patients who listened to music with RAS every day for a month without any gait training also displayed significant improvements in their gait velocity and step length.

To our knowledge, two RCTs have investigated gait training with the use of rhythmic music in patients with PD (de Bruin et al., 2010; Thaut et al., 1996). We have previously shown that stride length and walking velocity increase significantly when the results of these studies are pooled in a meta-analysis (de Dreu et al., 2012). This is consistent with the results of RAS/metronome studies.

7.7.2 Dance

The use of music in partnered dancing has an extensive history. Westbrook and McKibben (1989) were the first to investigate dance specifically as a possible intervention for people with PD. Subsequently, Hackney and associates investigated different aspects of partnered tango dancing as an intervention in PD (Earhart, 2009). Both partnered and non-partnered dance have been indicated as alternative therapies that increase physical function (e.g. gait speed, strength, balance) in people with other conditions, such as cardiac disease (Belardinelli et al., 2008), obesity (Shimamoto et al., 1998), and dementia.

Furthermore, dance classes for patients with dementia have been indicated as a way to stimulate social interaction between patients (Palo-Bengtsson and Ekman, 2002). Moreover, the intensity of dance can be sufficient to increase fitness, at least in patients with heart disease (Belardinelli et al., 2008).

Rhythmic dance classes may be a promising therapeutic intervention for people with PD, because they naturally combine cueing techniques, cognitive movement strategies, balance exercises, and physical exercise (as recommended by Keus et al., 2007) with group dynamics (which include social interaction, partnership in misfortune, and peer support) while focusing on the enjoyment and esthetics of moving to music instead of the current mobility limitations of the patient (de Dreu et al., 2012). However, if dance exercises require the learning of new skills (i.e. dance steps), they may present another challenge to facilitate motor control in PD.

In order to summarize the current literature, we pooled all of the studies investigating a form of therapy using whole body movements stimulated by music and dance in PD (de Dreu et al., 2012). Of these studies, two investigated gait training with music (De Bruin, 2010; Thaut, 1996), one investigated music therapy (Pacchetti et al., 2000), and three investigated "partnered" dance in patients with PD (Hackney and Earhart, 2009a, 2009b; Hackney et al., 2007). Since the publication of our review (de Dreu et al., 2012), one new RCT has been published (Duncan and Earhart, 2012), which investigated the effects of a 1-year program of tango dance classes and was included in the results that are described here.

A significant standardized mean difference (SMD) was found for the Berg Balance Scale in favor of RAS using music and dance (SMD (fixed): 0.894, 95% CI, 0.510–1.277; $Z = 4.566$; $P < 0.01$; $I^2 = 0\%$). The multiple stops, starts, and turns, as well as backwards walking, weight-shifting and multitasking during dance, may affect balance performance (de Dreu et al., 2012). This view is further supported by epidemiological studies which reported that healthy individuals who danced regularly during their life had better balance compared with people who did not dance regularly (Kattenstroth et al., 2010; Verghese, 2006; Zhang et al., 2008). This finding is important because most balance deficits in PD are resistant to anti-Parkinson medication (i.e. dopaminergic medication) (Grimbergen et al., 2004), and actual falls as well as the fear of falling greatly influence the individual and have a large socio-economic impact (Tinetti and Williams, 1997).

In addition, a significant mean difference (MD) was found for stride length [MD (fixed): 0.113, 95% CI, 0.037–0.189; $Z = 2.918$; $P < 0.01$; $I^2 = 9\%$]. This may be an important normalization of walking pattern in view of the diminished step length compared with that of healthy age-matched controls (Hausdorff et al., 2007; Willems et al., 2006). Furthermore, a significant and clinically meaningful improvement in walking velocity was found [MD (fixed): 0.127, 95% CI, 0.013–0.241; $Z = 2.179$; $P = 0.03$; $I^2 = 48\%$] (Perera et al., 2006).

Dual-task walking velocity increased significantly [MD (fixed): 0.171, 95% CI, 0.024–0.319; $Z = 2.218$; $P = 0.02$; $I^2 = 0\%$], reflecting an increased automaticity of walking (Rochester et al., 2010b). This is an important finding, as automaticity of movements is impaired in patients with PD, as reflected by a higher brain activity when they perform automatic tasks (Mentis et al., 2003).

The significant increase in performance during the Six-Minute Walk Test (6MWT) [MD (fixed): 46.306, 95% CI, 15.553–77.059; Z = 2.951; P < 0.01; I^2 = 0%] can be interpreted as a substantial and clinically meaningful cardiovascular improvement and an increase in physical capacity (Perera et al., 2006).

The effect of RAS with music and dance on the TUG test [MD (fixed): 2.221, 95% CI, 1.155–3.288; Z = 4.083; P < 0.01; I^2 = 0%] and the UPDRS-II [MD (random): 4.672, 95% CI, 0.570–8.774; Z = 3.631; P = 0.03; I^2 = 57%] indicates an increased level of ease in performance of gait and activities of daily living. This is promising evidence in view of the general lack of generalization in rehabilitation (Kwakkel et al., 2007). As described earlier, this could be related to the duration of the interventions and/or to the content of the therapy. Further research is warranted to determine the important factors involved in transfer to activities of daily living. Such knowledge might be transferable to rehabilitation for other neurological diseases. Rehabilitation interventions do not seem to affect basic symptomatology (Olanow et al., 2009). However, regular exercise may provide a neuroprotective effect through an up-regulation of brain-derived nerve growth factors (Ahlskog, 2011). The trend toward significance with regard to the UPDRS-III suggests that, when provided for a longer duration, such as 1 year (Duncan and Earhart, 2012), rehabilitative therapies may slow disease progression.

7.8 **Conclusion and recommendations for future research**

A number of studies that investigated RAS provided by a metronome were of high methodological quality. However, many had small sample sizes and lacked a dose-matched control intervention. Pooling of these phase II trials reveals strong evidence suggesting that RAS used in combination with gait training improves walking velocity and step length. Considering the relatively slow speed, small steps, and high cadence that a typical patient with PD normally displays, this could indicate a very important normalization of the walking pattern.

Future studies should aim to better understand the optimal cueing strategies for relieving pathological motor symptoms such as festination, freezing, rigidity, and bradykinesia, and to gain greater insight into the neurophysiological mechanisms that underlie training-induced changes in gait performance. Further optimization could be achieved by assessing the synchronization error between footfalls and the RAS provided in various forms (metronome, music, and others). To optimize therapies using RAS, dose–response studies with varying intensity and duration of RAS in combination with gait training, exercise therapy, or physical therapy are desirable.

Traditional partnered dance classes may provide an interesting framework that includes motivation, engagement, and enjoyable group dynamics which may foster peer support for the patient as well as the partner. Extended RAS therapy has been shown to have a wide range of effects, including an increase in balance (reflected by the BBS), stride length, and dual-task walking speed, and improved performance on the 6MWT, TUG, and UPDRS-II. A trend toward significance was observed with respect to walking speed and the UPDRS-III. Although the studies were of reasonably high methodological quality (with a score of 4–7 points on the PEDro scale), sample sizes were small, and there was a general lack of an intention-to-treat analysis (with the exception of the study by Duncan and Earhart, 2012)) and an adequate follow-up (with the exception of the study by Thaut et al., 1996). Allocation was concealed in only half the studies (de Bruin et al., 2010; Duncan and Earhart, 2012; Hackney and Earhart, 2009a, 2009b). Furthermore, as was the case with RAS, a major issue is the lack of application of dose-matched control interventions. Future high-quality trials should aim to address these shortcomings. To date it is unknown whether RAS affects motor performance through the use of adaptive movement strategies or through plasticity-induced reductions in the neurophysiological deficits.

Our meta-analysis of studies on the effects of extended RAS indicates a positive transfer to the activities of daily living domain, but to date not to the quality of life domain. Even though certain aspects of the therapy (e.g. group dynamics, peer support) might be expected to promote an increase in quality of life, effects at the participation level have yet to be demonstrated. Further research on this aspect, as well as on the possible effects of partnered dance on the burden of the caregiver/partner, is warranted.

This research synthesis showed that RAS can be provided to patients with PD using a metronome beat and/or a beat embedded within music. Music may have additional benefits, such as a (temporary) positive effect on mood (Blood and Zatorre, 2001). Furthermore, it will be important to investigate which aspects of music could contribute to optimal synchronization (Grahn, 2009; Teki et al., 2011) compared with a metronome beat.

Acknowledgments

This work was funded in part by the International Parkinson Fund (grant nr. IPF-VUmc-2010.1). We would like to thank A. S. D. van der Wilk and E. Poppe for their help with the meta-analysis.

References

Ahlskog, J. E. (2011). Does vigorous exercise have a neuroprotective effect in Parkinson disease? *Neurology, 77*, 288–94.

Ainsworth, B. E. et al. (2000). Compendium of physical activities: an update of activity codes and MET intensities. *Medicine and Science in Sports and Exercise 32*(9 Suppl.), S498–504.

Arias, P. and Cudeiro, J. (2008). Effects of rhythmic sensory stimulation (auditory, visual) on gait in Parkinson's disease patients. *Experimental Brain Research, 186*, 589–601.

Arias, P. and Cudeiro, J. (2010). Effect of rhythmic auditory stimulation on gait in Parkinsonian patients with and without freezing of gait. *PLoS ONE, 5*, e9675.

Baker, K., Rochester, L., and Nieuwboer, A. (2007). The immediate effect of attentional, auditory, and a combined cue strategy on gait during single and dual tasks in Parkinson's disease. *Archives of Physical Medicine and Rehabilitation, 88*, 1593–600.

Baker, K., Rochester, L., and Nieuwboer, A. (2008). The effect of cues on gait variability—reducing the attentional cost of walking in people with Parkinson's disease. *Parkinsonism & Related Disorders, 14*, 314–20.

Ball, J. M. (1967). Demonstration of the traditional approach in the treatment of a patient with parkinsonism. *American Journal of Physical Medicine 46*, 1034–6.

Belardinelli, R. et al. (2008). Waltz dancing in patients with chronic heart failure: new form of exercise training. *Circulation. Heart Failure*, 1, 107–14.

Bloem, B., Hausdorff, J., Visser, J., and Giladi, N. (2004). Falls and freezing of gait in Parkinson's disease: a review of two interconnected, episodic phenomena. *Movement Disorders*, 19, 871–84.

Blood, A. J. and Zatorre, R. J. (2001). Intensely pleasurable responses to music correlate with activity in brain regions implicated in reward and emotion. *Proceedings of the National Academy of Sciences of the USA*, 98, 11818–23.

Boso, M., Politi, P., Barale, F., and Enzo, E. (2006). Neurophysiology and neurobiology of the musical experience. *Functional Neurology*, 21, 187–91.

Brown, L. A. et al. (2009). Novel challenges to gait in Parkinson's disease: the effect of concurrent music in single- and dual-task contexts. *Archives of Physical Medicine and Rehabilitation*, 90, 1578–83.

Brown, L. A. et al. (2010). Obstacle crossing among people with Parkinson disease is influenced by concurrent music. *Journal of Rehabilitation Research and Development*, 47, 225–31.

Chaudhuri, K. R., Healy, D. G., and Schapira, A. H. V. (2006). Non-motor symptoms of Parkinson's disease: diagnosis and management. *Lancet Neurology*, 5, 235–45.

Covinsky, K. E., Hilton, J., Lindquist, K., and Dudley, R. A. (2006). Development and validation of an index to predict activity of daily living dependence in community-dwelling elders. *Medical Care*, 44, 149–57.

Cubo, E., Leurgans, S., and Goetz, C. G. (2004). Short-term and practice effects of metronome pacing in Parkinson's disease patients with gait freezing while in the 'on' state: randomized single blind evaluation. *Parkinsonism & Related Disorders*, 10, 507–10.

Cunnington, R., Windischberger, C., Deecke, L., and Moser, E. (2002). The preparation and execution of self-initiated and externally-triggered movement: a study of event-related fMRI. *Neuroimage*, 15, 373–85.

de Bruin, N. et al. (2010). Walking with music is a safe and viable tool for gait training in Parkinson's disease: the effect of a 13-week feasibility study on single and dual task walking. *Parkinson's Disease*, 2010, 1–9.

de Dreu, M. J. et al. (2012). Rehabilitation, exercise therapy and music in patients with Parkinson's disease: a meta-analysis of the effects of music-based movement therapy on walking ability, balance and quality of life. *Parkinsonism & Related Disorders*, 18, S114–19.

Debaere, F. et al. (2003). Internal vs external generation of movements: differential neural pathways involved in bimanual coordination performed in the presence or absence of augmented visual feedback. *NeuroImage*, 19, 764–76.

Duncan, R. P. and Earhart, G. M. (2012). Randomized controlled trial of community-based dancing to modify disease progression in Parkinson disease. *Neurorehabilitation and Neural Repair*, 26, 132–43.

Earhart, G. M. (2009). Dance as therapy for individuals with Parkinson disease. *European Journal of Physical and Rehabilitation Medicine*, 45, 231–8.

Ebersbach, G. et al. (1999). Interference of rhythmic constraint on gait in healthy subjects and patients with early Parkinson's disease: evidence for impaired locomotor pattern generation in early Parkinson's disease. *Movement Disorders*, 14, 619–25.

Elbers, R. G., Van Wegen, E. E. H., Verhoef, J., and Kwakkel, G. (2013). Is gait speed a valid measure to predict community ambulation in patients with Parkinson's disease? *Journal of Rehabilitation Medicine*, 45, 370–75.

Ellis, T. et al. (2005). Efficacy of a physical therapy program in patients with Parkinson's disease: a randomized controlled trial. *Archives of Physical Medicine and Rehabilitation*, 86, 626–32.

Ellis, T. et al. (2011). Which measures of physical function and motor impairment best predict quality of life in Parkinson's disease? *Parkinsonism & Related Disorders*, 17, 693–7.

Elston, J. et al. (2010). Do metronomes improve the quality of life in people with Parkinson's disease? A pragmatic, single-blind, randomized cross-over trial. *Clinical Rehabilitation*, 24, 523–32.

Enzensberger, W., Oberlander, U., and Stecker, K. (1997). [Metronome therapy in patients with Parkinson disease] [article in German]. *Nervenarzt*, 68, 972–7.

Freedland, R. L. et al. (2002). The effects of pulsed auditory stimulation on various gait measurements in persons with Parkinson's disease. *NeuroRehabilitation*, 17, 81–7.

Freeman, J. S., Cody, F. W., and Schady, W. (1993). The influence of external timing cues upon the rhythm of voluntary movements in Parkinson's disease. *Journal of Neurology, Neurosurgery & Psychiatry*, 56, 1078–84.

Fritz, T. et al. (2009). Universal recognition of three basic emotions in music. *Current Biology*, 19, 573–6.

Gauthier, L., Dalziel, S., and Gauthier, S. (1987). The benefits of group occupational therapy for patients with Parkinson's disease. *American Journal of Occupational Therapy*, 41, 360–65.

Giladi, N. and Nieuwboer, A. (2008). Understanding and treating freezing of gait in parkinsonism, proposed working definition, and setting the stage. *Movement Disorders*, 23(Suppl. 2), S423–5.

Grahn, J. A. (2009). The role of the basal ganglia in beat perception: neuroimaging and neuropsychological investigations. *Annals of the New York Academy of Sciences*, 1169, 35–45.

Grahn, J. A. and Brett, M. (2009). Impairment of beat-based rhythm discrimination in Parkinson's disease. *Cortex*, 45, 54–61.

Grimbergen, Y. A. M., Munneke, M., and Bloem, B. R. (2004). Falls in Parkinson's disease. *Current Opinion in Neurology*, 17, 405–15.

Hackney, M. E. and Earhart, G. M. (2009a). Effects of dance on movement control in Parkinson's disease: a comparison of Argentine tango and American ballroom. *Journal of Rehabilitation Medicine*, 41, 475–81.

Hackney, M. E. and Earhart, G. M. (2009b). Health-related quality of life and alternative forms of exercise in Parkinson disease. *Parkinsonism & Related Disorders*, 15, 644–8.

Hackney, M. E., Kantorovich, S., Levin, R., and Earhart, G. M. (2007). Effects of tango on functional mobility in Parkinson's disease: a preliminary study. *Journal of Neurologic Physical Therapy*, 31, 173–9.

Hausdorff, J. M. et al. (2007). Rhythmic auditory stimulation modulates gait variability in Parkinson's disease. *European Journal of Neuroscience*, 26, 2369–75.

Hayakawa, Y., Miki, H., Takada, K., and Tanaka, K. (2000). Effects of music on mood during bench stepping exercise. *Perceptual and Motor Skills*, 90, 307–14.

Howe, T. et al. (2003). Auditory cues can modify the gait of persons with early-stage Parkinson's disease: a method for enhancing parkinsonian walking performance? *Clinical Rehabilitation*, 17, 363–7.

Ito, N. et al. (2000). *Music Therapy in Parkinson's Disease: improvement of parkinsonian gait and depression with rhythmic auditory stimulation*. New York: Elsevier Science.

Jahanshahi, M. et al. (1995). Self-initiated versus externally triggered movements. I. An investigation using measurement of regional cerebral blood flow with PET and movement-related potentials in normal and Parkinson's disease subjects. *Brain*, 118, 913–33.

Kattenstroth, J., Kolankowska, I., Kalisch, T., and Dinse, H. (2010). Superior sensory, motor, and cognitive performance in elderly individuals with multi-year dancing activities. *Frontiers in Aging Neuroscience*, 2, 31.

Keus, S. H. et al. (2007). Evidence-based analysis of physical therapy in Parkinson's disease with recommendations for practice and research. *Movement Disorders*, 22, 451–60; quiz 600.

Krumhansl, C. L. (2000). Rhythm and pitch in music cognition. *Psychological Bulletin*, 126, 159–79.

Kwakkel, G., de Goede, C. J., and van Wegen, E. E. (2007). Impact of physical therapy for Parkinson's disease: a critical review of the literature. *Parkinsonism & Related Disorders*, 13(Suppl. 3), S478–87.

Large, E. W. and Palmer, C. (2002). Perceiving temporal regularity in music. *Cognitive Science, 26,* 1–37.

Laukka, P. (2006). Uses of music and psychological well-being among the elderly. *Journal of Happiness Studies, 8,* 215–41.

Lee, S. J. et al. (2012). The effects of visual and auditory cues on freezing of gait in patients with Parkinson disease. *American Journal of Physical Medicine & Rehabilitation, 91,* 2–11.

Lim, H. A., Miller, K., and Fabian, C. (2011). The effects of therapeutic instrumental music performance on endurance level, self-perceived fatigue level, and self-perceived exertion of inpatients in physical rehabilitation. *Journal of Music Therapy, 48,* 124–48.

Lim, I. et al. (2005). Effects of external rhythmical cueing on gait in patients with Parkinson's disease: a systematic review. *Clinical Rehabilitation, 19,* 695–713.

Lim, I. et al. (2010). Does cueing training improve physical activity in patients with Parkinson's disease? *Neurorehabilitation and Neural Repair, 24,* 469–77.

Lohnes, C. A. and Earhart, G. M. (2011). The impact of attentional, auditory, and combined cues on walking during single and cognitive dual tasks in Parkinson disease. *Gait & Posture, 33,* 478–83.

Lopopolo, R. B. et al. (2006). Effect of therapeutic exercise on gait speed in community-dwelling elderly people: a meta-analysis. *Physical Therapy, 86,* 520–40.

McIntosh, G. M., Brown, S. H., and Rice, R. R. (1997). Rhythmic auditory-motor facilitation of gait patterns in patients with Parkinson's disease. *Journal of Neurology, Neurosurgery, & Psychiatry, 62,* 22–6.

McIntosh, G.M., Rice, R.R., Hurt, C.P., and Thaut, M.H. (1998). Long-term training effects of rhythmic auditory stimulation on gait in patients with Parkinson's disease. *Movement Disorders, 13(Suppl. 2),* 212.

Madison, G., Gouyon, F., Ullen, F., and Hornstrom, K. (2011). Modeling the tendency for music to induce movement in humans: first correlations with low-level audio descriptors across music genres. *Journal of Experimental Psychology. Human Perception and Performance, 37,* 1578–94.

Marchese, R. et al. (2000). The role of sensory cues in the rehabilitation of parkinsonian patients: a comparison of two physical therapy protocols. *Movement Disorders, 15,* 879–83.

Martin, J. P. (1963). The basal ganglia and locomotion. *Annals of the Royal College of Surgeons of England, 32,* 219–39.

Mentis, M. J. et al. (2003). Enhancement of brain activation during trial-and-error sequence learning in early PD. *Neurology, 60,* 612–19.

Milat, A. J. et al. (2011). Prevalence, circumstances and consequences of falls among community-dwelling older people: results of the 2009 NSW Falls Prevention Baseline Survey. *New South Wales Public Health Bulletin, 22,* 43–8.

Miller, R.A., Thaut, M.H., McIntosh, G.C., and Rice, R.R. (1996). Components of EMG symmetry and variability in Parkinsonian and healthy elderly gait. *Electroencephalography and Clinical Neurophysiology, 101,* 1–7

Molinari, M. et al. (2003). Neurobiology of rhythmic motor entrainment. *Annals of the New York Academy of Sciences, 999,* 313–21.

Morris, M. E. (2006). Locomotor training in people with Parkinson disease. *Physical Therapy, 86,* 1426–35.

Morris, M. E., Iansek, R., Matyas, T. A., and Summers, J. J. (1994). The pathogenesis of gait hypokinesia in Parkinson's disease. *Brain, 117,* 1169–81.

Morris, M. E., Iansek, R., Matyas, T. A., and Summers, J. J. (1996). Stride length regulation in Parkinson's disease. Normalization strategies and underlying mechanisms. *Brain, 119,* 551–68.

Morris, M. E., Iansek, R., and Kirkwood, B. (2009). A randomized controlled trial of movement strategies compared with exercise for people with Parkinson's disease. *Movement Disorders, 24,* 64–71.

Nieuwboer, A. and Giladi, N. (2008). The challenge of evaluating freezing of gait in patients with Parkinson's disease. *British Journal of Neurosurgery, 22(Suppl. 1)*, S16–18.

Nieuwboer, A. et al. (2007). Cueing training in the home improves gait-related mobility in Parkinson's disease: the RESCUE trial. *Journal of Neurology, Neurosurgery, & Psychiatry, 78*, 134–40.

Nieuwboer, A., Rochester, L., and Jones, D. (2008). Cueing gait and gait-related mobility in patients with Parkinson's disease: developing a therapeutic method based on the international classification of functioning, disability, and health. *Topics in Geriatric Rehabilitation, 24*, 151–65.

Nieuwboer, A. et al. (2009). The short-term effects of different cueing modalities on turn speed in people with Parkinson's disease. *Neurorehabilitation and Neural Repair, 23*, 831–6.

Olanow, C. W., Stern, M. B., and Sethi, K. (2009). The scientific and clinical basis for the treatment of Parkinson disease (2009). *Neurology, 72(Suppl. 4)*, S1–136.

O'Shea, S., Morris, M. E., and Iansek, R. (2002). Dual task interference during gait in people with Parkinson disease: effects of motor versus cognitive secondary tasks. *Physical Therapy, 82*, 888–97.

Pacchetti, C. et al. (2000) Active music therapy in Parkinson's disease: an integrative method for motor and emotional rehabilitation. *Psychosomatic Medicine, 62*, 386–93.

Palo-Bengtsson, L. and Ekman, S.-L. (2002). Emotional response to social dancing and walks in persons with dementia. *American Journal of Alzheimer's Disease and Other Dementias, 17*, 149–53.

Perera, S., Mody, S. H., Woodman, R. C., and Studenski, S. A. (2006). Meaningful change and responsiveness in common physical performance measures in older adults. *Journal of the American Geriatrics Society, 54*, 743–9.

Pluijm, S. et al. (2006). A risk profile for identifying community-dwelling elderly with a high risk of recurrent falling: results of a 3-year prospective study. *Osteoporosis International, 17*, 417–25.

Rahman, S., Griffin, H. J., Quinn, N. P., and Jahanshahi, M. (2011). On the nature of fear of falling in Parkinson's disease. *Behavioural Neurology, 24*, 219–28.

Rochester, L. et al. (2009). Does auditory rhythmical cueing improve gait in people with Parkinson's disease and cognitive impairment? A feasibility study. *Movement Disorders, 24*, 839–45.

Rochester, L. et al. (2010a). Evidence for motor learning in Parkinson's disease: acquisition, automaticity and retention of cued gait performance after training with external rhythmical cues. *Brain Research, 1319*, 103–11.

Rochester, L. et al. (2010b). The effect of cueing therapy on single and dual-task gait in a drug naive population of people with Parkinson's disease in northern Tanzania. *Movement Disorders, 25*, 906–11.

Rubinstein, T. C., Giladi, N., and Hausdorff, J. M. (2002). The power of cueing to circumvent dopamine deficits: a review of physical therapy treatment of gait disturbances in Parkinson's disease. *Movement Disorders, 17*, 1148–60.

Shimamoto, H., Adachi, Y., Takahashi, M., and Tanaka, K. (1998). Low impact aerobic dance as a useful exercise mode for reducing body mass in mildly obese middle-aged women. *Applied Human Science, 17*, 109–14.

Studenski, S. et al. (2011). Gait speed and survival in older adults. *Journal of the American Medical Association, 305*, 50–58.

Suteerawattananon, M. et al. (2004). Effects of visual and auditory cues on gait in individuals with Parkinson's disease. *Journal of the Neurological Sciences, 219*, 63–9.

Teki, S., Grube, M., Kumar, S., and Griffiths, T. D. (2011). Distinct neural substrates of duration-based and beat-based auditory timing. *Journal of Neuroscience, 31*, 3805–12.

Thaut, M. H. (2005). The future of music in therapy and medicine. *Annals of the New York Academy of Sciences, 1060*, 303–8.

Thaut, M. H. et al. (1996). Rhythmic auditory stimulation in gait training for Parkinson's disease patients. *Movement Disorders, 11*, 193–200.

Thaut, M. H., Rathbun, J. A., and Miller, R. A. (1997). Music versus metronome timekeeper in a rhythmic motor task. *International Journal of Arts Medicine, 5,* 4–12.

Tinetti, M. E. and Williams, C. S. (1997). Falls, injuries due to falls, and the risk of admission to a nursing home. *New England Journal of Medicine, 337,* 1279–84.

Toyomura, A., Shibata, M., and Kuriki, S. (2012). Self-paced and externally triggered rhythmical lower limb movements: a functional MRI study. *Neuroscience Letters, 516,* 39–44.

van Wegen, E. et al. (2006a). The effect of rhythmic somatosensory cueing on gait in patients with Parkinson's disease. *Journal of the Neurological Sciences, 248,* 210–14.

van Wegen, E. et al. (2006b). The effects of visual rhythms and optic flow on stride patterns of patients with Parkinson's disease. *Parkinsonism & Related Disorders, 12,* 21–7.

Verghese, J. (2006). Cognitive and mobility profile of older social dancers. *Journal of the American Geriatrics Society, 54,* 1241–4.

Verghese, J., Wang, C., and Holtzer, R. (2011). Relationship of clinic-based gait speed measurement to limitations in community-based activities in older adults. *Archives of Physical Medicine and Rehabilitation, 92,* 844–6.

Von Wilzenben, H. D. (1942). *Methods in the Treatment of Postencephalic Parkinson's.* New York: Grune and Stratten.

Westbrook, B. K. and McKibben, H. (1989). Dance/movement therapy with groups of outpatients with Parkinson's disease. *American Journal of Dance Therapy, 11,* 27–38.

Westheimer, O. (2008). Why dance for Parkinson's disease. *Topics in Geriatric Rehabilitation, 24,* 127–40.

Willems, A. M. et al. (2006). The use of rhythmic auditory cues to influence gait in patients with Parkinson's disease, the differential effect for freezers and non-freezers, an explorative study. *Disability and Rehabilitation, 28,* 721–8.

Willems, A. M. et al. (2007). Turning in Parkinson's disease patients and controls: the effect of auditory cues. *Movement Disorders, 22,* 1871–8.

Zhang, J.-G. et al. (2008). Postural stability and physical performance in social dancers. *Gait & Posture, 27,* 697–701.

Chapter 8

Rhythmic Auditory Stimulation (RAS)

Corene P. Thaut and Ruth Rice

8.1 Definition

Rhythmic auditory stimulation (RAS) is a neurologic technique used to facilitate the rehabilitation, development, and maintenance of movements that are intrinsically biologically rhythmical. This primarily refers to gait. However, arm swing is also rhythmic when paired with walking. RAS uses the physiological effects of auditory rhythm on the motor system to improve the control of movement in rehabilitation of functional, stable, and adaptive gait patterns in patients with significant gait deficits due to neurological impairment (Thaut, 2005). Research has shown RAS to be effective in two different ways—first, as an immediate entrainment stimulus providing rhythmic cues during movement, and secondly, as a facilitating stimulus for training in order to achieve more functional gait patterns.

8.2 Target populations

The RAS technique can be used with a variety of populations who demonstrate deficits in their gait parameters, including (but not limited to) Parkinson's disease, stroke, traumatic brain injury, multiple sclerosis, cerebral palsy, and orthopedic patients.

RAS is a very effective technique in patients with *Parkinson's disease*, to address kinematic deficits that interfere with productive and safe gait. Typical characteristics may include flexed or stooped posture when standing and with gait, decreased range of motion (ROM), particularly with hip and knee motion, and reduced ankle dorsiflexion, decreased trunk and pelvis motion, decreased step length and decreased arm swing, toe walking with decreased heel strike, a shuffling gait pattern, an excessively slow gait or a very quick festinate gait pattern with increased speed to prevent falling forward, difficulty initiating gait, freezing, or changes in gait with difficulty turning or going through doorways, poor balance, and increased cadence related to small steps, but decreased velocity secondary to decreased stride length (O'Sullivan and Schmitz, 2007).

Stroke patients also display many deficits which can interfere with safety and proper gait kinematics. RAS can be used to address hypotonicity or decreased tone or spasticity and increased tone in unilateral upper or lower extremities, hemiparesis or weakness in unilateral upper or lower extremities, toe drag during the swing phase of gait, decreased coordination of movement patterns, poor balance, postural and trunk control, contractures and limited joint range of motion, uneven stride length between left and right, decreased weight bearing on the affected side, decreased cadence and stride length, decreased velocity, and decreased arm swing and heel strike unilaterally (O'Sullivan and Schmitz, 2007).

Patients with a *traumatic brain injury* also present with many similar characteristics to stroke patients. However, they often have bilateral involvement and more significant cognitive deficits. Neuromuscular impairments include abnormal tone, sensory impairments, poor motor control, impaired balance, and paresis (O'Sullivan and Schmitz, 2007). Depending on the patient's specific problems, RAS can be used to work on quality of gait, balance, velocity, cadence, stride length, strength, and endurance. It is important to recognize that increasing speed too much may increase upper and lower extremity tone.

Multiple sclerosis is another diagnosis that often presents with significant deficits in gait. RAS can be an effective technique for addressing unilateral and bilateral upper and lower extremity weakness, drop foot due to pretibial weakness, fatigue, poor balance, ataxic gait, spasticity, staggering, uneven steps with poor foot placement, and uncoordinated movements (O'Sullivan and Schmitz, 2007).

Orthopedic conditions such as total knee or hip replacements or other joint problems can also benefit from RAS to increase weight bearing on unilateral or bilateral lower extremities, increase ROM at the affected joints, and improve strength of the affected extremities.

8.3 Research summary

Since 1991, when Thaut and colleagues published the first in a series of research papers that would become the foundation for investigating the effects of rhythm on motor control of both the upper and lower extremities in normal and neurologically impaired subjects, basic science and clinical research supporting the use of music in the rehabilitation of movement have continued to grow rapidly. Recent studies looking at the effects of RAS on gait with Parkinson's disease (de Dreu et al., 2012; Kadivar et al., 2011), traumatic brain injury (Hurt et al., 1998), multiple sclerosis (Baram and Miller, 2007; Conklyn et al., 2010), spinal cord injuries (de l'Etoile, 2008), and spastic diplegic cerebral palsy (Baram and Lenger, 2012; Kim et al., 2011) continue to show the significant impact of rhythm on gait kinematics through better posture, more appropriate step rates (step cadence) and stride length, and more efficient and symmetric muscle activation patterns in the lower extremities during walking. A Cochrane review of music therapy for acquired brain injury (Bradt et al., 2010) suggested that RAS may be beneficial for improving gait parameters in stroke patients, including gait velocity, cadence, stride length, and gait symmetry, these conclusions being based on studies of RAS.

8.4 Therapeutic mechanisms

RAS is based on four neurological principles, namely rhythmic entrainment, priming, cueing of the movement period, and stepwise limit cycle entrainment.

Rhythmic entrainment is the ability of the motor system to couple with the auditory system and drive movement patterns. *Central pattern generators (CPGs)* are local spinal cord circuits that help to connect incoming sensory information to appropriate motor neurons that enable movement. The CPG is capable of producing coordinated movement of the limbs with no input from the brain. Therefore this magnet effect of auditory rhythm in synchronizing and entraining movement patterns occurs even at levels below conscious perception and without cognitive learning. A simple example of rhythmic entrainment can be seen when we are walking down a hallway, and someone wearing high heels (click, click, click) approaches from behind, simulating the sound of a metronome. Even when we are making a conscious effort, it is difficult not to fall into the same walking cadence as the approaching person.

Priming is the ability of an external auditory cue to stimulate recruitment of motor neurons at the spinal cord level, therefore resulting in entrainment of the muscle activation patterns in the legs during walking. In 1991, Thaut and colleagues conducted a study to analyze auditory rhythm as a time keeper for modifying the onset, duration, and variability of electromyography (EMG) patterns in the biceps and triceps during the performance of a gross motor task. The results indicated a decreased variability in muscle activity during a motor task when auditory rhythm was present, indicating a more efficient recruitment of motor units necessary in skilled movement. These results indicated that more efficient use of the muscles would result in the patient being able to perform a task for a longer period of time. In 1992, Thaut et al. investigated the effect of auditory rhythm on temporal parameters of the stride cycle and EMG activity in normal gait. In the rhythmic condition, subjects showed improved stride rhythmicity between the right and left lower extremities, delayed onset and shorter duration of gastrocnemius muscle activity, and increased integrated amplitude ratios for the gastrocnemius muscle. These results provided evidence of more focused and consistent muscle activity during push off when a rhythmic auditory cue is present due to a priming effect. Similar results were seen by Thaut et al. (1993) with hemiparetic gait and stroke patients.

An additional concept, *cueing of the movement period*, arose from a 1997 study of rhythmic entrainment and motor synchronization mechanisms. Evidence emerged that rhythmic motor synchronization is primarily driven by interval adaptation or frequency entrainment rather than event synchronization or phase entrainment between motor response and the rhythmic beat (Thaut et al., 1997). When using rhythm in movement cueing, this meant that time stability is enhanced by rhythmic synchronization throughout the whole duration and trajectory of the movement, and not just at the endpoints of the movement coincidental with the rhythmic beat. This is illustrated in the velocity profiles of the wrist joint during a tapping task between two targets, with and without rhythm, as shown in Figure 8.1.

A limit cycle is the step cadence or frequency in which a person's gait functions optimally. Limit cycles can change due to neurologic disease or injury, resulting in deficient gait patterns. *Step-wise limit cycle entrainment (SLICE)* is the process of entraining a patient's current limit cycle, and gradually through a stepwise progression modulating their step cadence to approximate premorbid movement frequencies. This process is accomplished through six steps which make up the protocol for RAS gait training.

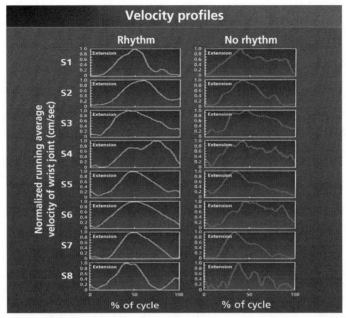

Fig. 8.1 Velocity profiles of the wrist joint during a tapping task between two targets, with and without rhythm.

8.5 **Clinical protocols**

8.5.1 **Principles of gait kinematics**

In order to understand how RAS can be used in the rehabilitation of gait, it is important to first have a basic understanding of normal gait kinematics. Human gait is beautifully simple and amazingly complex at the same time. Gait is one of our most basic functional independence activities. However, it is also something to which we do not give much thought until it goes wrong in some way. It is the ability that anyone wants back the most if they have lost it, but it can be a very complicated struggle to improve and regain.

The basic unit for gait is the "gait cycle", also called a "stride." This can be measured in both time and distance. The gait cycle is the sequence that each limb goes through repetitively as we ambulate (see Figure 8.2). Each lower extremity goes through alternating gait cycles during which the foot is on the ground, called the *stance phase*, and during which it is in the air, called the *swing phase* of gait. The stance phase accounts for approximately 60% of the gait cycle, and the swing phase accounts for approximately 40%.

A stride or full gait cycle begins when one foot hits the ground to start the stance phase, and ends after the stance and swing phase have been completed, when the same foot hits the ground again. During the gait cycle there are two occasions when both feet are on the ground, and this is called *double support time*. Each double support time accounts for approximately 10% of the gait cycle, with a total of 20% for both. This is the most stable portion of the gait cycle, so with any abnormal gait pattern there is usually an increase in

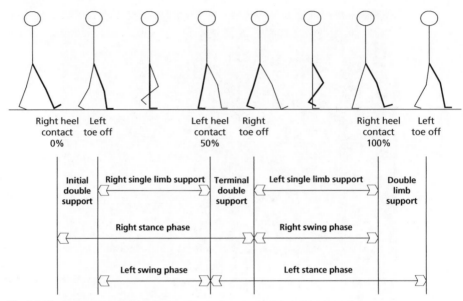

Fig. 8.2 The gait cycle (stride).

the double support time, with an effort by the body to improve stability and decrease the risk of falling.

Another component of gait is the *step*. A step is measured from the time when one foot hits the ground until the time when the other foot hits the ground. We count steps when we calculate cadence, or steps per minute (see Figure 8.3).

Two different sets of terminology are often used to describe the phases of gait, namely the traditional terminology and the terminology developed by the Ranchos Los Amigos Research and Education Institute Inc. (LAREI) of Ranchos Los Amigos National Rehabilitation Center (Pathokinesiology Service and Physical Therapy Department, 2001).

Weight acceptance includes the *initial contact and loading response* phase of gait. During this period, weight is rapidly loaded on to the outstretched leg and shock absorption occurs. This is the first double support time of the gait cycle, where both feet are in contact with the ground.

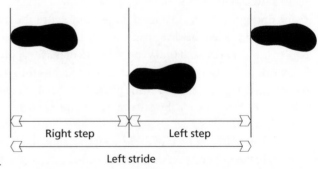

Fig. 8.3 Stride and step length.

Initial contact (known in traditional terminology as the "heel strike") refers to the beginning of stance, when the heel (normal gait) or other part of the foot (in altered gait) first makes contact with the ground.

Loading response (known in traditional terminology as "foot flat") refers to the phase during which weight is transferred to the outstretched leg and the foot is lowered to the ground. This phase continues until the other limb is lifted for swing.

Single limb support includes *mid stance and terminal stance* phases of gait. During this period the body moves forward over a single limb and continues until the opposite foot makes contact with the ground. Weight is then transferred on to the metatarsal heads, and the heel comes off the ground.

Mid stance (known in traditional terminology as "mid stance") begins as the other foot is lifted, and continues until the body is directly over the stance limb.

Terminal stance (known in traditional terminology as "heel off") refers to the phase in which the body continues to move ahead of the stance limb and weight is transferred on to the forefoot. This phase ends just prior to the other foot contacting the ground.

Swing limb advancement includes the *pre-swing, initial swing, mid swing,* and *terminal swing* phases. During this period the foot comes off the ground and weight is transferred to the opposite limb. The foot is moved from behind to in front of the body in preparation for the next heel strike.

Pre-swing (known in traditional terminology as "toe off") refers to the final phase of stance and the second double limb support time of the gait cycle. Weight is transferred to the contralateral limb, and this phase ends as the foot is lifted from the ground with the toe off.

Initial swing (known in traditional terminology as "acceleration") refers to the portion of swing as the foot is lifted and the thigh begins to advance and the knee progresses to maximum flexion of 60 degrees to assist clearing of the foot. This phase ends when the swinging foot is opposite the stance foot.

Mid swing (known in traditional terminology as "mid swing") begins as the swinging foot is opposite the stance limb. During this portion of swing the thigh continues to advance with the foot clearing the ground, and it ends when the tibia is vertical.

Terminal swing (known in traditional terminology as "deceleration") begins with the tibia vertical and ends just prior to initial contact. The knee extends during this phase in preparation for heel strike.

8.6 **RAS protocol steps**

RAS gait training consists of six steps. The amount of time spent on each step depends on the level of functioning of the client, but all steps should be considered and carried out in the following order:

1 assessment of current gait parameters

2 resonant frequency entrainment and pre-gait exercises

3 frequency modulation at increments of 5–10%

4 advanced gait exercises

5 fading of musical stimulus

6 reassessment of gait parameters.

8.6.1 Step 1: assessment of current gait parameters

Step 1 in an RAS gait training session always begins with a thorough assessment of the client's gait parameters. An assessment should include a 10-meter walk to calculate current cadence (in steps/minute), velocity (in meters/minute), and stride length (in meters). In addition, the therapist should evaluate gait kinematics, such as symmetry of gait, muscle weakness, trunk rotation, arm swing, posture, heel strike, toe off, single and double support time, and effective use of an assistive device.

Cadence refers to the number of steps that a person takes in a minute. This can be calculated simply by asking your client to walk for 30 or 60 seconds while counting the number of steps that they take. For those clients who fatigue quickly and are unable to walk for this amount of time, you may ask them to walk 10 meters while timing how long it takes them and how many steps they take. You may then calculate cadence by using the following formula: 60/time × number of steps.

Velocity is the speed at which someone walks, and it is measured in meters/minute or feet/minute (feet/minute divided by 3.281 = meter/minute). Velocity can also be calculated in the clinic by using the information collected in the 10-meter walk:

$$\text{velocity} = 60/\underline{\quad}\text{time (in seconds)} \times 10 \text{ meter (distance)}.$$

Stride length refers to the length of a stride on one side of the body, from the heel strike of one foot until the next time that the same heel hits the ground. Stride length can be calculated by dividing velocity by the cadence and multiplying by two (velocity/cadence × 2 = velocity).

In addition to the 10-meter walk and observation of gait, several standardized gait assessments, such as the Berg Balance Scale (Berg et al., 1992) and the Timed Up and Go test (Podsiadlo and Richardson, 1991), can be used to collect additional information related to gait deviations.

8.6.1.1 Common deviations of the ankle, knee, and hip

8.6.1.1.1 Ankle

Common deviations of the ankle related to weakness in the tibialis anterior may include foot slap (in which the foot slaps down to the floor) or foot flat (in which the foot is placed flat on the ground) during initial contact, and foot drop and/or toe dragging during the swing phase, which may result in compensation strategies such as increased hip and knee flexion, and hip hiking and circumduction to clear the foot.

Deviations related to weakness in the gastrocnemius and soleus include increased dorsiflexion and uncontrolled tibial advance during the stance phase, no push off when going into the swing phase, and no heel off and toe off as the whole foot may be lifted off the ground going into the swing phase.

Other deviations may occur due to limited ankle range of motion (less than 10 degrees of dorsiflexion and 15 degrees of plantar flexion), or if there is excessive tone in the ankle muscles (O'Sullivan and Schmitz, 2007).

8.6.1.1.2 Knee

Common deviations of the knee due to quadriceps weakness may include excessive knee flexion during initial contact through midstance. Compensations may include knee hyperextension produced by increased hip flexion, a forward lean at the trunk, and plantar flexion at the ankle. Quadriceps weakness also contributes to inadequate knee extension during terminal swing in preparation for initial contact.

Hamstring weakness may result in inadequate knee flexion, resulting in a toe drag during the swing phase of gait. Compensation patterns to assist clearance of the foot include increased hip flexion, hip hiking and circumduction, and vaulting on the opposite side (O'Sullivan and Schmitz, 2007).

8.6.1.1.3 Hip

Common deviations of the hip due to weakness in the gluteus maximus and hamstring include excessive hip flexion during the stance phase with a compensation of trunk backward lean to prevent further hip flexion; during the swing phase this weakness contributes to difficulty with placement of the leg in preparation for heel strike. Weakness in the gluteus medius may result in a Trendelenburg gait pattern in which the pelvis drops on the opposite side. Compensations may include a trunk lean or shift toward the side of the weakness. Weakness in the hip flexor muscles, primarily the iliopsoas, adductor longus, gracilis, and sartorius, may result in difficulty in initiating hip flexion when going into the swing phase, and result in hip hiking and circumduction to assist forward motion and clearing of the foot during the swing phase (O'Sullivan and Schmitz, 2007).

8.6.2 **Step 2: resonant frequency entrainment and pre-gait exercises**

Step 2 in RAS gait training involves adding a rhythmic cue through a metronome and/or music with a strong 2/4 meter, set at the same tempo as the client's internal cadence during their assessment. The therapist should use a metronome when doing RAS in order to make sure that the rhythmic cue is always driving the movement and that the therapist is not musically responding to fluctuation in the patient's speed. The metronome does not need to be audible to the patient, but must be audible to the therapist. Initially, the therapist may need to provide verbal cues to help the patient to entrain, but they should then fade their verbal cueing and allow the rhythmic auditory stimulus to drive the movement pattern. The therapist should observe any immediate effects that the rhythm may have on the gait kinematics, such as increased step length, symmetry, or changes in single and double support time.

In addition to resonant frequency entrainment, Step 2 also addresses specific kinematic deviations and compensation patterns related to muscle weakness through pre-gait exercises. These exercises are designed using *patterned sensory enhancement (PSE)* to address aspects of gait related to balance, strength and endurance, neuromuscular re-education, and development of normal kinematic patterns.

Typical pre-gait exercises may include a variety of movements that are performed both sitting and standing, such as weight shifting, marching, stepping forward and backward, trunk rotation and arm swing exercises with dowels, heel-to-toe rocking, long arc quads, and leg abduction/adduction. The amount of time spent on this step will depend on the patient's level of impairment and endurance. For patients who fatigue quickly, the therapist may spend the majority of the RAS gait training session doing pre-gait exercises, and very little time with the patient actually walking. For a higher-functioning patient, more focus may be put on the advanced adaptive gait exercises.

8.6.3 Step 3: frequency modulation at increments of 5–10%

As the therapist continues to shape the patient's gait patterns through pre-gait exercise in Step 2, the limit cycle (or natural cadence) will typically begin to increase. The patient is beginning to normalize their gait pattern, so they are able to walk faster. In Step 3 (frequency modulation), the therapist begins to speed up the rhythmic auditory cue in increments of 5–10% in order to see whether the patient can maintain the practiced gait pattern as they work to bring the patient's limit cycle to a more normal range.

In some instances, the therapist may need to slow the patient's cadence down in order to increase safety and create a more normalized pattern. This may be the case in a patient with Parkinson's disease who exhibits a normal or faster than normal cadence, with decreased stride length and velocity.

8.6.4 Step 4: advanced gait exercises

Steps 1 to 3 in RAS gait training address the most basic aspects of gait and mobility under controlled conditions. However, normal ambulation in everyday life may present many challenges, such as changing direction, speeding up and slowing down, walking on uneven surfaces, stopping and starting movement, walking around obstacles, walking up stairs, and walking with and without an assistive device. Step 4 involves creating exercises using RAS to practice those advanced gait situations that we encounter in everyday life.

Examples include the following:

1 walking with RAS through an obstacle course with different surfaces and objects to move around

2 walking forward when the music starts, and stopping when the music stops

3 walking backward to a rhythmic cue

4 walking on the beat to music that fluctuates in tempo

5 walking in a figure of eight to practice turning

6 walking outside on different surfaces (e.g. grass, ramps, sidewalk).

8.6.5 **Step 5: fading of musical stimulus**

The goal in Step 5 of RAS gait training is to begin to take the rhythmic auditory stimulus away, and see whether the patient can maintain the changes in their gait patterns without the music. This can be done by gradually fading the music and the metronome as the patient is walking. The therapist may need to give additional verbal cues if the patient has difficulty, or they may need to bring the rhythmic cue in and out several times as the patient is walking.

8.6.6 **Step 6: reassessment of gait parameters**

The final step in RAS gait training is to reassess the patient's gait parameters using the assessment tools from Step 1.

8.7 **Suggestions for implementing RAS with various populations**

8.7.1 **Stroke**

1 Instruct the patient to work on evenness of step length on each side, and emphasize hitting the heel on the beat on each side.

2 Emphasize the heel strike to improve a heel-to-toe gait pattern.

3 Encourage weightbearing as much as possible through the affected leg staying with the beat bilaterally. Ask the patient to work on decreasing gait deviations as appropriate.

4 Work on arm swing and trunk rotation.

5 Work on posture while walking, through the trunk and upper body, and pelvis/lumbar regions.

6 Push the velocity, but not at the expense of gait quality; you do not want to reinforce bad habits or increase tone.

7 Slowly progress the duration, to increase functional endurance.

8.7.2 **Parkinson's disease**

1 Instruct the patient to work on increasing stride length, and take bigger steps.

2 Emphasize the heel strike, and with a heel-to-toe gait pattern this will help to decrease toe walking.

3 Increase cadence if appropriate; the emphasis will more likely be on step length.

4 Instruct the patient in improvement of posture, but not at the expense of their balance; many also need balance training to improve stability and reduce their fall risk.

5 "Stop and go" rhythmic cueing can be used to work on initiation and coordination.

6 Work on improving arm swing and trunk rotation with gait.

7 Progress the duration of their program, to improve functional endurance.

8 Use RAS training to improve the patient's ability to walk through doorways, keeping to the beat.

9 Encourage staying to the beat and even going into a marching pattern if necessary to improve turns.

8.7.3 Multiple sclerosis

1 Keep the duration of walking time low, so as not to overtire the patient; work more on the quality of gait, depending on the patient's specific gait deviations.

2 Work on cadence, stride length, and even step length.

3 The goal should be to increase the efficiency and quality of the patient's gait, and improve balance as needed.

8.7.4 Traumatic brain injury

1 Depending on the patient's specific problems, it is usually necessary to work on quality of gait, balance, velocity (including cadence and stride length), and endurance.

2 Increasing speed too much may increase upper-extremity or lower-extremity tone; take this into account when progressing the patient's program.

3 These patients have many of the same needs as stroke patients, including an emphasis on heel strike and a heel-to-toe gait pattern, even weightbearing bilaterally, postural corrections, arm swing, trunk rotation, and improved control of movement patterns.

References

Baram, Y. and Miller, A. (2007). Auditory feedback control for improvement of gait in patients with multiple sclerosis. *Neurological Sciences, 254*, 90–94.

Baram, Y. and Lenger, R. (2012). Gait improvement in patients with cerebral palsy by visual and auditory feedback. *Neuromodulation, 15*, 48–52.

Berg, K. O., Wood-Dauphinee, S. L., Williams, J. I., and Maki, B. (1992). Measuring balance in the elderly: validation of an instrument. *Canadian Journal of Public Health, 83*(Suppl. 2), S7–11.

Bradt, J. et al. (2010). Music therapy for acquired brain injury. *Cochrane Database of Systematic Reviews, 7*, CD006787.

Conklyn, D. et al. (2010). A home-based walking program using rhythmic auditory stimulation improves gait performance in patients with multiple sclerosis: a pilot study. *Neurorehabilitation and Neural Repair, 24*, 835–42.

de Dreu, M. J. et al. (2012). Rehabilitation, exercise therapy and music in patients with Parkinson's disease: a meta-analysis of the effects of music-based movement therapy on walking ability, balance and quality of life. *Parkinsonism & Related Disorders, 18*(Suppl. 1), S114–19.

de l'Etoile, S. K. (2008). The effect of rhythmic auditory stimulation on the gait parameters of patients with incomplete spinal cord injury: an exploratory pilot study. *International Journal of Rehabilitation Research, 31*, 155–7.

Hurt, C. P., Rice, R. R., McIntosh, G. C., and Thaut, M. H. (1998). Rhythmic auditory stimulation in gait training for patients with traumatic brain injury. *Journal of Music Therapy, 35*, 228–41.

Kadivar, Z., Corcos, D. M., Foto, J., and Hondzinski, J. M. (2011). Effect of step training and rhythmic auditory stimulation on functional performance in Parkinson patients. *Neurorehabilitation and Neural Repair, 25,* 626–35.

Kim, S. J. et al. (2011). Changes in gait patterns with rhythmic auditory stimulation in adults with cerebral palsy. *NeuroRehabilitation, 29,* 233–41.

O'Sullivan, S. B. and Schmitz, T. J. (2007). *Physical Rehabilitation,* 5th edition. Philadelphia, PA: F. A. Davis Company.

Pathokinesiology Service and Physical Therapy Department (2001). *Observational Gait Analysis,* 4th edn. Downey, CA: Los Amigos Research and Education Institute, Inc, Rancho Los Amigos Rehabilitation Center.

Podsiadlo, D. and Richardson, S. (1991). The timed "Up & Go": a test of basic functional mobility for frail elderly persons. *Journal of the American Geriatrics Society, 39,* 142–8.

Thaut, M. H. (2005). *Rhythm, Music, and the Brain: scientific foundations and clinical applications.* New York: Routledge.

Thaut, M. H., Schleiffers, S., and Davis, W. B. (1991). Analysis of EMG activity in biceps and triceps muscle in a gross motor task under the influence of auditory rhythm. *Journal of Music Therapy, 28,* 64–88.

Thaut, M. H., McIntosh, G. C., Prassas, S. G., and Rice, R. R. (1992). Effects of auditory rhythmic pacing on normal gait and gait in stroke, cerebellar disorder, and transverse myelitis. In: M. Woollacott and F. Horak (eds) *Posture and Gait: control mechanisms. Volume 2.* Eugene, OR: University of Oregon Books. pp. 437–40.

Thaut, M. H., Rice, R. R., McIntosh, G. C., and Prassas, S. G. (1993). The effect of auditory rhythmic cuing on stride and EMG patterns in hemiparetic gait of stroke patients. *Physical Therapy, 73,* 107.

Thaut, M. H., Rice, R. R., and McIntosh, G. C. (1997). Rhythmic facilitation of gait training in hemiparetic stroke rehabilitation. *Journal of Neurological Sciences, 151,* 207–12.

Chapter 9

Patterned Sensory Enhancement (PSE)

Corene P. Thaut

9.1 Definition

Patterned sensory enhancement (PSE) is a technique that uses the rhythmic, melodic, harmonic, and dynamic–acoustical elements of music to provide temporal, spatial, and force cues for movements which reflect functional movements of activities of daily living, or the fundamental motor patterns underlying these activities. PSE is applied to movements that are not rhythmical by nature (e.g. most arm and hand movements, functional movement sequences such as dressing or sit-to-stand transfers). PSE uses musical patterns to assemble single discrete motions (e.g. arm and hand movements during reaching and grasping) into functional movement patterns and sequences. During a PSE exercise, the temporal, spatial, and muscular dynamics of a movement are trained through musical gestalt patterns that enhance and regulate the performance of the movement gestalts. PSE is often used to work toward goals to increase physical strength and endurance, improve balance and posture, and increase functional motor skills of the upper limbs (Thaut, 2005).

There are two ways in which PSE can be used in therapy. First, it can be used as a facilitator of simple repetitive exercises, which are done with a variety of populations to meet a wide range of goals (see Table 9.1). In simple exercise PSE, a musical pattern supporting the spatial, temporal, and force aspects of a movement is repeated in order to shape and facilitate an exercise movement repeatedly over time.

PSE can also be used to facilitate functional sequence patterns that consist of several discrete movements with different spatial parameters, timing aspects, and muscular dynamics. Examples of functional sequence patterns could include reaching, grasping, and lifting an object, opening a door using a handle, or moving from supine to standing position. Each one of these examples combines several smaller movements in order to complete a larger movement sequence. When doing a sequence PSE exercise, it is important that there is a consistent underlying timing structure which is cueing the movement.

9.2 Target population

PSE can be used with a variety of neurological and orthopedic populations, ranging from children to geriatric patients, in order to address goals related to physical strength and endurance, balance and posture, range of motion, and other functional motor skills of the upper and lower limbs.

Table 9.1 Examples of active range of motion exercises for the upper and lower extremities

Exercise	Movement	Description
Shoulder circles	Scapular elevation	Roll shoulders forward or backward in a circle
Shoulder raises	Scapular elevation	Shrug shoulders up and down
Shoulder squeezes	Scapular adduction	Pinch shoulder blades together without shrugging shoulders
Arm raises	Shoulder flexion	Lift arm over the head with thumb up and elbow straight
Arm circles	Shoulder abduction	Hold arms out to the sides at shoulder height. Move arms in a circle, clockwise
Arm raises to the side	Shoulder abduction	Lift arm out to the side with the palm up. Keep elbow straight. Do not lean to opposite side
Bicep curls	Elbow flexion/extension	Bend and straighten elbow
Marching	Hip flexion	Raise legs up and down while bending at the knee
Heel slides	Knee flexion/extension	Slide foot forward and backward
Long arc quads	Knee extension	From a sitting position, raise the leg up to full extension
Heel-to-toe rocking	Dorsiflexion/plantar flexion	Alternate raising and lowering the heel and toe
Side steps	Hip abduction/adduction	Pick up the foot and step to the side, keeping the knee pointing straight ahead
Postural alignment	Pelvic tilt/trunk extension/ cervical extension	While sitting in a chair, slump forward and then move to an upright sitting position

9.3 **Research summary**

Extensive research has been done that supports the use of rhythmic cueing to facilitate and organize motor performance in the upper and lower extremities (http://www.colostate. edu/depts/cbrm, accessed 1 July 2013). An early study by Thaut et al. (1991) showed that the use of a rhythmic cue for priming of the biceps and triceps during a gross motor task can be effective in modifying the onset, duration, and variability of electromyography (EMG) patterns, supporting priming and audio-spinal facilitation. It is also well documented that rhythmically cued hand/arm movements improve significantly in patients with Parkinson's disease when externally paced by auditory rhythm (e.g. Freeman et al., 1993; Georgiou et al., 1993). In a study by Peng et al. (2011), children with cerebral palsy exhibited increased knee extensor power, with smoother and faster movement, when performing a sit-to-stand exercise with PSE. There is no question that music's ability to temporally structure and regulate movement patterns makes it an effective tool for learning and training functional movement exercises in motor rehabilitation (Brown et al., 1993; Buetefish et al., 1995; Effenberg and Mechling, 1998; Goldshtrom et al., 2010, Luft et al., 2004; Pacchetti et al., 1998; Thaut et al., 2002; Whitall et al., 2000; Williams, 1993).

9.4 **Therapeutic mechanisms**

Although RAS is a technique aimed at biologically rhythmic movements, and PSE was developed for the rehabilitation, development, and maintenance of complex movements that are not intrinsically rhythmic, the neurologic mechanisms for RAS also apply to PSE. While PSE utilizes sensorimotor integration principles of auditory motor control through priming and timing (Paltsev and Elner, 1967; Rossignol and Melvill Jones, 1976), additional and more complex sensorimotor integration processes in the brain are being accessed than with RAS. In addition to using rhythm and timing to cue movement, as in RAS, PSE uses highly patterned structures in music to stimulate and facilitate patterned information processing that regulates and enhances the specific spatial, force, and temporal aspects of complex movements.

Although the exercises used in PSE are typically not rhythmic in nature, it is important to remember that consistent rhythmic repetition still results in the coupling of the motor system with the auditory system through rhythmic entrainment, and therefore drives the movement pattern. For this reason, it is of key importance that the therapist uses the metronome during PSE in order to ensure that the rhythm is always driving the movements, and that the music therapist is not just responding to the client's movements.

9.5 **Clinical protocols**

When implementing PSE, it is important not to think of the music as an accompaniment to the movement, but as a facilitator of the movement. This concept has been referred to in research as sonification, and involves using different components of sound to alter or change the user's perception of the sound, and in turn their perception of the underlying information that is being portrayed. Too often music therapists accompany themselves and their clients on the guitar or keyboard, providing pleasing background for a song or movement sequence. However, they miss the opportunity to capitalize on manipulating the varied elements of the music in order to musically create the movement by using the spatial, temporal, and force cues that are inherent in music. When musical cues are properly used to facilitate rather than accompany movement, clients are better able to organize and respond to motor expectations.

Due to the large pitch range, vast harmonic opportunities, and dynamic capabilities, the keyboard and autoharp are recommended as the most effective instruments for executing PSE in the clinical setting. The range and dynamic capabilities of the keyboard are particularly effective for facilitating complex functional PSE sequences.

9.5.1 **Types of cueing**

9.5.1.1 Spatial cues

One very important aspect of movement cued during PSE is the spatial component of the movement. There are four key elements in music that can influence the size and direction of a movement, namely *pitch*, *dynamics*, *sound duration*, and *harmony*.

9.5.1.1.1 Pitch

When a movement is on a vertical plane, pitch is an obvious element of music that can indicate the direction in which that movement is going. When pitch goes up the movement goes up, and when pitch goes down the movement goes down. Take the example of moving your arms up and down as in the shoulder flexion exercise shown in Figure 9.1.

Marching (see Figure 9.2), long arc quads (see Figure 9.3), and bicep curls (see Figure 9.4) are additional examples in which pitch can indicate a movement going up and down.

9.5.1.1.2 Dynamics

There are some movements for which pitch cannot accurately cue direction, but dynamics can be more effective in facilitating the spatial aspects. This is illustrated

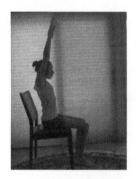
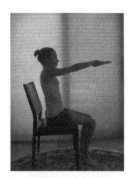

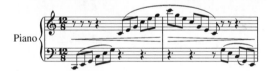

Fig. 9.1 Shoulder flexion exercise.

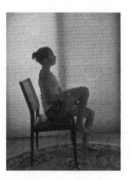

Fig. 9.2 Marching.

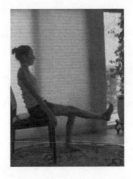

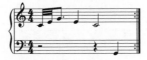

Fig. 9.3 Long arc quads.

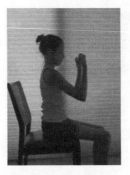

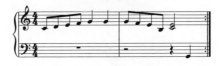

Fig. 9.4 Bicep curls.

in Figure 9.5, which demonstrates a movement going away from the body and back toward the body.

9.5.1.1.3 Sound duration

In addition to pitch and dynamics, the sound duration of notes can also have an impact on the spatial aspects of a movement. If the therapist would like to create a fluid movement, it would be most effective to use legato notes, whereas a jerky or rigid movement may be better cued with staccato notes.

9.5.1.1.4 Harmony

Harmony is an additional musical element that can have an impact on the spatial quality of a movement. Harmonies that are closer together give a feeling of spatially closer

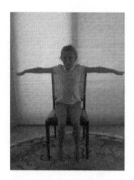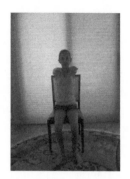

Fig. 9.5 Movement away from the body and back toward the body.

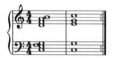

Fig. 9.6 Movement from closed to open.

movements, whereas movements that are more open would be better cued by more open harmonies. The example shown in Figure 9.6 could be used to cue a movement from closed to open.

9.5.1.2 Temporal cues

The temporal cues are probably the most important ones to consider when implementing PSE with a client. If the music does not accurately match the temporal structure of the movement, it will be difficult for the client to use any aspect of the music to facilitate their movement. The temporal structure of a movement can include four different aspects, namely *tempo* (or timing), *meter*, *rhythmic pattern*, and *form*.

9.5.1.2.1 Tempo

The first and most important thing for the therapist to do before adding music to any movement is to go through the movement with their client and identify the most effective tempo. This will require the therapist also to provide verbal cueing to enable the patient to understand the movement and the key aspects of it. Simple words such as "up and down", "side to side", or "in and out" can define important points in the movement and help to frame the timing structure. In addition to visual and verbal cues, it is important for the therapist to use a metronome at this point, in order to identify the starting tempo for the music. The simplest way to do this is to use a metronome with a tap function.

9.5.1.2.2 Meter

Every movement has a meter within the temporal structure. Some movements, such as skipping and weight shifting, are typically in 6/8, whereas other movements, such as marching or walking, may be in 2/4. With patients, the meter often changes, depending on the goal for the movement and how fast or slowly it is being carried out.

9.5.1.2.3 Rhythmic pattern

When cueing a movement, it is not necessary to provide a musical cue on every beat, but within the meter there may be a rhythmic pattern that best emphasizes the key aspects of the movement (e.g. shifting of weight, change in direction, or reaching a target endpoint). This is demonstrated in the weight-shifting movement shown in Figure 9.7. Although the movement is in 6/8, the rhythmic pattern is only providing a cue at the outer endpoints of the movement on beats 1 and 4, and at the point when the weight shifts from one side of the body to the other on beats 3 and 6.

9.5.1.2.4 Form

The final aspect of temporal structure that must be kept in mind when using PSE is *form*. Form refers to the structure of the whole temporal pattern that is being used to cue a movement. Some movements, particularly in functional-sequence PSE, may have multiple components that require different rhythmic structures. Perhaps raising the leg during a marching exercise takes 4 beats, whereas lowering the leg takes only 2 beats and then the patient needs 2 beats to rest.

Form can also refer to the bigger structure in a piece of music. Perhaps the therapist wants to incorporate two different movements into a song with ABA form. When the client hears the verse of the song with pattern number 1, they are cued to do bicep curls, and when the client hears pattern number 2 during the chorus they are cued to switch to a supination/pronation exercise.

9.5.1.3 Muscular dynamics/force

The final aspect of movement that the therapist is trying to cue through PSE is the muscular dynamics. It is often helpful to think of muscular dynamics in terms of the question "Where is the work for your client when they are doing a particular movement?". There are

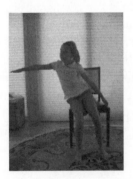
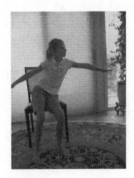

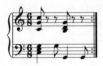

Fig. 9.7 Weight-shifting movement.

several aspects of music that influence how much force is behind a movement, including *tempo*, *dynamics*, and *harmony*.

9.5.1.3.1 Tempo

Tempo can have a big impact on the muscular dynamics of a movement as well as on how much force is behind the movement. However, it is important to weigh the potential advantages and risks of doing a movement at a fast or slow tempo. If the therapist is trying to get the client from a sitting position to a standing position, a fast forceful tempo may be most effective for cueing the muscles, whereas when cueing the patient to sit down again, a slow controlled tempo will probably be safer.

9.5.1.3.2 Dynamics

Dynamics can be a very effective way to create a feeling of increased force behind a movement. A crescendo can convey the feeling of increased muscle force, whereas a continuous loud dynamic may indicate the holding of the current position, with no additional force necessary. On the other hand, a decrescendo may create the feeling of a decrease in muscle force, and a continuous soft dynamic can convey the feeling of a resting position.

9.5.1.3.3 Harmony

A very effective way to create muscular tension in a movement is through tone clusters or unresolved harmonies. When a chord creates some tension in the harmony, it can cue the muscle to continue working until the harmony is resolved, at which point it cues the muscle to relax.

The musical illustrations in Figures 9.8 and 9.9 provide examples of the leg extension exercise with two different clients. The first example involves a client who is recovering from a double knee replacement (see Figure 9.8). The goal of the movement is to increase the range of motion at the knee, and therefore the most important aspect of the movement is the extension of the leg. In this case, the work for the client is going to be taking place while lifting the leg, and that is where the force cue needs to be emphasized in the music. The second example is a musical pattern that could be used in the rehabilitation of the lower extremities after a stroke (see Figure 9.9). The goal in this case is to increase muscular strength and control during both extension and flexion at the knee. Therefore a strong force cue will be essential to cue not only the lifting of the leg, but also a controlled return to the floor.

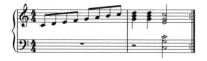

Fig. 9.8 Patient who has undergone double knee replacement.

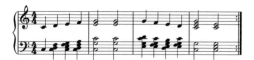

Fig. 9.9 Stroke patient.

9.6 **Helpful hints for practicing and implementing PSE**

PSE is a very complex technique that requires the therapist to think about many layers of musical structure, and how each aspect of the music can influence a movement. It is important to remember that PSE does not need to be complex in order to be successful. The following steps are recommended for implementation:

1 Go through the movement with your client and get an idea of their optimal tempo while tapping the tempo into the metronome.

2 Using the metronome, talk the client through the movement rhythmically, using simple verbal cues such as "up and down", "side to side", and "forward and back."

3 Maintain your verbal cues while slowly bringing the music in. Keep the music simple to begin with, and then gradually layer the music in order to cue the spatial, temporal, and force cues.

4 Fade out your verbal cues and let the music facilitate the movement.

References

Brown, S. H., Thaut, M. H., Benjamin, J., and Cooke, J. D. (1993). Effects of rhythmic auditory cueing on temporal sequencing of complex arm movements. In: *Proceedings of the Society for Neuroscience*, 227.2 (abstract). Washington, DC: Society for Neuroscience.

Buetefish, C., Hummelsheim, H., Denzler, P., and Mauritz, K. H. (1995). Repetitive training of isolated movements improves the outcome of motor rehabilitation of the centrally paretic hand. *Journal of Neurological Sciences*, *130*, 59–68.

Effenberg, A. O. and Mechling, H. (1998). Bewegung horbar machen-Warum? Zur Zukunftsperspektive einer systematischen Umsetzung von Bewegung in Klaenge [abstract in English]. *Psychologie und Sport*, *5*, 28–38.

Freeman, J. S., Cody, F. W., and Schady, W. (1993). The influence of external timing cues upon the rhythm of voluntary movements in Parkinson's disease. *Journal of Neurology, Neurosurgery, & Psychiatry*, *56*, 1078–84.

Georgiou, N. et al. (1993). An evaluation of the role of internal cues in the pathogenesis of Parkinsonian hypokinesia. *Brain*, *116*, 1575–87.

Goldshtrom Y, Knorr G, and Goldshtrom I (2010). Rhythmic exercises in rehabilitation of TBI patients: a case report. *Journal of Bodywork and Movement Therapies*, *14*, 336–45.

Luft, A. R. et al. (2004). Repetitive bilateral arm training and motor cortex activation in chronic stroke: a randomized controlled trial. *Journal of the American Medical Association*, *292*, 1853–61.

Pacchetti, C. et al. (1998). Active music therapy and Parkinson's disease: methods. *Functional Neurology*, *13*, 57–67.

Paltsev, Y. I. and Elner, A. M. (1967). Change in the functional state of the segmental apparatus of the spinal cord under the influence of sound stimuli and its role in voluntary movement. *Biophysics*, *12*, 1219–26.

Peng, Y.-C. et al. (2011). Immediate effects of therapeutic music on loaded sit-to-stand movement in children with spastic diplegia. *Gait Posture*, *33*, 274–8.

Rossignol S. and Melvill Jones G. M. (1976). Audio-spinal influence in man studied by the H-reflex and its possible role on rhythmic movements synchronized to sound. *Electroencephalography and Clinical Neurophysiology*, *41*, 83–92.

Thaut, M. H. (2005). *Rhythm, Music and the Brain: scientific foundations and clinical applications.* New York: Routledge.

Thaut, M. H., Schleiffers, S., and Davis, W. B. (1991). Analysis of EMG activity in biceps and triceps muscle in a gross motor task under the influence of auditory rhythm. *Journal of Music Therapy, 28,* 64–88.

Thaut, M. H. et al. (2002). Kinematic optimization of spatiotemporal patterns in paretic arm training with stroke patients. *Neuropsychologia, 40,* 1073–81.

Whitall, J. et al. (2000). Repetitive bilateral arm training with rhythmic auditory cueing improves motor function in chronic hemiparetic stroke. *Stroke, 31,* 2390–95.

Williams, S. M. (1993). Perceptual principles of sound grouping. In: *The Proceedings of SIGGRAPH '93: an introduction to data sonification (course notes 81).* Anaheim, CA: SIGGRAPH.

Chapter 10

Therapeutical Instrumental Music Performance (TIMP)

Kathrin Mertel

10.1 Definition

Therapeutical instrumental music performance (TIMP) is one of the three techniques in neurologic music therapy <NMT) that address motor rehabilitation. TIMP utilizes musical instruments to help patients to exercise impaired motor function and regain functional patterns of movement.

The choice of musical instruments, their spatial configurations, and therapeutically designed patterns for playing them all help to facilitate the (re)training of functional movement skills. TIMP is also useful for helping the patient to overcome unhealthy compensation strategies while increasing strength, endurance, and motor control.

The use of TIMP can help the therapist and patient to address appropriate ranges of motion, limb coordination, finger dexterity and grasp, flexion/extension, adduction/abduction, rotation, and supination/pronation in the upper extremities, among other goals.

10.2 Target populations

The majority of individuals who have neurological damage show a wide variety of motor impairment. These impairments can be manifested as paresis of one or more limbs, weakness, spasticity, ataxia, athetosis, tremor, and rigidity. These signs can result from various non-progressive disorders, including the following:

- traumatic brain injury (TBI), including polytrauma
- spinal cord injuries with paraplegia syndrome
- hypoxic brain damage
- ischemic or hemorrhagic strokes
- spina bifida
- ataxiate–langiectasia
- cerebral palsy
- poliomyelitis.

All of the disorders listed tend to include damage to the motor areas of the brain, and therefore result in impairments in movement and posture. It is important to recognize that the type of motor abnormality is related to the specific type of brain lesion. For instance, in spastic lesions, the pyramidal system within the central nervous system has been damaged, whereas in pure athetoid lesions only the extrapyramidal system is involved.

It is also important to note the distinction between central disorders caused by lesions to the central nervous system, which leave the peripheral nervous system (i.e. the nerves and muscles outside the brain and spinal cord) intact, and peripheral neuropathies, which are caused by damage to nerves in the peripheral nervous system, most commonly damage to nerve axons. Based on the type of lesion, movements may show different types of abnormalities. An understanding of the impairments associated with different lesions is essential when designing effective treatment programs.

Patients often show impaired balance, weak or reduced reflex patterns of movement, abnormal muscle tone, imbalance between muscle groups, and loss of selective muscle control and coordination.

Spasticity causes the muscles of the arms and legs to be tighter than normal, so they tend to contract with inappropriate strength when the patient attempts to stretch or move suddenly. Several important muscle reflexes are also disturbed, which leads to abnormal posture and movement patterns.

Patients with athetosis tend to show involuntary, purposeless movements of the limbs, as well as contortion of purposeful movements.

Patients with ataxia often suffer from balance impairment as well a disturbed sense proprioception (i.e. sense of the bodys position in space). Typically, these patients are unable to coordinate their movements, walk slowly with a swaying trunk and wide-based gait, and may keep their arms held out in an effort to maintain balance.

It should be noted that these signs do not usually occur in isolation, and patients tend to have some mixture of multiple types of disability. It is not uncommon for patients to show signs of both spasticity and athetosis. Furthermore, among other disabilities many patients with neurological problems also tend to have some degree of tremor and ataxia.

Another way to categorize the extent of motor impairment is according to which limbs are involved. The most common conditions are the following:

- monoplegia, in which one limb is involved
- hemiplegia, which affects one upper and one lower limb on one side of the body
- paraplegia, which immobilizes the lower limbs only
- diplegia major, which involves the lower limbs, with only minor involvement of the upper limbs
- triplegia, which is the involvement of three limbs, usually both lower limbs and one upper limb
- quadriplegia major, in which all four limbs are involved.

The majority of patients with cerebral damage suffer from multiple disabilities. In addition to some of the sensorimotor impairments mentioned earlier, mental retardation, seizures, and cognitive deficits such as distractibility, lack of concentration, and poor attention span are often seen. Another common and disturbing deficit is loss of sensation on areas of the body that were once innervated by the now damaged brain area. Depending on the location of the insult within the nervous system, paralysis of the bladder and bowel system may also be present. Finally, the majority of patients with acquired brain damage also need some form of speech therapy following resolution of the acute phase of damage.

Similar symptoms can be seen in patients suffering from neurodegenerative and other diseases, such as the following:

◆ inflammation of the brain, spinal cord, or peripheral nervous system

◆ tumors of the brain or spinal cord

◆ Parkinsons disease

◆ multiple sclerosis

◆ Huntington's disease

◆ muscular dystrophies.

In these conditions the course of the illness is often progressive, and deficits tend to worsen with time. Therefore these patients benefit more from a rehabilitative approach that is designed to preserve existing abilities and retard the progression of symptoms.

In addition to patients who have neurological disease or injury, candidates for rehabilitation with TIMP include patients in orthopedic rehabilitation, and individuals with any of the following:

◆ congenital hip dislocation

◆ arthrogryposis

◆ osteogenesis imperfecta

◆ thermal injuries

◆ acquired amputations.

In the case of amputee rehabilitation, therapy is geared toward helping to maximize the use of prosthetic devices and artificial limbs. Rather than restoring function, therapy often focuses on improving the ability to complete activities of daily living with the new prosthesis.

10.3 **Research summary**

Music communicates temporal sensory information to the brain that can have profound effects on development, learning, and recovery of function. Furthermore, music activates a large array of multiple neural networks in the brain that subserve motor, speech/language, and cognitive functions.

Research efforts have demonstrated that auditory perception of rhythm helps to prime and time the motor system. As far back as the 1960s and 1970s, researchers described a direct neural connection between the auditory and motor systems via connections from the brainstem to the spinal cord, namely the auditory reticulospinal pathway (Paltsev and

Elner, 1967; Rossignol and Melvill Jones, 1976). As the main element of chronometric organization in music, rhythm has the ability to enhance motor control, creating stable and well-defined templates for the temporal organization of motor responses.

Since the 1990s, numerous research projects have focused on elucidating the effect of auditory stimuli on motor functions. Thaut et al. (1997, 2002) described direct sensorimotor synchronization (entrainment) to auditor–yrhythmic patterns. This is hypothesized to occur because rhythm creates stable internal reference intervals and can be useful in helping to initialize and regulate motor movements.

Modern neuroimaging techniques have enabled various research groups to take a more detailed look at how music is neurally processed. It has been discovered that cognitive and motor learning experiences result not only in behavioral changes, but also in structural and functional alterations in the brain. Studies comparing musicians and non-musicians have documented how auditory rhythm is processed cortically and subcortically, in both parallel and distributed fashion. It is also known that musical training leads to plasticity in sensory and motor areas of the brain, with the degree of alteration being dependent on the intensity and duration of musical training (Gaser and Schlaug, 2003).

Other studies have provided deeper insight into rhythmic entrainment processes by studying synchronized adaptations of finger tapping to changing metronome frequencies (Hasan and Thaut, 1999; Stephan et al., 2002; Thaut and Kenyon, 2003; Thaut et al., 1998a, 1998b). The results of these investigations proved that the brain is able to adapt movements rapidly even to minimal tempo alterations. Most interestingly, the participants in these studies adapted their fingertapping *even if tempo changes were below the level of conscious perception*. In 2005, Molinari and colleagues reported that even cerebellar pathology fails to affect the capacity of auditory rhythms to entrain rhythmic motor responses. Similar findings were reported by Bernatzky et al. (2004), who found an improvement in the accuracy of arm and finger movements of patients with Parkinsons disease after listening to music.

It has been shown that listening as well as active instrumental music playing leads to the activation of widely distributed cortical and subcortical networks related to motor, sensory, and cognitive functions (Penhune et al. 1998; Platel et al. 1997; Schlaug and Chen, 2001). In summary, the temporal and spectral complexity of music has a profound influence on temporal information processing in the human brain (Harrington and Haaland, 1999; Rao et al., 2001).

Unlike gait patterns, which are rhythmic in nature and thought to be controlled by physiological pattern generators (Grillner and Wallen, 1985), most functional body movements are discrete, biologically non-rhythmic, and volitional. However, these movement patterns should also benefit from rhythmic cueing if it is appropriately organized. It has been recently shown that turning discrete reaching movements of the paretic arm in patients with stroke into cyclical continuous movements via rhythmic patterning and cueing leads to beneficial changes in motor control (e.g. decreases in trunk flexion accompanied by increases in trunk rotation closer to normal movement strategies) (Massie et al., 2012). Rhythmic patterning of movement facilitates repetition, which has been shown to be a key element of successful motor rehabilitation (Btefisch et al., 1995).

In 1982, Safranek et al. investigated the effect of auditory rhythm on muscle activation during arm movements. These researchers compared movement patterns with and without rhythmic stimulation, and used steady and unsteady beats. Their results showed a clear reduction in variability of muscle activity when moving to a steady beat instead of an unsteady beat or one without rhythm. These findings were later confirmed by Thaut et al. (2002). The latter study also looked at the effect of rhythmic cueing on spatiotemporal control of sequential reaching movements of paretic arms with and without rhythmic metronome cueing. Sequential movement repetitions showed an immediate reduction in variability of arm kinematics during rhythmic entrainment. Rhythm also produced significant increases in angle ranges of elbow motion, along with significant smoothing of movement in wrist joint acceleration and velocity profiles. Whitall et al. (2000) reported improved functional movement skills after a 6-week period of metronome-based home training of hemiparetic upper extremities (bilateral arm training with rhythmic auditory cueing, BATRAC), which were still evident in a controlled measurement taken 2 months later. Schneider et al. (2007) and Altenmüller et al. (2009) investigated the benefits of functional music training involving active musical instrument playing in an inpatient stroke rehabilitation program. After 3 weeks of musical training the patients showed a significant improvement in fine as well as gross motor skills with respect to speed, precision, and smoothness of arm movements, whereas almost no differences were seen in a control group who received conventional movement therapy. Improvements after musical training were accompanied by electrophysiological changes that were argued to be an indication of better cortical connectivity and enhanced activation of the motor cortex.

As well as the sensorimotor effects of therapeutic instrumental playing, music can facilitate additional supportive benefits for therapy, such as enhanced motivation and positive emotional states (Pacchetti et al., 2000).

10.3.1 Therapeutic mechanisms

Music has a multitude of neurological effects, and the act of playing music leads to the activation of widely distributed cortical and subcortical networks related to motor, sensory, and cognitive aspects of brain function (Penhune et al., 1998; Platel et al., 1997; Schlaug and Chen, 2001).

Research over the past 20 years has repeatedly shown that the use of music, especially rhythm, induces predictable neurological responses. By utilizing the rich connectivity between auditory and motor pathways via the reticular formation, rhythmic stimuli can trigger motor function and create stable and well-defined templates for the temporal organization of motor responses (Harrington and Haaland, 1999; Rao et al., 2001). This effect enables synchronization of movement and rhythm and entrains movement patterns, even at levels below conscious perception and without major cognitive effort.

Therapeutically playing a musical instrument stimulates and trains functional non-musical movement patterns that are used in daily life in an efficient and repetitive way. Music can serve as a strong sensory cue that temporally structures and regulates movement patterns. While playing an instrument, sound-induced priming of the motor system,

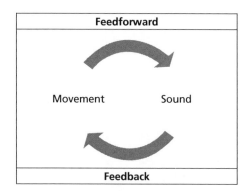

Fig. 10.1 Feedforward–feedback loop.

auditory feedback from playing the instrument, and entrainment via rhythmic cues create a feedforward–feedback loop (see Figure 10.1), which enables the patient to plan, anticipate, and execute their movements in a more efficient way. The sound feedback from playing an instrument creates meaningful "knowledge of result" feedback, while synchronizing the sound produced by the instrument to the external fixed rhythm cue creates a feedback–feedforward loop that facilitates the efficient (re)learning and execution of functional movement exercises in motor rehabilitation.

Structured playing of an instrument for (re)training a specific movement also fulfills at least five of the core principles of motor learning. These principles are repetition, task orientation, feedback, shaping (increasing the complexity of a task step by step), and motivation to do the exercise (see Figure 10.2). The repetitive, task-oriented movements that musicians make while practicing lead to demonstrable growth in sensorimotor and auditory brain regions, as well as strengthened connectivity between certain areas of the brain (Bermudez et al., 2009). The practicing of predefined movement patterns also strongly engages memory. Musical structure and metric organization of the musical activity are strongly linked to motor memory, and, as such, these higher-quality movement sequences are easily transferred into daily life.

Lastly, TIMP allows patients to practice in functional music-centered exercise groups in which the patients—while working on their individually designed exercises—work together by playing their instruments in a common musical structure, creating a musical piece (see Tables 10.1–10.7). This setting can generate feelings of accomplishment, collaboration, and enhanced motivation to work toward therapeutic goals, perhaps more so than during other types of individually separated physical exercise programs. Moreover, especially with young patients, group training also facilitates motor learning through watching and imitating other children.

10.4 **Clinical protocols**

As one can imagine, in a therapeutic setting the number of possibilities for instrumental set-up is almost limitless. Musical instruments can serve both to define the parameters of a desired movement and as targets to which movement can be directed. That is, the specific

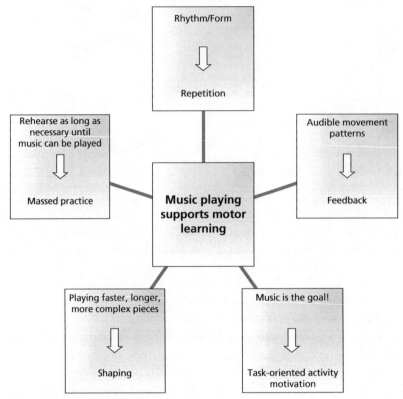

Fig. 10.2 Core principles of motor learning.

instrumental set-up visually defines parameters of the movement, but, as mentioned earlier, the patient also receives both auditory and kinesthetic feedback from successfully contacting the target instrument.

In summary, TIMP can be used in functional exercises that require the patient to move toward or alternate between several targets. This type of therapy allows the therapist to address functional needs of the patient, such as arm and leg flexion/extension, finger strength and dexterity, or strengthening of specific muscle groups, among other goals (see Tables 10.1–10.5).

The therapeutic appropriateness of instrument selection is based on a thorough assessment of the physical abilities and motor restrictions of the patient, as well as a kinematic analysis of the motor functions required to play different instruments. Due to injury or handicap, the patient is often unable to use bows, picks, or mallets in a traditional way. Therefore the therapist must adapt many musical instruments for ease of use on a patient-by-patient basis. Clark and Chadwick (1980) have written a comprehensive guide to the clinical adaptation of musical instruments for disabled populations. Elliot (1982) has provided an in-depth manual detailing the physical requirements (e.g. positioning, range of motion, involved muscle groups) for playing a wide variety of musical instruments. This

Table 10.1 Trunk exercises with the goal of strengthening, erecting, bending, and rotating the trunk

Movement	Instruments	Performance	Illustration
Flexion and extension of the trunk in a sitting position	1 standtom 1 cymbal/frame drum on a stand	Hold the mallet with both hands, bend forward and hit the drum in front of you, then stretch up and hit the cymbal standing behind you	
Rotation and erection of the trunk in a sitting and standing position	2 timpani 1 cymbal/frame drum on a stand	Stand between the instruments, hold the mallet with both hands, and hit the three instruments successively	
Rotation and erection of the trunk in a sitting position	1 standtom 1 cymbal/frame drum on a stand	Sit between the instruments, hold the mallet with both hands, hit the cymbal up next to you, and then cross the body in the midline and hit the drum on the other side	

Table 10.1 (continued)

Movement	Instruments	Performance	Illustration
Rotation and erection of the trunk in a standing position	1 standtom 1 cymbal/frame drum on a stand	Stand between the instruments, hold the mallet with both hands, hit the drum behind the body, and then hit the cymbal in front of you	
Rotation of the trunk in a sitting and standing position	2 congas (on a stand)	Stand or sit between the instruments and hit the drums with both hands or with the left hand on the right conga and vice versa, while crossing the body in the midline	
Bending down sideways in a sitting position	2 tone bars	Sit between the instruments and bend down on the left side and hit the tone bars on the floor, then bend down on the right side and hit the other tone bar on the floor	

Drawings by Maria Eckoldt.

Table 10.2 Exercises with a focus on balance and stand stability

Movement	Instruments	Performance	Illustration
Stand stability: "swinging" in a standing position		Stand between the two congas and shift your weight from one side to the other and play one conga on each side	
Balance/weight shifting: "swaying" in a sitting position	2 cymbals/frame drums on stands	Sit between the cymbals and shift your weight from one side to the other, lift up buttock and stretch up to hit the drum on each side	
Stand stability: "side stretch" in a standing position	2 frame drums/ 2 tambourines	Stand between the instruments and hit the drum/tambourine next to you alternately with your left and right foot	
Stand stability: swing back and forth in a standing position	1 timpani 1 cymbal on a stand	Stand in a stride position, hold the mallet in both hands, and hit the cymbal in front of you and then the timpani diagonally behind you	

Table 10.2 (continued)

Movement	Instruments	Performance	Illustration
Balance/weightshift/upper legs: "swinging" in a standing position	2 congas standing directly on the floor	Stand between the congas and swing from side to side; on each side bend your knee down and hit the drum	
Balance/arm stretch: "reaching" in a sitting position	2 frame drums on stands/ 2 timpani	Sit between the two instruments, and shift your weight from side to side and stretch out your arm to hit the instruments on each side	
Balance: stand stability on one leg	2 drums, different height 1 unstable underlay 1 footrest	Stand on the unstable underlay and place one foot on the footrest, hold the stick with both hands, then bend down to hit the drum on the floor, then stretch up and hit the drum in front of and above you	
Balance: strength and endurance	1 drum on stand 1 pair of bongos on stands shoulder high) Soft mat	Kneel down on one knee on the soft mat, then hit the drum in front of you with both hands and reach up to play the bongos in front of you	

Drawings by Maria Eckoldt.

Table 10.3 Specific rehabilitation of lower extremities, with a focus on hip movements

Movement	Instruments	Performance	Illustration
Hip flexion: "marching" in a sitting or standing position	1–2 tambourines (on stands)	Sit or stand with the instrument in front of you, then raise your leg and hit the tambourine with your knee (one side or alternately)	
Hip flexion / dorsi- plantar flexion: Heel-to-toe rocking in a standing position	1 tone bar per foot	Step forward over the tone bar and hit the floor with your heel, then step back over the tone bar and hit the floor with your toes; repeat with the opposite leg	
Hip flexion/ abduction/adduction: "step aside" in a sitting or standing position	2 tone bars	Sit or stand between the instruments and step alternately sideways over the tone bars	
Stretching of hip/ balance training: "taps" in a standing position	1 disco tap 1 tambourine on a stand	Stand in front of the tambourine and swing your foot forward to tap with your toes (disco tap) on the floor, then swing back and hit the tambourine with your heel (the tambourine can be raised up)	

Drawings by Maria Eckoldt.

Table 10.4 Specific rehabilitation of lower extremities, with a focus on leg, knee, and ankle movements

Movement	Instruments	Performance	Illustration
Knee extension, flexion: "heel slides" in a sitting position	1 rainmaker	Sit on the chair, place your feet on the rainmaker, and move it back and forth	
Knee extension: "stretch" in a sitting position	1 tambourine on a stand	Sit on the chair, raise your leg, and hit the tambourine with the tip of your foot	
Strengthening of upper leg/knee extension/flexion: mini-quads in a standing position	1 timpani/drum	Stand behind the timpani, hold the sticks with both hands, and bend your knees down to hit the drum, then stretch your knees	

Table 10.4 (continued)

Movement	Instruments	Performance	Illustration
Knee flexion in a standing position	1–2 tambourines on stands	Stand in front of the instruments, bend your knee to hit the tambourine with your heel, and stretch your knee again (either one side or alternately with both legs)	
Dorsiflexion: "toes up" in a sitting position	1–2 disco taps 1–2 tambourines on stands	Sit in a chair and attach a stick and a disco tap to one foot, then raise your toes to hit the tambourine and lower your foot to tap the disco tap (either with one foot or alternately)	
Dorsiflexion/plantar flexion in a sitting position	1–2 tone bars 1–2 tambourines on stands 1–2 stable footrests	Sit in a higher chair and place your feet/foot with heel(s) on the footrest. Attach sticks to the feet, then lower your toes to hit the tone bars under the footrest, and raise your toes to hit the tambourine above (either with one foot or alternately)	

Drawings by Maria Eckoldt.

Table 10.5 Specific rehabilitation of upper extremities, with a focus on shoulder, elbow, wrist, hand, and finger movements

Movement	Instruments	Performance	Illustration
Shoulder flexion: "arms up" in a sitting or standing position	2 timpani 2 cymbals on stands 2 cymbals in hands	Hold a cymbal in each hand and smash them together over your head Hold a drumstick in each hand and hit the lower drums next to you and then lift your arms up to hit the cymbals standing next to each side	
Shoulder extension: "move arms back" in a sitting or standing position	2 cymbals on stands 2 tambourines on stands	Hold a drumstick in each hand and hit the instruments standing behind you	
Shoulder extension/ flexion *Arm swing* in a sitting or standing position	4 cymbals/frame drums on stands	Hold a mallet in each hand and hit the instruments alternately in front of and behind you	

Table 10.5 (continued)

Movement	Instruments	Performance	Illustration
Elbow extension/flexion: "bicep curls" in a sitting or standing position	2 maracas	Move the maracas alternately up and down	
Elbow flexion/shoulder extension: "high bicep" curls in a sitting position	1 frame drum on a stand 1 cymbal on a stand	Lift your arms up, flex your elbow and hit the instrument behind you and then extend your elbow and hit the instrument standing in front of you	
Wrist pronation/supination: "pronation–supination" in a sitting or standing position	2 timpani 1 snare drum	Hold a drumstick in each hand and play simultaneously from the middle snare drum to the outer-standing timpani	
Wrist dorsiflexion: in a sitting position	1 pair of bongos on a stand 1 conga placed on the floor	Sit on a chair and place the instruments on one side of your body. Hit the conga with your flat open hand and raise your wrist up to reach and hit the bongo straight before	

Table 10.5 (continued)

Movement	Instruments	Performance	Illustration
Wrist dorsiflexion: in a sitting position	1–2 disco taps 1 table	Sit at the table and rest your forearms on it with your flat open hands toward the surface (and disco taps attached to your hands). Tap the disco taps by lifting only your hands up on the table. Your forearms must stay on the table surface (use either one hand or both hands alternately)	
Hand opening/closing Finger extension/flexion	1 guitar 1 table	Sit next to the table and rest one forearm close to the edge of the table. Place your hand so that the thumb points to the ceiling. Place the guitar upright on your legs with the strings by your hand on the table. Play the guitar by strumming the strings with the fingertips by opening and closing the hand	
Selective finger dexterity (without thumb)	1 guitar 1 table	Place the guitar in front of you on the table and pick each string with each finger; alternate the finger-picking patterns (e.g. 1-2, 1-2-3, 1-1-2-3-3, 1-4-2-3, etc.)This can also be done with your forearm close to the edge of the table and the guitar sitting upright on your legs	

Table 10.5 (continued)

Movement	Instruments	Performance	Illustration
Selective finger dexterity (all fingers)	1 piano or keyboard 1 table if needed	If you cannot hold your arm, rest it on a therapy table in front of the keyboard so that the fingers can easily reach the keys. Play one key per finger and try to play different finger combinations (e.g. 1-2-3-4-5, 1-3-2-4-3-5, 1-1-2-2-3-3-4-4-5-5, etc.)	
Grip (two and three fingers)	1 guitar/autoharp 3–4 tone bars 1 table	Place the guitar or autoharp on the table, hold the pick with your thumb, index, and middle finger (tripod grip), and strum the strings Place the tone bars on the table in front of you, hold the light mallet in your thumb and index finger, and hit the tone bars in various patterns	
Grip (holding pens)	1 autoharp 5–6 tone bars 1 table	Place the autoharp on a table in front of you, hold a drumstick like a pen, and strum the strings of the autoharp away from your body Place the tone bars directly in front of you on the table, hold a light mallet like a pen, and slide it over the tone bars from left to right	

Drawings by Maria Eckoldt.

Table 10.6 Example of a TIMP group session for five patients

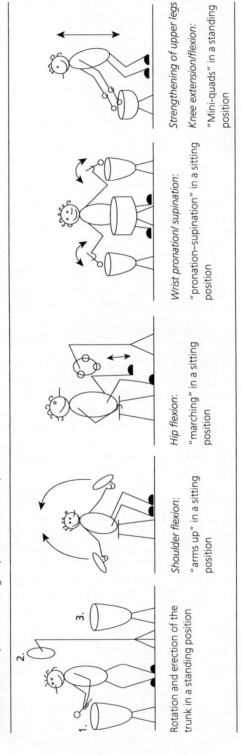

| Rotation and erection of the trunk in a standing position | *Shoulder flexion:* "arms up" in a sitting position | *Hip flexion:* "marching" in a sitting position | *Wrist pronation/ supination:* "pronation–supination" in a sitting position | *Strengthening of upper legs* *Knee extension/flexion:* "Mini-quads" in a standing position |

Drawings by Maria Eckoldt.

Table 10.7 Some examples of partner exercises

Patient 1	Exercise	Patient 2
• Weight shift in a sitting position • Stretching trunk • Shoulder extension • Elbow extension		• Weight shift in a standing position •Trunk erection •Shoulder extension •Elbow extension
• Shoulder extension • Elbow flexion and extension		• Mini quads (upper leg strengthening) •Shoulder extension • Elbow flexion and extension
• Leaning forward and back while sitting • Reaching through elbow flexion and extension		• Leaning forward and back while sitting • Reaching through elbow flexion and extension
• Grip: holding instrument with paretic and unimpaired hand		• Grip: practicing tripod grip on mallets and dorsiflexion of wrists

Drawings by Maria Eckoldt.

guide allows the therapist to match specific instruments with the individual abilities of the patient, as well as to select instruments based on specific therapeutic goals.

Percussion instruments are the most accessible group of musical instruments because they are easy to play, even for non-musicians. The wide range of percussion instruments offers a wide variety of sizes and sound timbres. Important for therapy considerations is the fact that all percussion instruments are played by the same basic arm/hand motions, which can be modified and altered in spatial configurations. The fact that these instruments are mostly non-pitched allows flexible arrangement in groups. Percussion instruments can be used to practice virtually all gross motor and fine motor functions. Keyboard applications in TIMP are particularly helpful for training finger, wrist, and arm control.

When using songs during exercises, it is helpful to select songs with a high degree of familiarity and structural simplicity. However, patients often wish to sing along with a familiar tune, which may interfere with their instrumental performance, especially in the case of children or patients who have attention problems. For such individuals, a simple repetitive melody with original lyrics may lead to a more effective interaction with the group and better functional performance for all of the participants. Also, it is important for the therapist to remain aware of the cognitive level of their patients. For some individuals, playing a musical instrument and listening to a song at the same time may be overwhelming. In this case, simply providing rhythmic structure with elements of PSE allows for a more effective therapy and a more enjoyable experience for the participant.

According to these principles, the design of TIMP exercises should be based on three elements:

- The *musical structure* is used to facilitate the organization of movement in time and space, as well as to mediate force dynamics. Therefore PSE mechanisms could be easily integrated into TIMP exercises. For instance, spatial cueing is considerably enhanced by setting up the instruments in a way that is specific to the needs of the patient.
- The *choice of instruments and the method of playing* both enhance therapeutically useful movements. Specific instruments may be more appropriate when focusing on a certain part of the body or when working on fine or gross motor skills.
- The *spatial arrangement and location* of the instruments facilitate desired paths of motion for the limbs as well as positions of the body.

TIMP exercises can be applied in a single or group setting, and offer an excellent opportunity for an interdisciplinary approach involving physiotherapists, occupational therapists, and neurologic music therapists. Ideally, the participants in any one group should be compatible in terms of their levels of actual rehabilitation needs and therapy tolerance (e.g. with regard to endurance). Each group can have a specific exercise focus. Session lengths will vary depending on recovery state, endurance, and levels of attention. Sessions should start with a warm-up before proceeding with TIMP exercises.

A *warm-up* could consist of singing a song with multiple verses, where different simple movements, such as bicep curls, shoulder rolls, or marching, are done to each verse. The warm-up procedure does not need an instrumental set-up; accompaniment on the keyboard or the autoharp using PSE principles is sufficient.

The TIMP *exercise part* can have one goal, on which the whole session is focused. Selection of specific exercises for a group setting should also be based on the steps of the transformational design model (TDM) (Thaut, 2005).

Some examples of group settings with thematic priority for single movements are shown in Tables 10.1–10.4.

10.4.1 **Specific rehabilitation of upper extremities**

Ischemic and hemorrhagic stroke are the most common causes of long-lasting hemiparesis. In children, cerebral palsy is still the leading cause of long-term disability. In most cases of hemiparesis the upper limb shows weakness and functional impairment and is more affected than the lower one. In the 1990s, Edward Taub developed *constraint-induced movement therapy (CIMT)*, which immobilizes the healthy extremity for several hours per day and leads to practice of movements of the impaired extremity (Taub et al., 1999). This procedure has been shown to lead to functional reorganization through repetitive, non-specific, but massed practice in the hemiparetic arm or hand. Even more rapid plastic adaptation when playing specific movement patterns on musical instruments was seen by Bangert et al. (2006). Such music performance is not restricted to cortical motor areas, but also involves auditory and integrative auditorysensorimotor circuits.

In TIMP exercises, timing, multi-joint coordination, and efficiency of movement can be integrated. Structured spatial and timing parameters of rhythmic auditory stimulation (RAS) while playing drive the patients feedforward planning mechanisms to produce rapid adjustments in movement within the task. According to Malcolm et al. (2008), CIMT in combination with RAS has an appreciable effect on kinematic variables of movement, with a substantial decrease in compensatory reaching strategies.

Strumming the autoharp provides an excellent method for developing wrist and arm control. For example, in order to address the fine motor skills of the hand, a child could strum the autoharp using a pick or a soft stick with their thumb, index, and middle finger (tripod grip). This exercise would be a creative way to help preschool children to build up the strength and endurance necessary for establishing writing skills.

A TIMP group session is also ideal for designing a full body workout in which all of the exercises can be built up like circuit training. In this context it is important to consider the patients needs and potential. The exercises selected can range from light to more challenging, or progress from the bottom part of the body to the top.

Rotation between the exercise stations can also be undertaken in a musical way. Instead of just walking from one chair to the next, the patients can collectively sidestep, step backward, walk while lifting the knees up high (like a stork), or walk on tiptoe with rhythmic accompaniment.

In a TIMP set-up, one of the exercises can be designed as a partner exercise between the participants. This also supports group interaction and motivates the patients to communicate with each other.

At the end of the TIMP exercise part, a short *cool-down* consisting of light movements such as shoulder rolls, ankle circles, or breathing pattern with PSE accompaniment can be used to conclude the session.

References

Altenmüller, E., Marco-Pallares, J., Muente, T. F. and Schneider, S. (2009). Neural reorganization underlies improvement in stroke-induced motor dysfunction by music-supported therapy. *Annals of the New York Academy of Sciences, 1169*, 395–405.

Bangert, M. et al. (2006). Shared networks for auditory and motor processing in professional pianists: evidence from fMRI conjunction. *NeuroImage, 30*, 917–26.

Bermudez, P. et al. (2009). Neuroanatomical correlates of musicianship as revealed by cortical thickness and voxel-based morphometry. *Cerebral Cortex, 19*, 1583–96.

Bernatzky, G.et al. (2004). Stimulating music increases motor coordination in patients afflicted by Morbus Parkinson. *Neuroscience Letters, 361*, 4–8.

Bütefisch, C., Hummelsheim, H., and Denzler, P. (1995). Repetitive training of isolated movements improves the outcome of motor rehabilitation of the centrally paretic hand. *Journal of Neurological Sciences, 130*, 59–68.

Clark, C. and Chadwick, D. (1980). *Clinically Adapted Instruments for the Multiply Handicapped*. St Louis, MO: Magnamusic-Baton.

Elliot, B. (1982). *Guide to the Selection of Musical Instruments with Respect to Physical Ability and Disability*. St Louis, MO: Magnamusic-Baton.

Gaser, G. and Schlaug, G. (2003). Brain structures differ between musicians and nonmusicians. *Journal of Neuroscience, 23*, 9240–45.

Grillner, S. and Wallen, P. (1985). Central pattern generators for locomotion, with special reference to vertebrates. *Annual Review of Neuroscience, 8*, 233–61.

Harrington, D. L. and Haaland, K. Y. (1999). Neural underpinnings of temporal processing: a review of focal lesion, pharmacological, and functional imaging research. *Reviews in the Neurosciences, 10*, 91–116.

Hasan, M. A. and Thaut, M. H. (1999). Autoregressive moving average modeling for finger tapping with an external stimulus. *Perceptual and Motor Skills, 88*, 1331–46.

Malcolm, M. P. et al. (2008). Repetitive transcranial magnetic stimulation interrupts phase synchronization during rhythmic motor entrainment. *Neuroscience Letters, 435*, 240–45.

Molinari, M. et al. (2005). Sensorimotor transduction of time information is preserved in subjects with cerebellar damage. *Brain Research Bulletin, 67*, 448–58.

Pacchetti, C. et al. (2000). Active music therapy in Parkinsons disease: an integrative method for motor and emotional rehabilitation. *Psychosomatic Medicine, 62*, 386–93.

Paltsev, Y. I. and Elner, A. M. (1967). Change in the functional state of the segmental apparatus of the spinal cord under the influence of sound stimuli and its role in voluntary movement. *Biophysics, 12*, 1219–26.

Penhune, V. B., Zartorre, R. J., and Evans, A. (1998). Cerebellar contributions to motor timing: a PET study of auditory and visual rhythm reproduction. *Journal of Cognitive Neuroscience, 10*, 752–65.

Platel, H. et al. (1997). The structural components of music perception: a functional anatomical study. *Brain, 120*, 229–43.

Rao, S. M., Mayer, A. R., and Harrington, D. L. (2001). The evolution of brain activation during temporal processing. *Nature Neuroscience, 4*, 317–23.

Rossignol, S. and Melvill Jones, G. (1976). Audio-spinal influence in man studied by the H-reflex and its possible role on rhythmic movements synchronized to sound. *Electroencephalography and Clinical Neurophysiology, 41*, 83–92.

Safranek, M. G., Koshland, G. F., and Raymond, G. (1982). The influence of auditory rhythm on muscle activity. *Physical Therapy, 2*, 161–8.

Schlaug, G. and Chen, C. (2001). The brain of musicians: a model for functional and structural adaptation. *Annals of the New York Academy of Sciences, 930*, 281–99.

Schneider, S., Schönle, P. W., Altenmueller, E., and Muente, T. F. (2007). Using musical instruments to improve motor skill recovery following a stroke. *Journal of Neurology*, *254*, 1339–46.

Stephan, K. M. et al. (2002). Conscious and subconscious sensorimotor synchronization–prefrontal cortex and the influence of awareness. *NeuroImage*, *15*, 345–52.

Taub, E., Uswatte, G., and Pidikiti, R. (1999). Constraint-Induced Movement Therapy: a new family of techniques with broad application to physical rehabilitation–a clinical review. *Journal of Rehabilitation Research and Development*, *36*, 237–51.

Thaut, M. H. (2005). *Rhythm, Music, and the Brain: scientific foundations and clinical applications*. New York: Routledge.

Thaut, M. H. and Kenyon, G. P. (2003). Fast motor adaptations to subliminal frequency shifts in auditory rhythm during syncopated sensorimotor synchronization. *Human Movement Science*, *22*, 321–38.

Thaut, M., McIntosh G. C., and Rice R. R. (1997). Rhythmic facilitation of gait training in hemiparetic stroke rehabilitation. *Journal of Neurological Sciences*, *151*, 207–12.

Thaut, M. H., Miller, R. A., and Schauer, M. L. (1998a). Multiple synchronization strategies in rhythmic sensorimotor tasks: period vs phase correction. *Biological Cybernetics*, *79*, 241–50.

Thaut, M. H., Hurt, C. P., Dragon, D., and McIntosh, G. C. (1998b). Rhythmic entrainment of gait patterns in children with cerebral palsy. *Developmental Medicine and Child Neurology*, *40*, 15.

Thaut, M. et al. (2002). Kinematic optimization of spatiotemporal patterns in paretic arm training with stroke patients. *Neuropsychologia*, *40*, 1073–81.

Whitall, J. et al. (2000). Repetitive bilateral arm training with rhythmic auditory cueing improves motor function in chronic hemiparetic stroke. *Stroke*, *31*, 2390–95.

Chapter 11

Melodic Intonation Therapy (MIT)

Michael H. Thaut, Corene P. Thaut,
and Kathleen McIntosh

11.1 Definition

Melodic intonation therapy (MIT) is a therapy technique that uses melodic and rhythmic elements of intoning (singing) phrases and words to assist in speech recovery for patients with aphasia. Functional phases or brief statements/utterances are sung or intoned by the patients, whereby the musical prosody should be modeled closely to the normal speech inflection patterns of the verbal utterance. The basic rationale for MIT emphasizes the use of rhythmic musical elements to engage language-capable regions of the undamaged right hemisphere. MIT was developed by a group of neurologic researchers in the early 1970s (Albert et al., 1973; Sparks et al., 1974; Sparks and Holland, 1976), and has been continually developed and adapted since then (Helm-Estabrooks and Albert, 2004).

11.2 Target populations

The majority of research in MIT has been conducted with expressive or Broca's aphasia. Therefore it is diagnostically recommended that patients with non-fluent Broca's aphasia will benefit from MIT. In addition, there is limited research showing that MIT will benefit other patient groups and speech disorders, such as patients with apraxia (Helfrich-Miller, 1994; Roper, 2003), autism spectrum disorder (Wan et al., 2011), or Down syndrome (Carroll, 1996).

The following patient criteria have been used to identify appropriate candidates for MIT (Helm-Estabrooks and Albert, 2004):

1 good auditory comprehension

2 facility for self-correction

3 significantly limited verbal output

4 reasonably functional attention span

5 emotional stability.

Patients with receptive aphasia (Wernicke's aphasia), transcortical aphasia, conduction aphasia, or other brain injuries that compromise the ability to read and comprehend language are not good candidates for MIT. Research about the inclusion of global aphasia in MIT is very limited and must be considered inconclusive (Belin et al., 1996).

11.3 **Research**

There are a significant number of research studies, starting in the mid-1970s, showing the efficacy of MIT with non-fluent expressive aphasia (Belin et al., 1996; Bonakdarpour et al., 2003; Boucher et al., 2001; Breier et al., 2010; Conklyn et al., 2012; Goldfarb and Bader, 1979; Hebert et al., 2003; Popovici, 1995; Racette et al., 2006; Schlaug et al., 2009; Seki and Sugishita, 1983; Stahl et al., 2011, 2013; Straube et al., 2008; Wilson, 2006; Yamadori et al., 1977; Yamaguchi et al., 2012). However, caution is needed, as most of these research studies were conducted with small sample sizes due to the fact that it is not easy to find homogenous study samples in aphasia research in terms of lesion site and symptom consistency. Several studies (e.g. Belin et al., 1996; Breier et al., 2010; Schlaug et al., 2009) have shown evidence for neuroplasticity induced by MIT, re-routing speech pathways from the damaged left hemisphere to the language-capable regions of the right hemisphere. Long-term MIT training may also show the reverse, reactivating left hemispheric speech circuitry (Belin et al., 1996; Schlaug et al., 2008). Modified MIT protocols have also been proposed and researched (Conklyn et al., 2012), showing positive outcomes. Recent research by Stahl et al. (2011) proposes that the element of rhythm may be as important as the element of melody, or more important than was originally thought.

11.4 **Therapeutic mechanisms**

There is evidence from brain imaging studies showing re-routing of speech pathways in the damaged left hemispheric to language-capable homologous right hemispheric regions. There is also evidence that long-term MIT may reactivate areas that control speech in the speech-dominant left hemisphere. The hemispheric shift was originally proposed as a putative mechanism by the originators of MIT in the early 1970s. The mechanism for the functional re-routing of speech pathways was thought to be triggered mainly by the use of melody and singing as core musical elements engaging predominantly the right hemisphere. However, recent studies suggest that the element of rhythm—using metronomic pacing, rhythmic hand tapping, and rhythmic speaking during MIT—may be just as or even more important for accessing right-hemispheric language resources.

The following elements of MIT may be regarded as the main mechanisms engaging preferentially right hemispheric networks for speech production:

◆ In melodic–rhythmic intonation, vocal output is slower than when spoken. Singing is characterized by syllables that are lengthened, chunked, and patterned, contributing to speed reduction in vocal output. The right hemisphere is better suited for processing slowly modulating signals. Thus translating spoken language into musical prosody preferentially activates right hemispheric language networks (Patel, 2008).

◆ Processing of music engages right hemispheric networks, thus helping to bypass damaged left hemispheric language networks (Seger et al., 2013).

◆ Rhythmic pacing and entrainment predominantly engage right hemispheric networks in the auditory, prefrontal, and parietal regions (Stephan et al., 2002).

♦ Left hand tapping activates right hemispheric language networks, as spoken language and arm gestures are controlled by the same motor control network (Gentilucci and Dalla Volta, 2008).

11.5 **Clinical protocols**

The original MIT protocol is divided into four progressive levels or stages. In Stage 1, the therapist hums the melody of an intoned utterance (a single word or short phrase) while aiding the patient in tapping the left hand to the rhythm and stress inflections of the selected melody. The rhythm and melody should follow the pitch and stress inflections of the spoken stimulus. At the beginning of Stage 2 the patient joins the therapist in humming. In subsequent steps the therapist first intones phrases and invites the patient to join in, and then fades. After fading the therapist intones the stimulus phrases and cues the patient to repeat them. Hand tapping continues throughout Stage 2. Stage 3 continues at the end of Stage 2, but the patient is required to wait for a designated period of a few seconds before repeating. At the last step the therapist intones a question about the information in the phrase with no hand tapping for the patient to appropriately respond to. At Stage 4, utterances are presented in a stepwise transition from intoning to "sprechgesang" (speech singing), to normal speech. Hand tapping is progressively faded and the final question about the information is not intoned (e.g. sentence: "I want a cup of coffee"—sentence question by therapist: "What do you want to drink?").

MIT applications are often modified to meet specific needs of patients. One important modification was proposed for children, in which Stage 1 is the same as in the adult model, Stage 2 follows Stage 3 in the adult model, and the final stage 3 follows Stage 4 of the adult model. However, signed English is used instead of hand tapping (Roper, 2003).

A shortened version of MIT in six steps or stages was recently developed, preserving the same hierarchical structure of the original MIT but compressing it into a shorter process for clinical efficiency (Thaut, 1999). The steps are as follows:

1 The therapist presents an intoned statement via humming while hand tapping with the patient. The patient listens to the presentation.

2 The therapist sings the intoned statement in several repetitions while hand tapping with the patient. The patient listens to the presentation.

3 The therapist sings and invites the patient to join in. The therapist and patient sing together with several repetitions. The therapist continues to aid the patient's hand tapping, but fades progressively as the patient shows more independent tapping motions.

4 The therapist fades during singing with the patient. Hand tapping continues.

5 The therapist sings first and then stops and cues the patient to respond by intoning independently. Hand tapping continues. The therapist may increase the "wait period" for the patient to respond after each repetition to exercise the ability to retrieve words.

6 The therapist asks one or more questions about the information in the exercise statement. The patient may respond by intoning or in normal speech. The therapist does not assist with hand tapping. The patient may or may not use tapping spontaneously.

The "sprechgesang" component is not explicitly included in this six-stage model, due to the frequent clinical observation that the patient's intonations are already narrowed in pitch and interval range and often resemble "sprechgesang" inflections. A second observation has been that at the final stage the verbal response of the patient tends to spontaneously follow more speech-like inflections due to the speech mode of the questions by the therapist. Therefore this model does not explicitly include separate practice steps at the final stage for moving "singing" to "sprechgesang" to "normal speech." Recent research suggests that maintaining accentuated stress and rhythm inflections may actually help the patient to continue to access speech capabilities (Stahl et al., 2011).

Typically the therapist sits in front of the patient and lightly holds the patient's left hand with the palm facing down. The other hand should be used with simple signs for "listen" and "respond." Several principles have been emphasized by the originators of MIT that should be carefully observed.

First, the linguistic materials that are used should follow careful progressions of length and difficulty, with the gradual withdrawal of the therapist's participation. Secondly, error correction should be limited to just one "retrial" or "back-up" trial. If it is still uncorrected, the item should be dropped. Insistence on repeated error correction will often lead to perseverance of error repetition and thus reinforce it. Thirdly, the therapist should pay careful attention to the timing and use of controlled latencies between stimulus presentation and patient response. Latencies should increase progressively to avoid reflexive habitual responses. Fourthly, in order to avoid practice effects that will diminish meaningful transfer into daily living, the therapist must provide an appropriate variety of meaningful material so that the same statements are not used over and over again in each therapy session. Fifthly, the verbal output of the therapist outside of using the practice material should be extremely restrained. Exuberant praise or verbal feedback will lead to stress and disruption for patients with expressive aphasia. A smile or nod of the head for a correct response is adequate and more effective. Sixthly, MIT requires a high frequency of therapy sessions, preferably daily—or twice daily in the early stages of recovery—over several weeks. If restrictions or limitations on therapy access exist, it is critical to train caregivers, partners, or other family members to function as assistants in a continuum of care from inpatient to outpatient to home settings. Lastly, repetition is at the core of MIT as an efficient training device. However, the use of repetition must be qualified by Principle 2 (error correction) and Principle 5 (variety of material).

References

Albert M, Sparks R W, and Helm N (1973). Melodic intonation therapy for aphasics. *Archives of Neurology, 29,* 130–31.

Belin P et al. (1996). Recovery from nonfluent aphasia after melodic intonation therapy. *Neurology, 47,* 1504–11.

Bonakdarpour B, Eftekharzadeh A, and Ashayeri H (2003). Melodic intonation therapy in Persian aphasic patients. *Aphasiology, 17,* 75–95.

Boucher V, Garcia J L, Fleurant J, and Paradis J (2001). Variable efficacy of rhythm and tone in melody-based interventions: implications for the assumption of a right-hemisphere facilitation in non-fluent aphasia. *Aphasiology, 15,* 131–49.

Breier J, Randle S, Maher I M, and Papanicolaou A C (2010). Changes in maps of language activity activation following melodic intonation therapy using magnetoencephalography: two case studies. *Journal of Clinical and Experimental Neuropsychology, 32,* 309–14.

Carroll D (1996). *A study of the effectiveness of an adaptation of melodic intonation therapy in increasing communicative speech of young children with Down syndrome.* Unpublished dissertation. Montreal: McGill University.

Conklyn D et al. (2012). The effects of modified melodic intonation therapy on nonfluent aphasia: a pilot study. *Journal of Speech, Language, and Hearing Research, 55,* 463–71.

Gentilucci M and and Dalla Volta R (2008). Spoken language and arm gestures are controlled by the same motor control system. *Quarterly Journal of Experimental Psychology, 61,* 944–57.

Goldfarb R and Bader E (1979). Espousing melodic intonation therapy in aphasia rehabilitation: a case study. *International Journal of Rehabilitation Research, 2,* 333–42.

Hebert S, Racette A, Gagnon L, and Peretz I (2003). Revisiting the dissociation between singing and speaking in expressive aphasia. *Journal of Neurology, 126,* 1838–51.

Helfrich-Miller K R (1994). Melodic intonation therapy with developmentally apraxic children. *Seminars in Speech and Language, 5,* 119–26.

Helm-Estabrooks N and Albert M (2004). *Manual of Aphasia and Aphasia Therapy.* Austin, TX: PRO-ED Publishers.

Patel A (2008). *Music, Language, and the Brain.* Oxford: Oxford University Press.

Popovici M (1995). Melodic intonation therapy in the verbal decoding of aphasics. *Revue Romaine de Neurologie et Psychiatrie, 33,* 57–97.

Racette A, Bard C, and Peretz I (2006). Making nonfluent aphasics speak: sing along! *Brain, 129,* 2571–84.

Roper N (2003). Melodic intonation therapy with young children with apraxia. *Bridges: Practice-Based Research Synthesis, 1,* 1–7.

Schlaug G, Marchina S, and Norton A (2008). From singing to speaking: why singing may lead to recovery of expressive language function in patients with Broca's aphasia. *Music Perception, 25,* 315–23.

Schlaug G, Marchina S, and Norton A (2009). Evidence for plasticity in white-matter tracts of patients with chronic Broca's aphasia undergoing intense intonation-based speech therapy. *Annals of the New York Academy of Sciences, 1169,* 385–94.

Seger C et al. (2013). Corticostriatal contributions to musical expectancy perception. *Journal of Cognitive Neuroscience, 25,* 1062–77.

Seki K and Sugishita M (1983). Japanese-applied melodic intonation therapy for Broca's aphasia [article in Japanese]. *No to Shinkei, 35,* 1031–7.

Sparks R W and Holland A L (1976). Method: melodic intonation therapy for aphasia. *Journal of Speech and Hearing Disorders, 41,* 287–97.

Sparks R W, Helm N, and Albert M (1974). Aphasia rehabilitation resulting from melodic intonation therapy. *Cortex, 10,* 313–16.

Stahl B et al. (2011). Rhythm in disguise: why singing may not hold the key to recovery from aphasia. *Brain, 134,* 3083–93.

Stahl B et al. (2013). How to engage the right brain hemisphere in aphasics without even singing: evidence for two paths of speech recovery. *Frontiers in Human Neuroscience, 7,* 1–12.

Stephan K M et al. (2002). Conscious and subconscious sensorimotor synchronization: cortex and the influence of awareness. *NeuroImage, 15,* 345–52.

Straube T et al. (2008). Dissociation between singing and speaking in expressive aphasia: the role of song familiarity. *Neuropsychologia, 46,* 1505–12.

Thaut M H. (1999). *Training Manual for Neurologic Music Therapy*. Fort Collins, CO: Center for Biomedical Research in Music, Colorado State University.

Wan C Y et al. (2011). Auditory motor mapping training as an intervention to facilitate speech output in non-verbal children with autism: a proof of concept study. *PLoS One*, 6, e25505.

Wilson S J (2006). Preserved singing in aphasia: a case study of the efficacy of melodic intonation therapy. *Music Perception*, 24, 23–6.

Yamadori A, Osumi Y, Masuhara S, and Okubo M (1977). Preservation of singing in Broca's aphasia. *Journal of Neurology, Neurosurgery, & Psychiatry*, 40, 221–4.

Yamaguchi S et al. (2012). Singing therapy can be effective for a patient with severe nonfluent aphasia. *International Journal of Rehabilitation Research*, 35, 78–81.

Chapter 12

Musical Speech Stimulation (MUSTIM)

Corene P. Thaut

12.1 Definition

Musical speech stimulation (MUSTIM) is a neurologic music therapy (NMT) technique for non-fluent aphasia, that utilizes musical materials such as songs, rhymes, chants, and musical phrases to simulate prosodic speech gestures and trigger automatic speech (Thaut, 2005). In many patients with aphasia, non-propositional reflexive speech is unaffected, and overlearned musical phrases or songs can be used to stimulate spontaneous speech output. MUSTIM is an appropriate technique to select for patients who do not meet the criteria to be good candidates for melodic intonation therapy (MIT), due to decreased cognition or to dementia-related primary progressive aphasia. MUSTIM can also be an appropriate follow-up technique for patients who are beginning to show increased functional language after MIT and are ready to increase their spontaneous output of propositional speech.

12.2 Target populations

Patients who have experienced a left hemisphere stroke or brain injury frequently suffer from some level of non-fluent aphasia which results in disrupted spontaneous expression of speech. Although many of these patients never recover speech despite intensive treatment, it has been observed that many patients with non-fluent expressive aphasia retain the ability to sing familiar melodies and words (Yamadori et al., 1977). MUSTIM is an NMT intervention designed for people with some form of non-fluent aphasia who still have the ability to produce non-propositional reflexive speech by accessing undamaged subcortical thalamic speech circuitry. Appropriate candidates for MUSTIM have some type of non-fluent aphasia, such as Broca's or primary progressive aphasia, accompanied by difficulty with cognition. Candidates are also typically unable to follow the complexity of MIT with good functional carryover. This may be due to a stroke, or to diffuse traumatic brain injury, or related to Alzheimer's disease or dementia. Other suitable candidates for MUSTIM are patients with Broca's aphasia who have progressed with MIT and are beginning to increase their functional use of language outside of the sentences practiced in MIT sessions. In this case, MUSTIM can be an excellent compensatory strategy for stimulating the initiation of spontaneous functional word or phrase utterances.

12.3 **Research summary**

Numerous studies support the use of singing and intoning to trigger non-propositional speech in people who present with non-fluent aphasia (Basso et al., 1979; Cadalbert et al., 1994; Lucia, 1987; Yamadori et al., 1977). Straube et al. (2008) found that singing helped word phrase production in some patients with severe expressive aphasia, probably due to the association of melody and text in long-term memory. In a case study conducted by Yamaguchi et al. (2012), the results suggested that singing can be an effective treatment for severe non-fluent aphasia in rehabilitation therapy even when a patient presents with significant cognitive impairment.

It is not disputed among researchers that there are strong similarities but also distinct differences between neural activation patterns in musical and non-musical speech tasks (Brown et al., 2006; Patel, 2003, 2005; Stewart, 2001). Brown et al. (2006) directly compared brain activation patterns during improvised melodic and linguistic phrases. The two tasks revealed activation in nearly identical functional brain areas, with some differences seen in lateralization tendencies, with the language task favoring the left hemisphere. Brown and colleagues further described parallel systems for music and language when generating complex sound structures (phonology), but distinctly different neural systems for informational content (semantics). In addition, Patel (2005) compared performance on syntactic priming tasks in language with harmonic priming tasks in music. Although the participants in the study performed poorly on both priming tasks, it was concluded that further research comparing the relationship between performance on the musical and non-musical priming task and the severity and variation of the deficits among aphasic patients is needed.

12.4 **Therapeutic mechanisms**

The results of a study by Ozdemir et al. (2006) suggested a bi-hemispheric network for vocal production during both singing and intoned speech, with additional right-lateralized activation of the superior temporal gyrus, inferior central operculum, and inferior frontal gyrus during singing. This may offer an explanation for the clinical observation that patients with non-fluent aphasia due to left hemisphere lesions are able to sing the text of a song even though they are unable to speak the same words.

12.5 **Clinical protocols**

MUSTIM can be implemented at many different levels of complexity depending on the goal and the level of functioning of the patient. These may include filling in words or phrases to familiar songs, filling in words to common phrases put to music, or practicing phrases that can be completed with many different responses.

The simplest application of MUSTIM is through the use of a familiar song, in which the therapist sings a phrase, leaving out words at the end of the phrase for the patient to fill in—for example, "My Bonnie Lies Over the (Ocean)." This can progress to the therapist alternating lines in the song, with the therapist singing the first musical phrase and the patient singing the second musical phrase, and then progress to having the patient initiate the first phrase and the therapist singing the second phrase. The final step would be to have the patient sing the entire song with or without musical accompaniment, and without assistance from the therapist. The goals in this example of MUSTIM could be (1) to maintain as much verbal output as possible for as long as possible with a patient with dementia, or (2) to encourage any spontaneous output during the early stages of expressive aphasia rehabilitation after a stroke or brain injury.

A second application of MUSTIM is the practicing of common, overlearned sentences with obvious completions, in order to help the patient to get started with a sentence with the intention that they will independently complete it. The melodies used should mimic the natural prosody and inflection of the sentence (e.g. a question may be presented through an upward arpeggio or a scale). Examples of sentences might include "How are you (today)?", "My name is (John)", or "Thank you very (much)" (see Figure 12.1). The goal in presenting MUSTIM through familiar phrases is to work toward the patient's independent automatic completion of familiar sentences when musically cued.

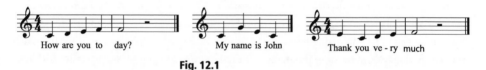

Fig. 12.1

A third application of MUSTIM is to present sentences that have many different possible endings. The sentence is presented through a melody in order to get the patient started, and they have the opportunity to respond in several different ways. A typical example might be "I would like to (go outside)" (see Figure 12.2). This level of MUSTIM allows the patient to choose from many different responses, and involves the initiation of propositional speech.

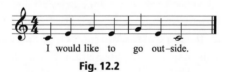

Fig. 12.2

A variation on the previous MUSTIM application would be to ask the patient a question to which there are two different musical responses—for example, "I want_____" or "I don't want _____." Each of the responses should begin with a different musical phrase in order to make it easier for the patient to initiate and distinguish between the two answers. The question asked by the therapist might be "Do you want something to eat?", to which the patient could respond "I want something to eat" or "I don't want something to eat" (see Figure 12.3).

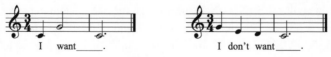

Fig. 12.3

In summary, MUSTIM is a technique designed specifically for expressive non-fluent aphasia in order to stimulate spontaneous non-propositional speech, or as a compensatory strategy to help higher-functioning aphasia patients to initiate intentional propositional speech. MUSTIM can be implemented at various levels of complexity, depending on the needs and goal of the patient.

References

Basso, A., Capitani, E., and Vignolo, L. A. (1979). Influence of rehabilitation on language skills in aphasic patients. *Archives of Neurology*, *36*, 190–96.

Brown, S., Martinez, M. J., and Parsons, L. M. (2006). Music and language side by side in the brain: a PET study of the generation of melodies and sentences. *European Journal of Neuroscience*, *23*, 2791–803.

Cadalbert, A., Landis, T., Regard, M., and Graves, R. E. (1994). Singing with and without words: hemispheric asymmetries in motor control. *Journal of Clinical and Experimental Neuropsychology*, *16*, 664–70.

Lucia, C. M. (1987). Toward developing a model of music therapy intervention in the rehabilitation of head trauma patients. *Music Therapy Perspectives*, *4*, 34–9.

Ozdemir, E., Norton, A., and Schlaug, G. (2006). Shared and distinct neural correlates of singing and speaking. *NeuroImage*, *33*, 628–35.

Patel, A. D. (2003). Rhythm in language and music: parallels and differences. *Annals of the New York Academy of Sciences*, *999*, 140–43.

Patel, A. D. (2005). The relationship of music to the melody of speech and to syntactic processing disorders in aphasia. *Annals of the New York Academy of Sciences*, *1060*, 59–70.

Stewart, L., Walsh, V., Frith, U., and Rothwell, J. (2001). Transcranial magnetic stimulation produces speech arrest but not song arrest. *Annals of the New York Academy of Sciences*, *930*, 433–5.

Straube, T. et al. (2008). Dissociation between singing and speaking in expressive aphasia: the role of song familiarity. *Neuropsychologia*, *46*, 1505–12.

Thaut M H (2005). *Rhythm, Music, and the Brain: scientific foundations and clinical applications*. New York: Routledge.

Yamadori, A., Osumi, Y., Masuhara, S., and Okubo, M. (1977). Preservation of singing in Broca's aphasia. *Journal of Neurology, Neurosurgery, & Psychiatry*, *40*, 221–4.

Yamaguchi S et al. (2012). Singing therapy can be effective for a patient with severe nonfluent aphasia. *International Journal of Rehabilitation Research*, *35*, 78–81.

Chapter 13

Rhythmic Speech Cueing (RSC)

Stefan Mainka and Grit Mallien

13.1 Definition

In *rhythmic speech cueing (RSC)*, speech rate control via auditory rhythm is used to improve temporal characteristics such as fluency, articulatory rate, pause time, and intelligibility of speaking. Speech rate can be the primary therapeutic focus as in fluency disorders like stuttering, or the tempo of speech can take on a mediating role for articulatory precision and thus speech intelligibility. In RSC the patient speaks to an auditory stimulation. This is presented as a metronome pulsed signal, a rhythmic pattern (played live with an instrument or synthesizer), or in the form of a more complex musical piece. Tempo is the most important factor for the therapeutic power of the technique. It has to be set precisely according to available research data and the specific therapeutic goal.

There are two modes of acoustically cueing speech production, namely metric and patterned cueing. In metric cueing a pulsed auditory stimulation is used (usually produced by a metronome). The patient is asked to match either one syllable or one full word to one beat. In patterned cueing the patient reproduces a pre-structured rhythmic sentence at a given tempo (e.g. as a rhyme or as in singing a song). In contrast to metric cueing, the syllables (and pauses) here are not of equal duration. There can be longer and shorter syllables, as in the song *Oh When the Saints go Marching in*.

13.2 Target populations

The main clinical indication for RSC is dysarthria. This is a neurological motor speech impairment characterized by slow or hastened, weak, uncoordinated movements of the articulatory muscles. It results in reduced speech intelligibility and leads to communicative difficulties. Social isolation and depression can develop as a consequence. RSC has been shown to be effective for patients with Parkinson's disease, in which dysarthria is a very common feature. Speaking in patients with Parkinson's disease often becomes soft (hypophonia), with monotone prosody, harsh voice, and a disturbed articulation. In patients with left-sided symptom dominance an additional tendency toward speech hastening can be observed (Flasskamp et al., 2012; Hammen et al., 1994; Yorkston et al., 1990). This phenomenon is also called *festination of speech*, and is associated with festination of gait (smaller shuffling and accelerating steps) (Moreau et al., 2007) (see Figure 13.1). The festination of speech in Parkinson's disease can be worsened by deep brain stimulation

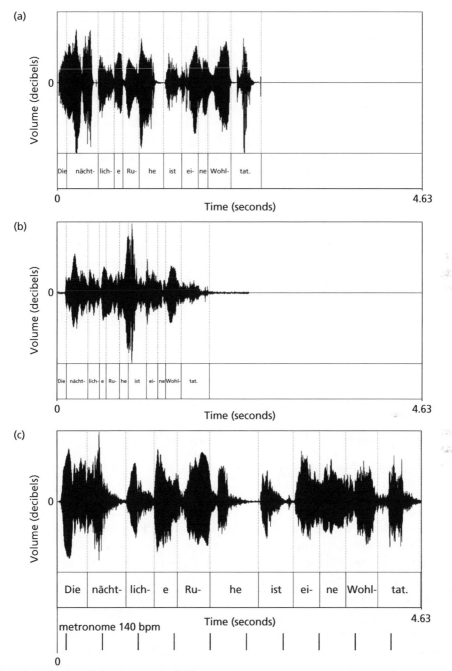

Figure 13.1 Temporal distribution of syllables in reading speech, comparing (a) normal speech in a healthy 74-year-old woman, (b) dysarthric speech in a 69-year-old woman with Parkinson's disease, and (c) dysarthric speech under the influence of rhythmic stimulation in the same patient as in (b). Please also listen to 🎵 Audio Samples 13.1, 13.2, and 13.3.

(Tripoliti et al., 2011). It is noteworthy that the patients themselves are frequently unaware of their acceleration in speech rate and their slurred unclear speech. This lack of awareness is so profound that the neuropsychologist George Prigatano classified it as anosognosia (Prigatano et al., 2010).

The combination of hypokinetic dysarthria, speech hastening, and unawareness, and thus inability to correct or compensate for the speech problems, often leads to extremely poor levels of intelligibility in this patient group (compare normal speech and Parkinsonian dysarthric speaking in ◑ Audio Samples 13.1 and 13.2). This can be effectively treated with RSC, which spontaneously leads to much slower and more intelligible speech (Hammen et al., 1994; Thaut et al., 2001; see Figure 13.1 and listen to ◑ Audio Sample 13.3). When festination of speech is absent or subsidiary, the dysarthria in Parkinson's disease would be better treated with vocal intonation therapy (VIT) (see Chapter 15).

Other forms and etiologies of dysarthria can also be considered for RSC, namely ataxic and spastic dysarthria or mixed dysarthria (for clinical descriptions, see Duffy, 2005). These can occur after traumatic brain injuries and degenerative neurological diseases. Even though speech rate is often already reduced in these dysarthrias, speech rate control techniques work best in slowing down these patients (Pilon et al., 1998; van Nuffelen et al., 2010; Yorkston et al., 1990).

A third indication for RSC is in people with stuttering. Stuttering often occurs as a problem of disturbed fluency where articulation is mostly undisturbed. It has been shown that singing can overcome disfluency in people with stuttering (Glover et al., 1996). Just as effective as other rate control techniques is metric cueing (Ingham et al., 2009, 2012).

Finally, there is evidence from one randomized controlled trial for a solid therapeutic effect on apraxia of speech (AOS) (Brendel and Ziegler, 2008).

13.3 **Research summary**

There is class III evidence for severe dysarthria in Parkinson's disease. Michael Thaut and colleagues conducted an experimental trial with 20 patients with Parkinson's disease who had severe to mild forms of dysarthria. They found a significant improvement among initially poorly intelligible participants (with intelligibility of less than 60%).

Cueing was most efficient at 60% of the habitual speaking rate. The best cueing modus was one syllable per beat (listen to ◑ Audio Sample 13.4). Furthermore, the study results indicated that in patients with Parkinson's disease who had mild to moderate dysarthric symptoms, RSC seemed to give a limited benefit (Thaut et al., 2001).

Several studies on different rate control techniques have demonstrated that slowing down is effective for various types of dysarthria (ataxic, spastic, and mixed type), despite the fact that nearly all of these forms exhibit a reduced speech rate. Furthermore, it has been shown that mildly to moderately impaired speakers do not benefit from a rate control technique (Hammen et al., 1994; Pilon et al., 1998; van Nuffelen et al., 2010; Yorkston et al., 1990). So far there are only limited data available comparing RSC and other types of rate control techniques.

Pilon and colleagues conducted a study of three traumatic brain injury patients with mixed dysarthria. They compared RSC (metric cueing word by word at the reduced pacing rate of 80%) with singing at an equally reduced pace and the pacing board (a small board with five marked sections for the patient to tap with each word). In this small study, RSC caused the largest improvements in intelligibility.

Although the advantages and disadvantages of RSC in the treatment of ataxic, spastic, and mixed dysarthria remain unclear, it should be considered an effective therapeutic option in this patient group.

For people with stuttering it has been shown that RSC is as effective as other fluency-inducing techniques in the form of metric cueing (one syllable per beat) to improve fluency. Cueing rate was set at the self-chosen tempo in the range of 90–180 bpm (Ingham et al., 2009, 2012). These stimulation frequencies most probably led to a slowing down in speech rate. Normal speech rates in reading are in the range of 200–360 syllables per minute (Breitbach-Snowdon, 2003).

Singing is also effective for people with stuttering. Glover et al. (1996) demonstrated a reduction in dysfluency after the instruction to sing. However, those authors point out that there was no confirmation that the participants were actually singing. Clearly, though, the instruction to sing had an impact on speaking behavior. This worked equally well when comparing a normal rate with a fast rate. Thus for singing it might not be essential to slow down the tempo when practicing with people with stuttering.

Brendel and Ziegler (2008) were able to show a significant effect on AOS. In a randomized controlled trial, 10 post-stroke patients with mild to severe AOS trained in a cross-over design with RSC. The control intervention consisted of various established AOS techniques. RSC was performed as metrical cueing with stimulation rates ranging from 60 to 240 syllables per minute. The RSC tempo was set according to the patients' speaking capacity, and started at a very low value and was eventually speeded up, if the progress of the patient allowed this. The metrical pacing showed superior improvements in speech rate, fluency, and segmental accuracy (Brendel and Ziegler, 2008).

13.4 **Therapeutic mechanisms**

When considering the therapeutic mechanisms for RSC, a distinction should be made between the treatment of dysarthria and dysfluency. In dysarthria, slowing down is clearly the main impact in terms of functional gains in intelligibility. In Parkinson's disease, RSC seems to compensate for the lack of ability to precisely perceive and regulate the speaking pace. The rhythmic stimulus serves as a stable time anchor to which the patient can adjust. Secondly, as speaking is a very complex sensorimotor function of numerous muscles, the rhythmic structure facilitates better coordination of the articulatory muscles. In that sense the speech motor function shows the same sensitivity to rhythmic entrainment as can be seen in gross or fine motor functions. In other words, acoustic rhythm seems to facilitate a better motor programming in the process of speaking. This certainly holds for all forms of dysarthria in which muscle functions are impaired.

There are several hypotheses as to why slowing down in particular is so effective for dysarthria. Apart from the sharpness of articulation due to optimized speech motor performance, it could also be that there is more time for listeners to analyze the somewhat unclear speech.

In patients with dysfluency, especially in stuttering and AOS, RSC might lead to an optimal coordination of breath and voice, due to the temporal regulation of the speech act. Furthermore, the acoustic rhythmic stimulation (even in a purely mental condition and in uncued singing) seems to stabilize the fluency of speaking.

13.5 **Therapy procedure**

13.5.1 **Start with diagnosis and assessment**

Before starting the training it is essential to define the speech pathology. Measuring the extent of dysarthria or dysfluency is a complicated matter. Several assessments are available, such as the Frenchay Dysarthria Assessment (Enderby, 1983), the UNS (Breitbach-Snowdon, 2003), and the Munich Intelligibility Profile (MVP) (Ziegler and Zierdt, 2008). However, the majority of clinicians use a descriptive form and estimate the severity of the symptom.

It is also important to look at the etiology and thus at the process and the perspective of the clinical symptom.

Then the therapist should take into account the views of the patient. How do they experience their speech pathology? Do they want to improve their speech? That is, having assessed the objective needs for therapy we need to look at the subjective aspects and also the personal communicative resources (i.e. the social environment) of the patient. When starting exercise therapy, the therapist needs to ensure that the patient is willing and able to participate in this treatment, as it is crucial to establish a high degree of compliance with the treatment. For this purpose it can be effective to record the speech of the patient and to play it back to them. This gives the patient an opportunity to perceive their own speaking more objectively.

When the symptoms have been thoroughly assessed, the therapeutic goal can be decided according to the clinical symptom.

Clinical example

A 67-year-old man has been suffering from Parkinson's disease for 12 years with left-sided dominant motor symptoms. He notices that his wife and close relatives often do not understand him straight away, so that they have to ask him to repeat what he has said. His voice is a little monotonous, and his speech rate is considerably increased, with slurred unclear articulation. When confronted with a recording of his own speech he is startled by how fast and unclear it is. After this experience he is willing to try out speech training with RSC in order to slow down his speaking to improve its intelligibility. (A similar problem of reduced intelligibility due to Parkinsonian dysarthria was experienced by the woman in 🔊 Audio Sample 13.2.)

When assessing speech problems, three questions need to be addressed.

1 *Is it a form of altered speech due to a neurologic disease?* Although there is an abnormal speaking rate or fluency, it is possible that this is the unaltered natural manner of speech of this person.

2 *Does the altered speech pattern cause any objective or subjective problem for the patient?* Does the patient want to change their way of speaking or are they experiencing communication problems (even though they might not relate these to their way of speaking)?

3 *Does the prognosis of the symptom justify initiating therapy?* In terms of etiology and assessment, how would we expect the phenomenon to develop? Is it expected to become worse, will it merely stay the same, or is it intermittent and therefore likely to resolve without any treatment?

If all three questions can be answered in the affirmative, the patient should be referred for therapy.

13.5.2 **Define the goal**

Once the speech pathology has been thoroughly described, the goal has to be determined. We know from research data that RSC can be used merely to improve intelligibility, sharpness of articulation, and speech fluency. So in this step, according to the findings of the assessment, we define a clear and realistic aim. This step must involve the patient, as we want to adjust the aim to their needs and wishes.

13.5.3 **Assess the natural speech rate and/or fluency**

Having defined the therapeutic goal we need to look at the actual temporal characteristics of the patient's speech. The only reliable way to assess a person's habitual speech rate is to record their free and consecutive speaking for 1 minute and then count the syllables while listening to the recording. However, in most cases this procedure is unsuitable for clinical practice. It is quite difficult to get a patient to speak freely and without pauses for 1 minute. Of course it is possible to assess speech rate by giving the patient a reading task. However, reading is from a functional perspective quite different to free speaking. There is no intention during the act of reading, but instead there is a visual stimulus that can influence speech rate to a large extent, whereas it is the rate of free speaking that has to be addressed by RSC, and it is this that needs to be assessed. The same is true for fluency, so both the rate and fluency of free speaking should be thoroughly observed and described. Eventually a recording could be made to support and provide a record of this observation (and subsequently monitor compliance.)

13.5.4 **Decide whether RSC is an effective means of achieving the therapeutic goal**

During the first two RSC sessions it should be ascertained whether RSC can be effectively applied to treat the speech pathology. Here again it is essential to take into consideration the clinical goal. If the goal was to improve fluency in a person with stuttering in order to achieve a more normalized speech pattern, the impact of RSC on this will need to be tested. This would involve assessing the influence of rhythmic stimulation on the fluency of this patient. In the case of the Parkinsonian patient in ♩ Audio Sample 13.2, it would be necessary to improve the articulation and intelligibility of their speech. We can find out whether this could be achieved by testing the patient's speaking under RSC conditions (listen to ♩ Audio Sample 13.3).

First, however, we need to test the patient's rhythmic entrainment ability. Here the patient should be asked to follow a comfortably paced beat with the hand. This could be done with the metronome set to 100 bpm. If audio–motor entrainment is markedly impaired, RSC will not be effective and therefore would not be tried out. In the next step the tempo and mode of stimulation need to be defined. Here the therapist should rely on research data. In a person with stuttering we would first try out metric cueing with one syllable per beat. The stimulation frequency should be set at a comfortable pace, but slower than the patient's natural speaking rate. During the first session it is usually easier to start with a reading task, such as a rhyme or poem. However, we also want to find out whether free speaking changes under the influence of RSC. The easiest way to do this is to ask the patient simple questions that can be answered without having to think about them. (It is helpful to explain to the patient that we are only looking at their manner of speaking, not the content of their speech.) If the speech does not change sufficiently, the mode and /or tempo of stimulation should be adjusted.

The simplest mode of stimulation is *metric cueing*, in which each syllable is matched to one beat from the metronome. The following is an example of metric cueing (listen to ♩ Audio Sample 13.4 to find out how this sounds):

To–day   I   want to go shop – ping in the ci – ty. Listen to the audio sample.
•   •   •   •   •   •   •   •   • • •   •   → spoken rhythm
′   ′   ′   ′   ′ ′   ′   ′   ′ ′ ′   ′   → rhythmic stimulation (beat = 0)

In *patterned cueing*, syllables of longer and shorter duration are rhythmically displaced according to the rhythmic pattern of normal speech. The following is an example of patterned cueing (quarter and eighth) (listen to ♩ Audio Sample 13.5):

To–day   I   want to go shop –ping in the ci –ty.
•   ○   ○   •   • ○   ○   ○   • • ○   ○   → spoken rhythm
    ′   ′   ′   ′ ′   ′   ′   ′ ′ ′   ′   → rhythmic stimulation (beat = 0)

The following is an example of patterned cueing (triplets) (listen to ♩ Audio Sample 13.6):

To –day   I   want to go shop –ping in the ci –ty.
•   ○   •   •   • •   ○   •   ○   • • • → spoken rhythm
/   ′   / ′   / ′   / ′   / ′   /   → rhythmic stimulation (beat = ′ / or 3)
    3   3   3   3   3

Although the speech pattern can display a complex rhythm, the rhythmic structure of the stimulus will stay the same to allow rhythmic (motor) entrainment.

After finding the optimal mode of stimulation, the cueing frequency or tempo of stimulation should be adjusted to identify the optimal stimulation rate.

The key question remains whether free speaking can be effectively altered according to the therapeutic goal (see Figure 13.1). Only when this has been established beyond doubt and the stimulation frequency has been defined can we start systematic RSC training. If there is no significant therapeutic change in speaking, an alternative rate control technique should be applied (e.g. pacing board, alphabet board, delayed auditory feedback).

13.6 **Five-step training scheme**

A systematic training scheme is recommended. This is derived from an evidence-based hierarchical training scheme, and it builds up from cued reading to free speaking in every session (Ramig et al., 2001).

13.6.1 **Preliminary practice: tapping to rhythmic stimulation**

The patient taps with their better hand to rhythmic stimulation. Here rhythmic entrainment is initiated. The patient can experience the effect of rhythm on their movement. As always in auditory–motor coupling, it is important not to synchronize every tap to every beat, but rather to let the movement become entrained to the given tempo. This should be already set to the RSC training frequency. This training step can be omitted if initiation of rhythmic entrainment is not an issue.

13.6.2 **Read pre-structured material to rhythmic cueing**

The patient is asked to read in the defined tempo and mode text material that is optimally structured for their speaking ability. Accordingly, a poem, rhyme, or song text could be used in which the phrases are fairly short and easy to reproduce with RSC. If appropriate, the patient can maintain tapping with the stimulation.

13.6.3 **Read routine phrases to rhythmic cueing**

At this stage the patient is still reading, but is now practicing phrases and sentences that occur as part of their normal daily routine. The lists used here can be individually designed for the patient's needs. If appropriate, the patient can maintain tapping with the stimulation.

13.6.4 **Speak freely to rhythmic cueing**

The patient should speak freely to rhythmic stimulation. This usually works best when the therapist is asking very simple questions (e.g. "What time did you get up this morning?", "What is the weather like today?", "What did you have for breakfast?"). If possible the patient can also give a monologue on a chosen topic. Another option is to read out headlines from a newspaper and ask the patient to comment on them. For the majority of patients this is the most important step in RSC training. Therefore it should be given more time than the other training steps in the session.

13.6.5 **Transfer of the functional change**

The patient is asked to speak freely without rhythmic stimulation, but maintaining the improved quality of speaking according to the therapeutic goal. The therapist should also suggest some transfer exercises to be carried out after therapy (e.g. the patient could be instructed to go to the nurse and ask for a cup of tea while maintaining the good speech quality).

13.7 **General tips and tricks**

1 Usually a metronome is used for RSC, as it allows accurate control of the tempo. The metronome should have a pleasant and loud sound. The loudness is important because the therapist also wants the patient to speak loudly (in most cases), so the stimulation should be clearly audible throughout. A mechanical metronome is also acceptable. In general, "seeing the beat" is an advantage, due to sensory integration. However, sound and loudness are more important and should be given priority.

2 In the patterned cueing mode the overall speaking rate will be higher than in metric cueing, due to the number of short syllables. Therefore the tempo of stimulation needs to be slower than in the metric cueing mode.

3 For the patterned cueing mode the idea of *sing-song* can be helpful. Usually when people are asked to do sing-song by themselves they achieve some kind of steady rhythmic pattern, such as ′/ ′ / or ′// ′ //. Often this steady pattern is carried out with a fixed prosodic interval (usually a fourth or a third). Through the idea of sing-song the patient can be enabled to engage in free speaking with a steady patterned cueing.

4 If hand tapping is continued during Steps 2 and 3, note that this should be done rather silently. The sound of tapping should not confound the rhythmic stimulus.

5 Look at the patient's capacity to do self-training. Only for Steps 4 and 5 might a training partner be needed. Ideally the training partner should be introduced to the RSC procedure by the therapist.

6 If no partner is available for self-training, the patient can read out the headlines from a newspaper and then freely comment on them.

13.8 **Therapeutic application in patients with Parkinson's disease**

It has already been mentioned that for patients with Parkinson's disease we mainly use RSC to improve intelligibility. For this, Parkinsonian patients need to be slowed down to at least 60% of their habitual speech tempo. Due to their impaired self-perception (e.g. "My wife doesn't understand me anymore, but I don't really know why") it seems to be essential to exaggerate all aspects of speaking, so we practice extra slowly, even slower then we want the patient to speak in daily routine. Usually the loudness improves to a similar extent while practicing RSC. Furthermore, the training must be intense (Farley et al., 2008; Fisher et al., 2008); 5 days a week for at least 15 minutes is essential. This high training frequency can usually only be achieved through extra home training, so self-perception and compliance are of great importance. Frequent audio recordings can help the patient to work on these aspects. As Parkinson's disease is a degenerative disease, it is recommended that the patient has therapy holidays (of 1 to 2 months) between these ongoing intense training periods.

13.9 **Therapeutic application in patients with spastic, ataxic, or mixed dysarthria**

As mentioned earlier, RSC can be effective in spastic or ataxic dysarthria by slowing these patients down, even though their speech might be slowed already. In order to establish good compliance, the goal of treatment must be carefully explained to the patient, as there is a risk that they may feel that they are in fact getting worse because of the additional slowing of their speech. A training frequency of three to four sessions a week is recommended.

13.10 **Therapeutic application in patients with stuttering**

The mode and tempo of cueing are not clearly indicated by research data, so it is worth trying out several frequencies (even up to the patient's habitual speech rate, which might be around 240 syllables per minute). The training mode should be one syllable per beat initially (metric cueing), but might be altered to one word per beat to achieve the optimal effect on fluency.

References

Breitbach-Snowdon, H. (2003). *UNS: Untersuchung Neurologisch bedingtes Sprech- und Stimmstörungen.* Köln: ProLog.

Brendel B and Ziegler W (2008). Effectiveness of metrical pacing in the treatment of apraxia of speech. *Aphasiology, 22*, 77–102.

Duffy, J. R. (2005). *Motor Speech Disorders: substrates, differential diagnosis, and management*, 2nd edition. St Louis, MO: Elsevier Mosby.

Enderby, P. (1983). *Frenchay Dysarthria Assessment.* Austin, TX: Pro-Ed.

Farley B G, Fox C M, Ramig L O, and McFarland D H (2008). Intensive amplitude-specific therapeutic approaches for Parkinson's disease: towards a neuroplasticity-principled rehabilitation model. *Topics in Geriatric Rehabilitation, 24*, 99–114.

Fisher, B. E. et al. (2008). The effect of exercise training in improving motor performance and corticomotor excitability in people with early Parkinson's disease. *Archives of Physical Medicine and Rehabilitation, 89*, 1221–9.

Flasskamp A, Kotz S A, Schlegel U, and Skodda S (2012). Acceleration of syllable repetition in Parkinson's disease is more prominent in the left-side dominant patients. *Parkinsonism & Related Disorders, 18*, 343–7.

Glover H, Kalinowski J, Rastatter M, and Stuart A (1996). Effect of instruction to sing on stuttering frequency at normal and fast rates. *Perceptual and Motor Skills, 83*, 511–22.

Hammen V L, Yorkston K M, and Minifie F D (1994). Effects of temporal alterations on speech intelligibility in parkinsonian dysarthria. *Journal of Speech and Hearing Research, 37*, 244–53.

Ingham R J et al. (2009). Measurement of speech effort during fluency-inducing conditions in adults who do and do not stutter. *Journal of Speech, Language, and Hearing Research, 52*, 1286–301.

Ingham R J et al. (2012). Phonation interval modification and speech performance quality during fluency-inducing conditions by adults who stutter. *Journal of Communication Disorders, 45*, 198–211.

Moreau C et al. (2007). Oral festination in Parkinson's disease: biomedical analysis and correlation with festination and freezing of gait. *Movement Disorders, 22*, 1503–6.

Pilon M A, McIntosh K W, and Thaut M H (1998). Auditory vs visual speech timing cues as external rate control to enhance verbal intelligibility in mixed spastic-dysarthric speakers: a pilot study. *Brain Injury, 12*, 793–803.

Prigatano G P, Maier F, and Burns R S (2010). Anosognosia and Parkinson's disease. In: G P Prigatano (ed.). *The Study of Anosognosia*. Oxford: Oxford University Press. pp. 159–69.

Ramig L O, Sapir S, Fox C, and Countryman S (2001). Changes in vocal loudness following intensive voice treatment (LSVT) in individuals with Parkinson's disease: a comparison with untreated patients and normal age-matched controls. *Movement Disorders, 16*, 79–83.

Thaut M H, McIntosh K W, McIntosh G C, and Hoemberg V (2001). Auditory rhythmicity enhances movement and speech motor control in patients with Parkinson's disease. *Functional Neurology, 16*, 163–72.

Tripoliti E et al. (2011). Effects of subthalamic stimulation on speech of consecutive patients with Parkinson disease. *Neurology, 76*, 80–86.

Van Nuffelen G et al. (2010). Effect of rate control on speech production and intelligibility in dysarthria. *Folia Phoniatrica et Logopaedica, 62*, 110–19.

Yorkston K M, Hammen V L, Beukelman D R, and Traynor C D (1990). The effect of rate control on the intelligibility and naturalness of dysarthric speech. *Journal of Speech and Hearing Disorders, 55*, 550–60.

Ziegler W and Zierdt A (2008). Telediagnostic assessment of intelligibility in dysarthria: a pilot investigation of MVP-online. *Journal of Communication Disorders, 41*, 553–77.

Chapter 14

Oral Motor and Respiratory Exercises (OMREX)

Kathrin Mertel

14.1 Definition

OMREX is a technique for addressing the improvement of articulatory control, respiratory strength, and function of the speech apparatus. Musical materials and exercises, mainly through sound vocalization and wind instrument playing, are applied to enhance articulatory control and respiratory strength and function of the speech apparatus.

14.2 Target populations

Speech disturbances occur in different forms and can stem from neural impairment, delays or problems with sensory faculties (visual or hearing impairment), problems with motor faculties that affect speech production, or more general developmental problems.

Impairments in communication are very common following various types of neurological damage, including the following.

- *Traumatic brain injury (TBI)* is a major cause of death and lifelong disability that presents with a broad spectrum of severity. Head injuries can cause widespread damage to the brain, which may result in many complex physical, linguistic, cognitive, social, and behavioral changes for the individual.

- *Strokes* are broadly classified as being ischemic or hemorrhagic. Ischemic strokes are caused by blockage within the arterial system of the brain, resulting in a lack of blood supply, which leads to tissue death. This is the most common type of stroke, thought to account for around 80% of strokes. Hemorrhagic strokes result from the rupture of a blood vessel within the brain, which leads to local tissue destruction, and they account for around 20% of strokes. Strokes are typically followed by persistent impairments of movement (paresis or frank paralysis) and/or of speech and cognitive abilities, depending on the specific anatomical site of the insult.

Dysarthria refers to a group of motor speech impairments that result from damage to the neurological areas that control the muscles used for speech. Due to the underlying damage, muscles of the tongue, lips, and face do not respond in the normal way, and speech often becomes quiet, slurred, or unintelligible. These muscular deficits can affect the range, timing, speed, and steadiness of oral movement coordination (Abbs and DePaul, 1989, cited in Tamplin, 2008).

In a systematic Cochrane review, Sellars et al. (2002) estimated the prevalence of dysarthria following stroke to be 20–30%, and the prevalence of dysarthria following TBI to be 10–60%. The characteristics of dysarthria include limited verbal intelligibility, decreased vocal intensity and range, abnormal rate of speech, and poor prosody. Patients with dysarthria tend to speak slowly, with slurred speech, and often in a monotonous, nasal voice. The overall flow and phrasing of speech may be affected due to difficulties in coordinating breathing and speaking.

Symptoms of dysarthria are also prominent in patients with Parkinson's disease or Huntington's disease:

- Huntington's disease is a relatively rare hereditary neurological disorder with an onset usually between 35 and 45 years of age. The characteristic symptom of this disease is chorea, or involuntary jerking movements that involve the entire body and interfere severely with normal activities of daily life. Swallowing and speech are frequently affected later in the course of the disease.

- Parkinson's disease is a more common neurodegenerative disease with a higher prevalence in the older age groups, and an average age of onset of 60 years. The most common initial symptom is a tremor, usually in one hand, that is worse at rest and improves slightly with intention. As the disease progresses, debilitating problems such as poverty of movement (difficulty with initiating and maintaining steady movements) begin to occur. Speech is also eventually affected, with individuals displaying varying degrees of slurring, poor articulation, or inappropriate acceleration of speech.

Both Parkinson's disease and Huntington's disease involve different parts of the basal ganglia, an area deep within the brain that plays a critical role in controlling movements, especially in initiating, maintaining, and sequencing movement patterns.

Neurological impairments such as thvose mentioned earlier can also result in *dyspraxia*— that is, a disturbance in the ability to sequence spoken language. In dyspraxia the brain is unable to coordinate complex motor actions (such as speech) despite normal muscle strength and sensation. Treatment of dyspraxic symptoms includes encouraging automatic or reflex-like speech, as well as direct work on articulation and sequencing of sound.

Symptoms of dysarthria and dyspraxia can also be seen in patients with *brain tumors*. Tumors may compress critical areas of the brain, alter blood flow and prevent sufficient oxygen delivery, or directly damage cerebral areas involved in speech.

Developmental disorders, as well as delays in or problems with sensory faculties such as *hearing impairment*, may contribute to speech and language delay.

14.2.1 Other disorders that affect speech motor and respiratory function

14.2.1.1 Muscular dystrophy

This is a progressive muscular degeneration that can be genetically linked or sporadic, and is characterized by a wasting of muscle cells and their replacement by fat and fibrous tissue.

Early signs of the disease include awkward and clumsy movements, poor posture, and tiptoeing. Muscle weakness almost always develops in a proximal-to-distal fashion, with the trunk and muscles of the upper legs and arms being affected first. Late in the course of the disease the hands, neck, and face can be affected. Nine major types of muscular dystrophy have been described, the most common type being X-linked Duchenne muscular dystrophy (DMD). Onset is typically between the ages of 3 and 5 years, although rarely symptoms may appear as late as 10 or 11 years of age. Most patients with DMD exhibit lower than average IQ, but retain normal behavioral, bowel, and sexual function. Around a third of patients who are severely affected may have behavioral, visual, speech, and more severe cognitive impairment as well. The disease is progressive, and eventually the heart and breathing muscles are affected. This makes the patient vulnerable to overwhelming lung infection and cardiac failure, and death usually occurs by 30 years of age.

14.2.1.2 Down syndrome

This is the most common chromosomal disorder and cause of mental retardation. There are multiple ways in which Down syndrome can develop, but around 95% of cases are known as trisomy 21, in which the condition results from the presence of all or part of an extra copy of chromosome 21. Down syndrome is associated with a substantial decrease in cognitive ability as well as with a particular set of facial characteristics, and associations with heart defects, leukemia, and early-onset Alzheimer's disease. Among affected individuals, language and communication skills tend to vary widely. Individuals with Down syndrome typically have an oversized tongue, leading to difficulty with speech articulation and pronunciation. A high incidence of mild hearing loss that is difficult to detect can contribute to delayed language skills. Individualized speech therapy is suggested to target specific speech errors, increase speech intelligibility, and in some cases encourage advanced language and literacy (Kirk et al., 2005).

14.2.1.3 Chronic obstructive pulmonary disease (COPD)

This is caused by chronic bronchitis (inflammation of the airways and a productive cough for 3 months over a period of two consecutive years), emphysema (terminal airway destruction, discussed later in this chapter), or most often a combination of both diseases. This combination results in a not entirely reversible airflow limitation that is continuous and progressive. The symptoms of COPD are productive cough, worsening dyspnea, and exercise intolerance. As the disease worsens, the patient experiences severe impairment in activities of daily living, due to progressive dyspnea, fatigue, and depression. Although medical treatment exists, the only two interventions that have been shown to slow the course of the disease are smoking cessation and supplemental oxygen administration (Bonilha et al., 2009).

14.2.1.4 Emphysema

This is a pathological and permanent enlargement of the distal portions of the respiratory tree within the lung. This enlargement is accompanied by destruction of the alveolar walls. Emphysema causes two problems: it decreases the surface area available for air exchange and it compromises the structural integrity of the lung. Patients with emphysema lack sufficient functional lung tissue to support efficient gas exchange, and therefore suffer from a lack of oxygen and a build-up of carbon dioxide in their blood. The destruction of lung architecture results in airway narrowing and decreased elastic recoil of the lung, both of which hinder effective breathing. This combination of problems results in shortness of breath, wheezing, and a productive cough (from coexisting chronic bronchitis). Smoking is the main cause of emphysema, and prolonged exposure to air pollutants and enzyme deficiency are secondary and less common causes (Engen, 2005).

14.3 **Research**

The overall role of neurologic music therapy (NMT) in language and speech disorders is to help the patient to develop spontaneous and functional speech, as well as to improve speech comprehension. More specifically, NMT can facilitate an improvement in motor control and muscular coordination (both of which are essential for articulation), respiratory capacity, speech fluency, vocalization, and sequencing of speech sounds, as well as speech rate and intelligibility.

NMT includes several speech therapy techniques that use musical materials to remediate speech and respiratory deficiencies. Respiratory dysfunction can negatively affect speech quality by reducing both the volume of speech and the length of phonation. Respiration plays a fundamental role in producing vocalizations, whether they be sounds, speech, or singing. Singing in particular requires close control of one's breathing, as it involves strong diaphragm contractions for deep inspirations, followed by controlled contractions of the diaphragm and other expiratory muscles against partially closed vocal cords during expiration.

The positive effect of singing on respiratory control has been studied in patients suffering from chronic respiratory deficits. Engen (2005) evaluated patients with emphysema after they had participated in 12 singing classes over a 6-week period, and found a significant increase in their intensity of speech and duration of counting numbers. Furthermore, their breathing patterns changed from a pathological "clavicular" dominance to a normal "diaphragmatic" dominance after the intervention. These findings were replicated 4 years later by Bonilha et al. (2009) in a study of patients with COPD. The researchers assigned half of the participants to 24 singing classes that included respiratory and vocalization exercises specifically designed for COPD patients, and the other half to a control group that produced handicrafts. This study also found that singing was able to produce transitory changes in pressure–volume relationships of the respiratory system. Specifically, the participants showed an increase in inspiratory capacity and a decrease in expiratory reserve volume, and these changes became evident after only a short session of singing. Finally, the singing group also exhibited small improvements in maximal expiratory pressure compared with the control group. There is a need for additional studies designed to better define the potential role of singing or specific wind instrument playing as a new tool for pulmonary rehabilitation as well.

Not only pulmonary deficits, but also to an even greater extent neurological impairments affect speech production, respiratory capacity, and breathing coordination. Tamplin

(2008) conducted a pilot study to investigate the effect of vocal exercises on intelligibility and speech naturalness for people with dysarthria due to TBI or stroke. In individual music therapy sessions a wide range of musical exercises, involving oral motor and respiratory exercises (OMREX), was applied. Some of their results after 24 music therapy sessions showed enhanced use of respiratory capacity and support, which was expressed by fewer pauses in the post-treatment sentences. Due to improved respiratory capacity, the patients were also able to speak more words per phrase and showed more natural speech rhythms than before treatment.

As one can imagine, the act of producing the sounds required to speak full sentences requires nuanced oral motor control and coordination of the lips, tongue, and jaw, as well as control of voice dynamics. The characteristics of orofacial movements during speech are largely determined by the phonetic requirements of specific utterances. Oral movements also vary systematically with the prosodic aspects of speech, such as rate and intensity.

McClean and Tasko (2002) described the general orofacial muscle activity. Motor control processes involve controlling output from motor neurons which are either tonic (co-activation of agonist and antagonist muscles) or phasic (pulse-like reciprocal activation of antagonist muscles) in nature. Among others, McClean and Clay (1995) were able to measure this tonic and phasic activity of orofacial muscles by using electromyography. Speech prosody (rate and intensity) influences the acoustics of any given sentence, which leads to variance in the converging input of the motor neurons that innervate the orofacial muscles.

Impairments in the oral motor production aspects of speech can be caused by a multitude of different insults to many different brain areas. Within the last decade, a considerable body of research, spearheaded by Thaut and colleagues, has supported the notion that rhythmic auditory stimulation (RAS) facilitates priming and timing of the motor system (McIntosh et al., 1996; Thaut et al., 1991, 1992, 1994, 1995, 1996). Since this is possible, it may be suggested—and indeed has already been documented by Thaut et al. (2001)—that RAS can also be used to stimulate the speech motor system to help to organize oral motor behavior and prime the motor neurons that innervate the orofacial muscles.

The pilot study by Tamplin (2008) mentioned earlier also supports the positive effect of a strong rhythmic beat on oral motor performance which resulted in improved speech intelligibility in dysarthric patients. Tamplin also documented a carryover effect that led to an increase in functional communication by some of the participants following the music therapy intervention.

Currently there is little evidence-based research on effective, appropriate, or specific clinical treatment techniques for improving the quality of speech production. Even for high-prevalence speech pathology, such as dysarthrias, most research has been focused on the classification of different types of dysarthria by reference to their neuroanatomic location as well as in relation to the assessment and classification of dysarthria severity.

It should be emphasized that any generalization of the results from most of the studies that have been described here should be approached with caution. The majority of the data were obtained either for a limited number of participants or in the absence of a control group. Further research into the effect of specific musical oral motor and respiratory applications will require studies with a larger number of participants, investigations within different clinical populations, and studies that replicate key findings. All of this will be necessary in order to clearly articulate the relationship between rhythmic entrainment and oral motor control and the effect of singing and wind instruments on respiration. A comprehensive summary of the therapeutic effects of singing in patients with neurologic disorders has been provided by Wan et al. (2010).

14.4 **Therapeutic mechanisms**

Both speech and singing involve the use of muscles of respiration and articulation, and contain elements of rhythm, pitch, dynamics, tempo, and diction. It is not surprising, then, that speech and singing share many of the same neural mechanisms, which can influence each other in a therapeutic process.

With its intrinsically motivating and encouraging character, music often facilitates the creation of voluntary sound production. Van der Merwe (1997) states that musical exercises in which speech movement patterns are mimicked or practiced are more likely to cause the neural adaptation necessary to improve speech precision than are simple resistance exercises focused on building oral muscle strength.

The use of songs in therapy can help to improve speech pathologies resulting from a wide range of neurological impairments, and songs are easily adapted to the appropriate developmental age of the patient. While using songs during therapy, the patient—regardless of age—will experience the use of words, vocabulary, speech melody, and other fundamental characteristics of language in an enjoyable way. Utilizing songs in therapy can also enhance concentration skills and memory performance.

While singing, a clear rhythmic cue is provided from the song that helps to stimulate and organize motor function of the oral muscles. This rhythmic cue is especially strong while singing single syllables or sounds, and supplies an organized and highly repetitive frame through the song presentation. In singing, the word production rate is slower than in spoken language, and rhythmic and melodic speech inflections are more pronounced. Both factors help to exercise oral motor control more efficiently. The neurologic music therapist is able to use and adapt the musical exercises with regard to principles of motor learning. Special singing exercises can be used that support and shape oral fine motor skills in order to enhance coordination of the lips, tongue, and movements of the jaw. Such improvements can result in better articulation and intelligibility of dysarthric speech. Rhythm in singing not only acts as a timekeeper for motor control and execution, but also helps to organize breathing patterns and cue verbal output. Singing can have the added benefit of assisting the development of general respiratory function, which can improve the patient's ability to complete activities of daily living and enhance their quality of life.

Research by Bonilha et al. (2009) has shown that controlled breathing, as is utilized when singing or playing wind instruments, can rapidly promote transitory changes in pressure–volume relationships of the respiratory system. Longer contraction of abdominal muscles during expiration causes increased abdominal pressure, resulting in more forceful expulsion of air, and helps to improve the training and efficiency of these muscles for singing and speech. In order to generate extended musical sounds, singing and wind instrument playing demands a greater amount of respiratory work, mostly on the part of the expiratory muscles. Finally, professional singers often perform respiratory and vocal exercises in order to improve respiratory coordination. Exercises similar to these could be a practical and enjoyable way of training respiratory function in a therapeutic setting.

14.5 **Clinical protocols**

Singing and playing wind instruments serve to help to define the parameters of a desired oral movement as well as to improve pulmonary function. Patients receive auditory and kinesthetic feedback when they sing or play wind instruments. Therapeutic singing and breathing exercises on wind instruments may reduce excess muscle tension, increase respiratory capacity, and improve articulatory accuracy through their ability to train and strengthen the involved muscle groups.

The act of playing music serves as a highly motivating tool to encourage participation in rehabilitation therapy, and has a high rate of spontaneous transfer to real-world language production.

14.5.1 **Improving oral motor functions**

Well-controlled and precise oral movement is a necessity for the production of understandable speech. Although these movements are learned throughout childhood, those who develop dysarthria must in many ways relearn these movements and plan and execute them volitionally. Singing can be used in therapy for the training of oral motor skills, as well as for increasing awareness and functional use of the lips, tongue, jaws, and teeth (see Table 14.1).

Table 14.1 Oral motor exercises on vowel and consonant combinations

	Mouth position	**Sound**
Labiodental consonant	Upper lip and upper front teeth	W, F
Bilabial consonant	Upper and lower lips (closed)	B, P, M
Velar consonant	Back part of tongue, soft palate	G, K, CH, NG
Palatal consonant	Front part of tongue, hard palate	J, CH
Dental consonant	Tip of tongue, upper front teeth	S, T, D, N
Uvular consonant	Back part of tongue, palatine uvula	NG, R
Vowel	Jaw open	A
	Lips broadly open	E
	Lips open, back part of tongue	I
	Lips round	O, U

The foundational oral motor skills involved in speech production are appropriate muscle tone and strength, coordination of speech-related muscle groups, proper range of motion of the jaw and tongue, controlling the speed of syllable combination, and *dissociation*, which is the ability to move structures (such as the tongue and jaw) independently of each other.

14.5.2 Some suggestions for practicing oral motor functions

- Singing songs or melodies using only one vowel as lyrics to help to shape awareness of jaw, lip, or tongue position:
  - open jaw: singing "a"
  - lips rounded: singing "o"
  - lips closed: singing "m"
  - tip of tongue up: singing "l"
  - back of tongue up: singing "g."
- Singing songs or melodies using single syllables as lyrics to practice single movements of the jaw, lips, or tongue:
  - lifting up tip of tongue: singing "la" with constant open jaw
  - opening/closing lips and jaw: singing "ma", "ba"
  - lifting up back of tongue: singing "ga", "ki"
  - moving lower lip: singing "fe", "wi."
- Singing songs or melodies using syllable combinations as lyrics to practice movement combinations of the jaw, lips, and tongue:
  - lips and tip of tongue: singing "so-sa-se-sa"
  - tip of tongue and jaw: singing "ta-ti-ta-ti"
  - lips, tip of tongue, and jaw: singing "du-ba-du-ba"
  - lower lip and jaw: singing "fi-fa-fi-fa"
  - tip and back of tongue: singing "se-ge-le-ge."

These exercises should start at a tempo at which the patient is able to correctly pronounce the target sound or syllable, and can then be gradually accelerated.

It is worth noting that Bonilha et al. (2009) observed an increase in coughing leading to expectoration of larger amounts of sputum following vocal exercises in their patients with COPD. It is reasonable from this observation to suggest that singing (a type of vocal exercise) may also improve bronchial hygiene, and may have the potential to elicit the cough reflex and the mobilization of respiratory secretions toward the upper airways. This positive effect seen with COPD patients could be also beneficial for severely impaired patients of other types in early rehabilitation who are struggling with weak cough reflexes and mucous congestion.

Patients with quadriplegia may also benefit from the application of OMREX therapy. If their disabilities are severe enough, many of these patients must learn to operate a wheel-chair by using a device that responds to mouth movements. Some individuals have developed these oral skills to the point where they can successfully participate in the workforce in computer-based or administrative jobs. Obviously the ability to accomplish any of these tasks requires exceptionally well-developed oral motor skills. For patients like these who wish to develop such skills, using a mouth stick to play cymbals, triangles, or small hand drums arranged in a specific way (as in TIMP exercises) can be an appropriate way to begin this training.

14.5.3 Using OMREX with children

The application of OMREX in children with various impairments is similar to that in adults. Children with autism or hearing difficulties tend to show deficits in expressive and receptive communication skills. Music therapy can encourage expressive (singing, speaking) and receptive (listening, understanding signs and gestures) language.

Children suffering from developmental disorders, muscular dystrophy, and dysarthria often lack the ability to completely close their mouth, and may as a result exhibit profuse drooling (myofunctional disorder). Playing wind instruments such as the recorder or harmonica is an ideal method for encouraging the child to close their lips for more extended periods of time. Exercises directed at facilitating lip closure would also improve the child's ability to pronounce fundamental sounds such as "p" and "ma." The song *Old MacDonald Had a Farm,* with its frequent incorporation of idealized animal noises, provides an enjoyable and useful way for children to practice the basic sounds of speech. Nearly all children like to sing, and utilizing therapeutic singing encourages prolonged voicing and use of multiple tones. Singing songs with simple combinations of syllables in place of lyrics can help to improve articulatory control. In this way, children develop awareness of the mouth and speech articulators, and learn the movements that are needed to make speech sounds (rounding lips, tongue movements, etc.).

It is important to remember that the primary goal in articulation exercises is to improve intelligibility and develop sufficient sound distinction, rather than to correct voice quality.

Music therapy sessions using OMREX may be held in an individual setting or among small groups of patients who are working toward similar goals.

14.5.4 Improving respiratory control

OMREX provides a variety of possibilities for addressing the needs of patients who have pathologic or dysfunctional respiratory control. As described earlier, rhythm and music can be included in an exercise to help to set appropriate rates of breathing frequency and depth. This inclusion of rhythm then enhances the ability of the exercise to address breath strength and control. Respiratory strength can be improved by consciously inspiring and expiring following the cues of a presented rhythm. Wind instruments such as the recorder, harmonica, or melodica can be used for breathing exercises to improve vocal strength, exercise laryngeal function, increase respiratory capacity, and refine oral motor function.

Some examples of wind instruments that can be readily used for OMREX will now be briefly discussed.

The *recorder* can be used for:

◆ maintaining mouth closure

◆ practicing controlled breathing patterns (inhale/exhale)

◆ prolonged exhalation

◆ establishing the ability to blow (for children).

The *harmonica* can be used for:

◆ coordination of breathing patterns (inhale/exhale)

◆ strengthening closure of the mouth and lips

◆ supporting sucking ability (for children)

◆ prolonged inhalation and exhalation

◆ practicing and supporting diaphragmatic breathing.

The *melodica* (played through a mouth tube) can be used for:

◆ maintaining mouth closure

◆ strengthening the lips

◆ prolonged exhalation

◆ practicing and supporting diaphragmatic breathing.

The *kazoo* can be used for:

◆ strengthening the voice

◆ promoting use of the voice

◆ maintaining mouth closure

◆ strengthening the lips

◆ voice modulation.

14.5.5 Suggestions for practicing breathing patterns on wind instruments

14.5.5.1 Controlled conscious inhalation and exhalation (see Figure 14.1)

The patient listens to a melody played or sung by the therapist and, following the end of the short piece, receives a predefined cue, inspires deeply, and blows a continuous breath into the flute. This process can then be repeated multiple times.

14.5.5.2 **Sustaining sounds on wind instruments for prolonged exhalation (see Figure 14.2)**

For this exercise the patient can play the flute or the melodica to a simple musical line sung or played by the therapist. The length of the breath that the patient must exhale into the instrument can be modified at the discretion of the therapist, perhaps by instructing the patient to continue blowing for as long as the therapist is playing a single chord on the piano.

When a melodica is used, the patient can be instructed to exhale for as long as the melody is being played by the therapist. The point of such an exercise is to gradually increase

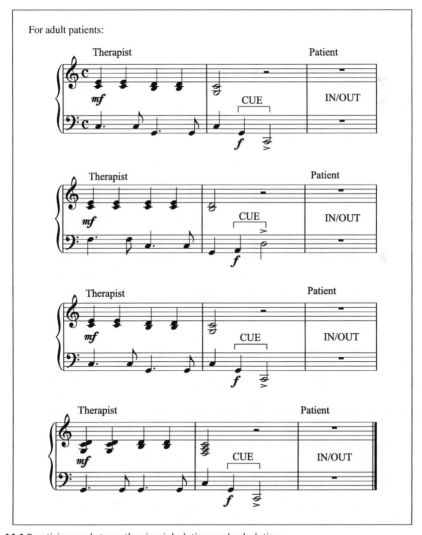

Fig. 14.1 Practicing and strengthening inhalation and exhalation.

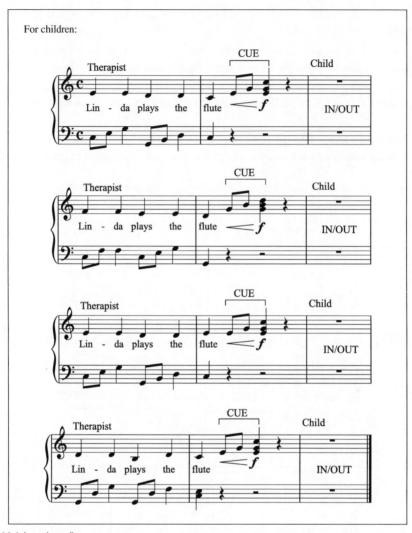

Fig. 14.1 (continued)

the length of time for which the patient is able to exhale under voluntary control, with the goal of allowing pronunciation of longer sentences or multisyllabic words.

14.5.5.3 Coordination of inhalation and exhalation

The harmonica is probably the ideal instrument for practicing coordinated inhalation and exhalation, as the patient is able to clearly hear the duration and strength of their attempts.

14.5.5.3.1 Single equal inhalation/exhalation (see Figure 14.3)

The patient listens to a melody played or sung by the therapist and, following the end of the melody, receives a predefined cue to inspire for the duration of 2 beats of tempo and then

Teach the patient to play three different pitches on the recorder, or use colored stickers to mark the keys of the melodica for this exercise:

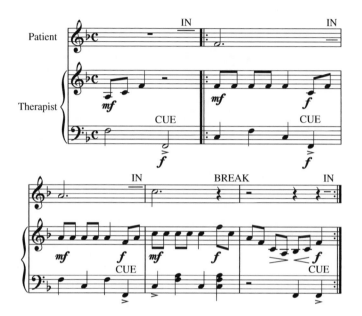

For longer exhaling gradually slow down the tempo of accompaniment.

For children:
This exercise can be easily turned into a fantasy game. Use a toy mouse and various drums or a xylophone. The story can be that the mouse goes for a walk and has to cross the street by jumping from one stone (drum, tone bar on the xylophone) to the next (drum, tone bar on the xylophone). While the mouse is jumping its way to the other side, the child has to play a sustained tone on the flute to support the mouse.

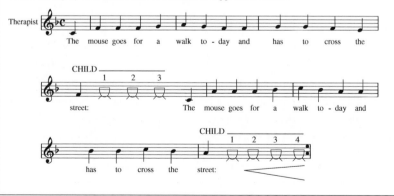

Fig. 14.2 Practicing longer exhalation.

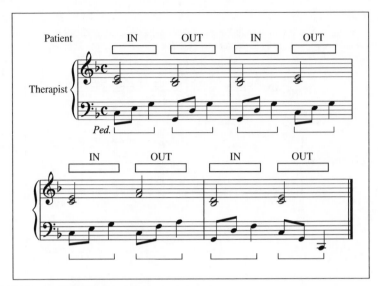

Fig. 14.3 Single equal inhalation/exhalation.

blow a continuous breath, also of 2 beats, into the harmonica. Again, this exercise can be modified in many ways to meet the individual needs of the patient.

14.5.5.3.2 **Breathing patterns (see Figure 14.4 and Table 14.2)**

The harmonica is ideally suited to aid the training of diaphragmatic breathing. The patient is instructed to inhale and exhale through the instrument in rhythmic patterns—an action that requires short and intense contractions of the diaphragm. By using this instrument, a rhythmic pattern (produced by the alternation of inhalation and exhalation) can be embedded within a broader musical structure.

The patient and the therapist can play together or alternately in the exercises described above.

1 *Playing together*: the patient (on the harmonica) and the therapist (on the piano) play one rhythmical pattern together (e.g. on the base of 2 beats breathing in and 2 beats breathing out) while the therapist plays a short melody in accompaniment.

2 *Alternate structure*: the patient is instructed to execute a certain breathing pattern (e.g. breathing in twice then breathing out twice), after which the therapist echoes the structure on the piano by playing two chords for breathing in and two chords for breathing out (structures like this can be easily modified for various breathing patterns).

14.5.5.3.3 **Coordination of nose and mouth breathing (see Figure 14.5 and Table 14.3)**

Obviously exercises for the coordination and training of breathing can also be applied to nose and mouth breathing. The difference is that for exercises like these, a flute or recorder is a better choice of instrument.

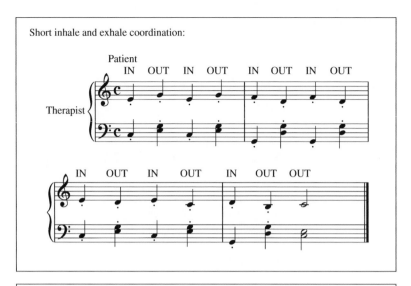

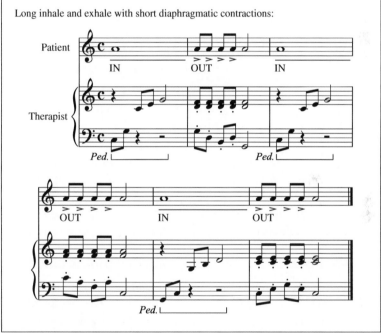

Fig. 14.4 Practicing breathing patterns.

Table 14.2 Practicing breathing patterns

Therapist plays the same chords for inhale and exhale on the piano:	Patient on harmonica (inhale and exhale through the mouth):
C – G – C – G	In – Out – In – Out
C C – G G	In – In Out – Out
C C C – G G G	In – In – In Out – Out – Out
C C__ – G G__	In In__ – Out Out__
C C C__ – G G G_	In In In__ – Out Out Out__

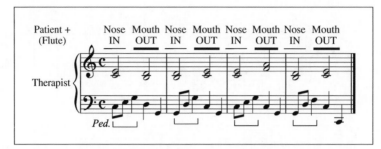

Fig. 14.5 Practicing coordination of nose and mouth breathing.

Table 14.3 Practicing coordination of nose and mouth breathing

Therapist plays the same chords for inhale and exhale on the piano:	Patient on instrument (inhales through the nose and exhales through the mouth):
C – G – C – G	In – Out – In – Out
C C – G G	In – In Out – Out
C C C – G G G	In – In – In Out – Out – Out
C C__ – G G__	In In__ – Out Out__
C C C__ – G G G__	In In In__ – Out Out Out__

All of the examples of exercises for breathing coordination or breathing patterns that have just been described can be applied here in the same way, except that breathing is directed through the nose.

Training in breathing patterns can be given in individual settings as well as in group settings, according to the patient's health circumstances or cognitive prerequisites.

14.5.6 **Combinations of breath control and oral motor functions**

In the exercises that have been mentioned so far, sound quality produced by the instrument was largely controlled by the force and rate of breathing, which is mainly dependent on diaphragmatic and abdominal muscle contraction. However, as those who play wind instruments already know, sound *articulation* is mainly achieved through tongue and lip movements. This allows rhythmic patterns to be played during a constant exhaled breath by interrupting the airstream using movements of the tongue. Playing a wind instrument in this way not only helps to shape and strengthen tongue movements, but also serves to train the many muscles responsible for lip movement, as these must close tightly around the instrument while playing a rhythmic melody (see Figures 14.6 and 14.7).

Therapeutic exercises that address breath control and oral motor function can be set up in a similar way to many of the exercises that have just been described.

The patient will receive immediate and continuous feedback about their breathing and oral motor abilities by learning how to play different rhythmic patterns at faster tempos, or repeating one pattern multiple times during one long breath.

Patient has to take a long breath in through the nose, and plays the rhythmic pattern through tongue movements while exhaling intothe recorder or melodica:

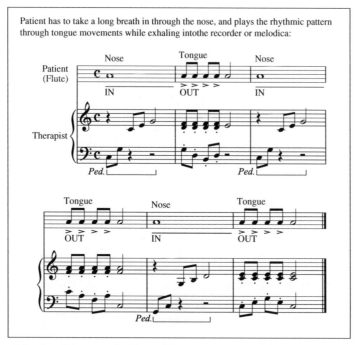

Fig. 14.6 Practicing breathing coordination and tongue movements: I.

In this exercise the patient practices short but deep inhaling through the nose and plays rhythmic patterns with the tongue. For this exercise, the tempo can be speeded up for faster tongue movements.

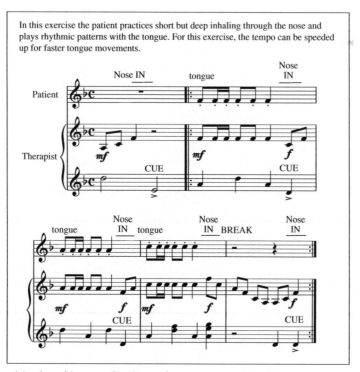

Fig. 14.7 Practicing breathing coordination and tongue movements: II.

References

Bonilha, A. G., Onofre, F., Prado, M. Y. A., and Baddini Martinez J. A. (2009). Effects of singing classes on pulmonary function and quality of life of COPD patients. *International Journal of Chronic Obstructive Pulmonary Disease*, 4, 1–8.

Engen, R. L. (2005). The singer's breath: implications for treatment of persons with emphysema. *Journal of Music Therapy*, 42, 20–48.

Kirk, S. A., Gallagher, J. J., Anastasiow, N. J., and Coleman, M. R. (2005). *Educating Exceptional Children*, 11th edition. Boston, MA: Houghton Mifflin.

McClean, M. D. and Clay, J. L. (1995). Activation of lip motor units with variations in speech rate and phonetic structure. *Journal of Speech and Hearing Research*, 38, 772–82

McClean, M. D. and Tasko, S. M. (2002). Association of orofacial with laryngeal and respiratory motor output during speech. *Experimental Brain Research*, 146, 481–9.

McIntosh, G. C., Thaut, M. H. and Rice, R. (1996). Rhythmic auditory stimulation as entrainment and therapy technique in gait of stroke and Parkinson's disease patients. In: R Pratt and R Spintge (eds) *MusicMedicine. Volume II.* St Louis, MO: MMB Music, Inc. pp. 145–52.

Sellars, C., Hughes, T., and Langhorne, P. (2002). Speech and language therapy for dysarthria due to nonprogressive brain damage: a systematic Cochrane review. *Clinical Rehabilitation*, 16, 61–8.

Tamplin, J. (2008). A pilot study into the effect of vocal exercises and singing on dysarthric speech. *NeuroRehabilitation*, 23, 207–16.

Thaut, M. H., Schleiffers, S., and Davis, W. B. (1991). Analysis of EMG activity in biceps and triceps in an upper extremity gross motor task under the influence of auditory rhythm. *Journal of Music Therapy*, 28, 64–88.

Thaut, M. H., McIntosh, G. C., Prassas, S. G., and Rice, R. R. (1992). Effect of rhythmic auditory cuing on temporal stride parameters and EMG. Patterns in hemiparetic gait of stroke patients. *Neurorehabilitation and Neural Repair*, 7, 9–16.

Thaut, M. H., Brown S., Benjamin, J., and Cooke, J. (1994). Rhythmic facilitation of movement sequencing: effects on spatio-temporal control and sensory modality dependence. In: R Pratt and R Spintge (eds) *MusicMedicine. Volume II.* St Louis, MO: MMB Music, Inc. pp. 104–9.

Thaut, M. H., Rathburn, J. A., and Miller R. A. (1995). Music versus metronome timekeeper in a rhythmic motor task. *International Journal of Arts Medicine*, 5, 4–12.

Thaut, M. H., McIntosh, G. C., and Rice R. R. (1996). Rhythmic auditory stimulation in gait training for Parkinson's disease patients. *Movement Disorders*, 11, 193–200.

Thaut, M. H., McIntosh, G. C., McIntosh, K. W., and Hömberg, V. (2001). Auditory rhythmicity enhances movement and speech motor control in patients with Parkinson's disease. *Functional Neurology*, 16, 163–72.

Van der Merwe, A. (1997). A theoretical framework for the characterization of pathological speech sensorimotor control. In: M R McNeil (ed.) *Clinical Management of Sensorimotor Speech Disorders.* New York: Thieme Medical Publishers, Inc. pp. 93–5.

Wan, C. Y., Rueber, T., Hohmann, A., and Schlaug, G. (2010). The therapeutic effect of singing in neurological disorders. *Music Perception*, 27, 287–95.

Chapter 15

Vocal Intonation Therapy (VIT)

Corene P. Thaut

15.1 Definition

Vocal intonation therapy (VIT) is the use of vocal exercises to train, maintain, develop, and rehabilitate aspects of voice control due to structural, neurological, physiological, psychological, or functional abnormalities of the voice apparatus. This includes aspects of vocal control such as inflection, pitch, breath control, timbre, and dynamics. Many exercises implemented in VIT are designed similarly to those exercises that a choir director would use to warm up and practice vocal control with a choir. Therapeutic application may also include relaxation exercises incorporating the head, neck, or upper trunk, and diaphragmatic breathing (Thaut, 2005).

15.2 Target populations

There are a wide range of reasons why a patient may present with an abnormality of vocal quality. Congenital disorders, such as a cleft palate, can lead to hypernasality. A motor vehicle accident may result in injuries to the vocal apparatus. The natural aging process can lead to loss of vocal fold elasticity, resulting in restricted pitch range and a hoarse or breathy tone quality. Neurologic impairments such as Parkinson's disease can lead to decreased loudness, breathy vocal quality, and short phonation time. Other neurologic impairments, including cerebral palsy and stroke, can result in a lack of the muscle control that is necessary for good breath support, which can affect several aspects of vocal control, such as pitch range, inflection, and intensity of vocal output. Physiological abnormalities, such as are seen in thyroid disease, can lead to voice changes such as reduced loudness and a decreased pitch range. Psychogenic voice disorders such as anxiety states and conversion reactions can also result in voice changes, such as a high-pitched voice. Functional voice disorders without any obvious anatomical or neurological difficulties are also common, and can present with symptoms such as a hoarse, husky, or rough voice, with a low and limited pitch range (http://www.sltinfo.com/voice-disorders.html, accessed 25 June 2013).

15.3 Research summary

Numerous studies have reported positive effects resulting from the use of vocal exercises and training in patient populations who commonly present with voice disorders, such as those with Parkinson's disease (DeStewart et al., 2003; Haneishi, 2001; Ramig et al., 1994;

Tautscher-Basnett et al., 2006), traumatic brain injury (Baker et al., 2005), multiple sclerosis (Wiens et al., 1999), hearing impairment (Bang, 1980; Darrow, 1986, 1991), and spinal cord injuries (Johansson et al., 2011; Tamplin et al., 2013).

In additional studies investigating the effects of singing in patients with neurologic disorders, Sabol et al. (1995) found that vocal function exercises improved coordination of laryngeal function and vocal fold vibration. Ramig et al. (2001) investigated the long-term effects of an intensive voice therapy program (Lee Silverman Voice Treatment, LSVT) and found positive improvements in vocal production parameters such as duration of sustained vowel phonation and fundamental frequency range, even 12 months after the termination of treatment. In addition, DeStewart et al. (2003) found that, when using LSVT, voicing in the low register helped to minimize strain on the laryngeal muscles. When investigating dysarthric speakers, Bellaire et al. (1986) suggested modifications of breath patterning to increase the naturalness of speech, while Tamplin (2008) suggested that a program of vocal exercises and singing might facilitate more normative speech production.

15.4 **Therapeutic mechanisms**

Due to the biological similarities between singing and speaking, as well as the shared and distinct neural networks, research examining the use of singing to treat speech–motor abnormalities associated with various neurological conditions has been of increasing interest over the years (Ozdemir et al., 2006; Wan, 2010). The ability to sing is something that humans are born with, and it is as natural as speaking, with no formal training being necessary. Babies at an early age begin to produce melodic vocalizations that are precursors to speech and music intonation (Welch, 2006). Due to this innate universal musical ability, singing can be a valuable tool for engaging the auditory–motor feedback loop in the brain more intensely than other music-making activities, such as instrumental playing (e.g. Bangert et al., 2006; Kleber et al., 2010).

Because singing and speaking use the same vocal mechanisms to produce sound, singing can be an effective tool for addressing specific aspects of vocal control in therapy. Singing directly stimulates the musculature associated with respiration, phonation, articulation, and resonance. It also requires a higher level of vocal control (Natke et al., 2003) and dynamic contrast (Tonkinson, 1994) than speaking. In addition, Wiens et al. (1999) have suggested that singing increases respiratory muscle strength.

15.5 **Clinical protocols**

VIT exercises used by neurologic music therapists often resemble the exercises used by a good voice coach or choir director to address aspects of vocal control such as breath control, inflection, pitch, timbre, and dynamics. However, since normal speech does not use the same level of breath control, pitch range, and dynamic contrast as singing, adaptations are often necessary.

Accompanying VIT exercises on the piano can significantly enhance the experience by providing preparatory time cues, enhancing vocal and pitch support, creating relaxation and tension cues, supporting dynamic changes, and motivating the patient to engage in the vocal exercises (Thaut, 2005).

15.5.1 **Breath control**

Good breath control is necessary for every aspect of vocal output. Therefore, in order to produce a good-quality sound, it is necessary to understand how to use breath support to influence vocal quality. When a patient has such control and understands how to use their diaphragm to support their vocal output, this can have a major impact on inflection, pitch, timbre, and dynamics. The exercise shown in Figure 15.1 allows the patient to physically feel whether they are using their diaphragm while singing.

15.5.2 **Inflection**

After a traumatic brain injury, it is not uncommon for patients to experience a monotone voice or limited prosody. In Parkinson's disease, lack of laryngeal control can also result in limited prosody. When creating VIT exercises for these patients, it is important to use a small range of notes, which simulate normal speech inflection. This can be done by practicing simple phrases or sentences while gradually increasing the range of inflexion. The VIT exercises in Figure 15.2a–d are examples of how to address inflexion in speech.

15.5.3 **Pitch**

Often a patient with limited or no prosody also presents with a lower pitch range than normal. In this case it is necessary for the therapist to first match the patient's current pitch, and then gradually modulate it to a more normal range (see Figure 15.3).

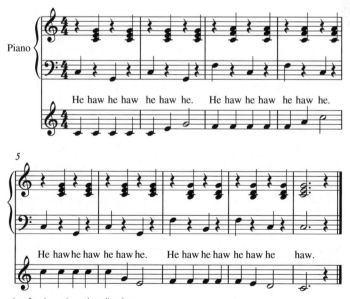

Fig. 15.1 Exercise for locating the diaphragm.

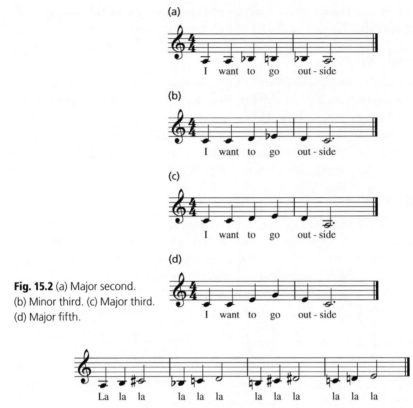

Fig. 15.2 (a) Major second.
(b) Minor third. (c) Major third.
(d) Major fifth.

Fig. 15.3 Pitch modulation exercise.

15.5.4 **Dynamics**

Breath support plays an important role in the control of dynamics or intensity during speech production. The exercises shown in Figure 15.4 require the patient to modulate their dynamics while singing a sound or phrase with a crescendo and decrescendo.

15.6 **Summary**

Vocal intonation therapy is a technique in NMT that trains, maintains, develops, and rehabilitates aspects of voice control that are affected by structural, neurological, physiological, psychological, or functional abnormalities of the voice apparatus. Due to the strong biological and neurological similarities between singing and speaking mechanisms, there

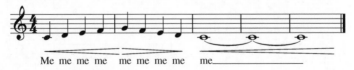

Fig. 15.4 Dynamic exercise.

is substantial research evidence supporting the basic mechanisms and clinical application of singing as a therapeutic intervention to address vocal issues related to inflection, pitch, breath control, timbre, and dynamics in a variety of neurological populations.

References

Baker, F., Wigram, T., and Gold, C. (2005). The effects of a song-singing programme on the affective speaking intonation of people with traumatic brain injury. *Brain Injury*, *19*, 519–28.

Bang, C. (1980). A world of sound and music. *Journal of the British Association for Teachers of the Deaf*, *4*, 1–10.

Bangert M et al. (2006). Shared networks for auditory and motor processing in professional pianists: evidence from fMRI conjunction. *NeuroImage*, *30*, 917–26.

Bellaire, K., Yorkston, K. M., and Beukelman, D. R. (1986). Modification of breath patterning to increase naturalness of a mildly dysarthric speaker. *Journal of Communication Disorders*, *19*, 271–80.

Darrow, A. A. and Starmer, G. J. (1986). The effect of vocal training on the intonation and rate of hearing-impaired children's speech: a pilot study. *Journal of Music Therapy*, *23*, 194–201.

Darrow, A. A. and Cohen, N. S. (1991). The effect of programmed pitch practice and private instruction on the vocal reproduction accuracy of hearing-impaired children: two case studies. *Music Therapy Perspectives*, *9*, 61–5.

DeStewart B J, Willemse S C, Maassen B A, and Horstink M W (2003). Improvement of voicing in patients with Parkinson's disease by speech therapy. *Neurology*, *60*, 498–500.

Haneishi, E. (2001). Effects of a music therapy voice protocol on speech intelligibility, vocal acoustic measures, and mood of individuals with Parkinson's disease. *Journal of Music Therapy*, *38*, 273–90.

Johansson K M, Nygren-Bonnier M, Klefbeck B, and Schalling E (2011). Effects of glossopharyngeal breathing on voice in cervical spinal cord injuries. *International Journal of Therapy and Rehabilitation*, *18*, 501–12.

Kleber B et al. (2010). The brain of opera singers: experience-dependent changes in functional activation. *Cerebral Cortex*, *20*, 1144–52.

Natke U, Donath T M, and Kalveram K T (2003). Control of voice fundamental frequency in speaking versus singing. *Journal of the Acoustical Society of America*, *113*, 1587–93.

Ozdemir E, Norton A, and Schlaug G (2006). Shared and distinct neural correlates of singing and speaking. *NeuroImage*, *33*, 628–35.

Pillot C and Vaissiere J (2006). Vocal effectiveness in speech and singing: acoustical, physiological and perceptive aspects. Applications in speech therapy [article in French]. *Revue de Laryngologie Otologie Rhinologie*, *127*, 293–8.

Ramig L O, Bonitati C M, Lemke J H, and Horii Y (1994). Voice treatment for patients with Parkinson's disease: development of an approach and preliminary efficacy data. *Journal of Medical Speech-Language Pathology*, *2*, 191–209.

Ramig L et al. (2001). Intensive voice treatment (LSVT®) for patients with Parkinson's disease: a 2-year follow-up. *Journal of Neurology, Neurosurgery, & Psychiatry*, *71*, 493–8.

Sabol J W, Lee L, and Stemple J C (1995). The value of vocal function exercises in the practice regimen of singers. *Journal of Voice*, *9*, 27–36.

Tamplin J (2008). A pilot study into the effect of vocal exercises and singing on dysarthric speech. *NeuroRehabilitation*, *23*, 207–16.

Tamplin J et al. (2013). The effect of singing on respiratory function, voice, and mood after quadriplegia: a randomized controlled trial. *Archives of Physical Medicine and Rehabilitation*, *94*, 426–34.

Tautscher-Basnett A, Tomantschger V, Keglevic S, and Freimuller M (2006). *Group therapy for individuals with Parkinson's disease focusing on voice strengthening*. LSVT poster,

Fourth World Congress on Neurorehabilitation, 16 December 2006. http://www.epda. eu.com/en/parkinsons/in-depth/managing-your-parkinsons/speech-language-therapy/ where-can-i-get-more-information/?entryid2=8383.

Thaut M H (2005).*Rhythm, Music, and the Brain: scientific foundations and clinical applications*. New York: Routledge.

Tonkinson S (1994). The Lombard effect in choral singing. *Journal of Voice*, 8, 24–9.

Wan C Y, Rüber T, Hohmann A, and Schlaug G (2010). The therapeutic effects of singing in neurological disorders. *Music Perception*, 27, 287–95.

Welch G F (2006). Singing and vocal development. In: G McPherson (ed.) *The Child as Musician: a handbook of musical development*. New York: Oxford University Press. pp. 311–29.

Wiens M E, Reimer M A, and Guyn H L (1999). Music therapy as a treatment method for improving respiratory muscle strength in patients with advanced multiple sclerosis: a pilot study. *Rehabilitation Nursing*, 24, 74–80.

Useful websites

Speech and Language Therapy Information. http://www.sltinfo.com

Chapter 16

Therapeutic Singing (TS)

Sarah B. Johnson

16.1 Definition

Therapeutic singing (TS) refers to the more generalized use of singing activities for a variety of therapeutic purposes. Therapeutic singing addresses a wide spectrum of functions in a more general and undifferentiated way than the other NMT techniques utilized in speech and language rehabilitation (Thaut, 2005). It can be implemented with individual clients or groups of patients across all ages and diagnoses. This technique can synthesize a range of specific speech, language, respiratory control, and vital capacity goal areas into an integrated therapeutic experience, thus providing follow-up exercise to other specific techniques such as oral motor and respiratory exercises (OMREX), rhythmic speech cueing (RSC), and vocal intonation therapy (VIT). Through participation in the creation of the musical experience, therapeutic singing can reinforce therapeutic goals targeted earlier within a session, as well as providing an opportunity for assessment of the patient's translation of these individualized elements into a functional task. Therapeutic singing can also be utilized as a physical exercise technique that addresses needs in global vocal and respiratory strengthening and endurance, without specific therapeutic goals in speech/language training. Because TS allows direct engagement in musical creation, it can be "a very success-oriented technique, thus providing important motivational input in tandem with functional enhancements to the client" (Thaut, 2005, p. 176).

16.2 Target populations

When defining the populations for which therapeutic singing might be most effective, one might ask who *cannot* benefit from the thoughtful application of this process. Therapeutic singing can be adapted to serve a broad spectrum of clients with varied needs. The following categories are by no means all-inclusive. \However, therapeutic singing has been successfully used by neurologic music therapists in the past with many of these populations, and is presented here to assist the therapist in determining who may benefit from the clinical application of this technique.

16.2.1 **Neurologically impaired populations**

These include, for example:

- patients who have experienced a cerebroascular accident (CVA), to reinforce goals for addressing aphasia, apraxia, and dysarthria
- patients with traumatic brain injury (TBI), to reinforce goals for addressing aphasia, apraxia, dysarthria, decreased pacing, volume control, and prosody
- patients with Parkinson's disease (PD) and PD-related syndromes, to reinforce goals for addressing dysarthria, decreased vital capacity, and volume control, and for improving pacing of speech
- patients with multiple sclerosis, to reinforce goals for addressing dysarthria, decreased pacing, volume control, prosody, and decreased vital capacity
- patients with Guillain-Barré syndrome and other neurologically based diseases and/or syndromes, to reinforce goals for addressing decreased vital capacity and volume control.

16.2.2 **Physically impaired populations**

These include, for example:

- patients with respiratory diagnoses such as chronic obstructive pulmonary disease (COPD), emphysema, or asthma, to reinforce goals for increasing vital capacity and volume of vocal output
- debilitated patients recovering from cardiac or other major surgery, and multiple trauma patients who may have been on ventilators or had extended ICU stays, to reinforce goals for increasing vital capacity, vocal output, and volume
- patients with spinal cord injuries with impaired respiratory function, to reinforce goals for increasing vital capacity and volume, and for assisting with the pacing of breathing.

16.2.3 **Hospice patients**

Therapeutic singing has been successfully used in these populations to maintain respiratory capacity.

16.2.4 **Aging adults and/or dementia populations**

Therapeutic singing has been successfully used in these populations to maintain verbal output and respiratory capacity.

16.2.5 **Pediatric/developmental populations**

These include, for example:

- developmentally delayed children and multiply handicapped children to reinforce goals for addressing speech delays, verbal apraxia, and articulation

* children on the autism spectrum, to reinforce goals for increased vocalizations and engagement in therapy
* children with hearing impairments and/or cochlear implants, to reinforce goals for improving verbal output, articulation, volume, and prosody.

16.3 **Research**

Because TS by definition "refers to an unspecific use of singing activities" (Thaut, 2005), there has been very little research that has focused exclusively on its *singular* effectiveness. This multidimensional technique does not necessarily lend itself to quantitative research studies. However, the evidence of the success of individualized NMT speech/language techniques, in combination with therapeutic singing, leads to the postulation that therapeutic singing can positively contribute to the transformation of patients' communication skills and/or address goals to increase their respiratory function.

Beginning in the 1950s, music therapists, as well as other professionals in the area of speech and language rehabilitation, began to document case studies and observations of the effectiveness of singing in facilitating speech for people with aphasia, apraxia, language delays, and other speech disorders (Cohen, 1994). In the ensuing decades, much of the research on the use of music in speech and language rehabilitation centered on diagnostic or technique-specific studies. For example, the combined use of other techniques, such as OMREX, RSC, and VIT, has been increasingly documented in the literature for patients with Parkinson's disease (DiBenedetto et al., 2009; Ferriero et al., 2013; Haneishi, 2001; Pilon et al., 1998; Tamplin 2008a, 2008b; Tamplin and Grocke, 2008; Thaut et al., 2001;).

There has been a resurging interest in the 1970s speech therapy technique known as *melodic intonation therapy (MIT)*, resulting in an emerging body of newer research supporting the use of MIT for improving expressive aphasia in neurologic rehabilitation (Conklyn et al., 2012; Schlaug et al., 2008; Wilson et al., 2006).

Although paired with vocal exercises, a pilot study examining the effects of therapeutic singing on dysarthria following TBI or stroke drew conclusions to "suggest that a program of vocal exercises and singing may facilitate more normative speech production" (Tamplin, 2008b, p. 207). Cohen (1992) also demonstrated improvements in a variety of the elements of speech through group singing with brain-injured patients. Baker et al. (2005) investigated the effect of therapeutic singing on affective speaking intonation for patients who had sustained a TBI. Although their data were drawn from only four case studies, they deemed that vocal range and the affective intonation styles of the patients were enhanced.

Singing has also been shown to be a building block for developing speech and language with handicapped children and children with autism spectrum disorder (Hairston, 1990; LaGasse, 2009; Lim, 2010; Miller and Toca, 1979; Wan et al., 2010). Another pediatric-based study, by Darrow and Starmer (1986), explored the effects of vocal training with hearing-impaired children. Although the singing in these studies may technically be considered to be more in the category of *developmental speech and language through music (DSLM)*, the studies are cited here to emphasize the effectiveness of the therapeutic application of singing with patients of all ages and with varied diagnoses.

Therapeutic singing is also a technique that can address goals for respiratory health, physical strengthening, coping with pain, and promoting emotional and social well-being in numerous settings. For example, the use of singing to address respiratory function has been shown to be effective in several studies (Bonilha et al., 2009; Lord et al., 2010; Wiens et al., 1999), and it may also be useful in targeting purposeful improvements in respiratory function for patients with spinal cord injuries (Tamplin et al., 2011). In addition, Kenny and Faunce (2004) have suggested that active singing may enhance the ability to cope with chronic pain.

Over the past decades, there has been a varied body of case study and small sample research that has examined the effectiveness of music interventions with diverse populations, such as patients with dementia, or those who are receiving hospice care. Often these music applications included interventions that might be interpreted as "therapeutic singing", although they were not identified as specific techniques. Many of these studies highlight the inherent richness of the musical experience of singing, and reinforce the concept that therapeutic singing can reach out to patients on social and emotional levels to increase their engagement in therapy as well as improving their quality of life.

16.4 **Therapeutic mechanisms**

Therapeutic singing is a powerful and accessible tool that can facilitate a wide range of therapeutic outcomes in the development and rehabilitation of speech and language. Speaking and singing "are natural pathways for human expression" (Cohen, 1994, p. 8). Songs incorporate musical elements such as tempo, melody, rhythm, and dynamics, as well as language. Singing is related to speech in its compositional organization. "Singing involves the fusion of music and language along a continuous spectrum" (Baker and Tamplin, 2006, p. 141). In the use of popular, pre-composed songs, the predictability of the musical structure and form can assist patients in improving their voice prosody (Baker and Uhlig, 2011). The rhythmic components of singing, and the way in which syllables are "chunked" together to form words, also contribute to the efficacy of singing in speech and language rehabilitation (Davis et al., 2008, p. 164).

Wan et al. (2010) maintain that, from infancy, humans demonstrate the ability to sing. She and her colleagues feel that because there are behavioral similarities between singing and speaking, as well as evidence of shared neural networks for both tasks, there is therapeutic evidence for demonstrating the "therapeutic effects of singing, and how it can potentially ameliorate some of the speech deficits associated with conditions such as stuttering, Parkinson's disease, acquired brain lesions, and autism" (Wan et al., 2010, p. 287).

Additionally, with the improved capabilities for brain imaging in recent years, scientists are able to visually demonstrate the neural processes that contribute to the process of singing. For example, Ozdemir et al. (2006) and Brown et al. (2006) demonstrated the shared bilateral hemispheric processing of singing and speech in functional MRI and PET studies.

In the development and support of the respiratory system, therapeutic singing promotes strengthening and control of the muscles used for breathing, thus increasing lung capacity. Baker and Tamplin (2006) also suggest that patients improve in their ability to organize breathing and phonating with the rhythm of the music, and therefore can increase their participation in therapy. Baker describes the effectiveness of "song-based singing voice work" for increasing breath control and support when utilized with patients with quadriplegia. The use of structured purposeful singing, in combination with other vocal therapy techniques, has been shown to be an effective therapeutic tool (Baker and Uhlig, 2011, pp. 154–6).

16.5 **Clinical applications**

Therapeutic singing is perhaps one of the most widely used NMT techniques, and yet it may generally be one of the least effectively implemented. There is huge potential for this technique to be interpreted as a "sing-along", or as mere entertainment for patients. The vast potential to elicit meaningful, functional benefits for patients through therapeutic singing often falls short. It is therefore essential that it is incorporated into therapy sessions with specific thought and intention.

The following clinical examples demonstrate the use of therapeutic singing in an NMT collaborative session with speech therapy, a TS group on an acute neurorehabilitation unit with a variety of patient diagnoses, another NMT/speech therapy collaboration focused on respiratory strengthening in a patient extremely weakened by critical illness, and a pediatric stroke patient.

16.5.1 **Clinical scenario for TS in an adult individual NMT/speech session**

Patient diagnosis: Multisystems atrophy with ataxic dysarthria.

Targeted areas to be addressed through therapeutic singing:

1 decreased respiratory support and coordination of breath

2 decreased rate of speech

3 coordination of speech production.

Sessions with this patient included other techniques, such as OMREX and RSC. However, therapeutic singing proved to be the most effective intervention for improving his functional communication.

Therapeutic singing was utilized in the following ways:

1 *As a vocal "warm-up" to prime the vocal system for the session.* For example, the song *Oh, What a Beautiful Morning,* by Richard Rodgers and Oscar Hammerstein, promoted vital capacity and breath support through the melodic contour and flowing style of the phrases, particularly in the chorus.

2 *To facilitate timing and coordination of breath control.* For example, the well-known song *Country Roads,* by John Denver, was frequently used with this patient. The 3- to

4-syllable, symmetrical phrases of the chorus provide a natural and predictable space in which to promote a deep and controlled breath. The end word or syllable of each phrase also extends for several beats, thus requiring sustained vocalization.

To visually encourage and facilitate the patient's participation more effectively, the lyric sheets were designed with an arrow extending out to the far right-hand side of the page following the last word of the phrase:

…roads --→

…home --→

3 *To facilitate pacing of functional speech.* One of the patient's goals was to be able to speak an entire sentence (5–6 syllables in length) on one breath; he usually spoke 1–2 syllables at a time, separated by short, shallow breaths. The speech therapist developed a list of functional phrases within the 5- to 6-syllable range, and the NMT created corresponding musical phrases with these sentences, which were then sung in a call-and-response format. The musical structure of these composed phrases provided prosodic and temporal cues, as well as a structured placement for breathing. For example, "Please pass me my laptop" was sung in a 6/8 meter, with emphasis on the syllables "please", "pass", and "lap." The melodic contour of the sung sentence imitated the ebb and flow of natural speech.

4 *To utilize targeted phonemes within a naturally occurring setting.* Although the patient was generally comprehensible in conversational speech, another goal for him was to improve the intelligibility of a small number of targeted blends, such as /ch/. The initial portion of the song *Chattanooga Choo Choo,* by Henry Warren, provided an excellent opportunity for the functional use of /ch/, and the song also "tolerated" the slower tempo required by this patient without losing the rhythmic integrity of the lyric, or the style of the song.

When targeting specific phonemes within a song, we would use a bold typeface, colored font, highlighting, and/or underlining for the targeted sound throughout the song sheet, to visually assist the patient in remembering to overemphasize the sound within the song.

16.5.2 Clinical scenario for TS in an adult NMT/speech-focused group session

Patient diagnosis: Parkinson's disease, CVA, and TBI.

Targeted areas to be addressed through therapeutic singing:

1 decreased intelligibility

2 decreased respiratory support and coordination of breath (volume).

These patients were all seen individually by a singing therapistST, and had also been seen initially in NMT/ST combined sessions. They were then incorporated into a therapeutic singing group session which met once a day.

Therapeutic singing was utilized in the following ways:

1 *As a vocal "warm-up" to prime the vocal and respiratory systems for the session* (as stated in the individual session description).

2 *To increase breath control and vocal output.* Songs that require good breath control through slow extended phrases were utilized. Patients would sing as a group with musical facilitation on the autoharp by the NMT. The patients' focus was on sustaining their vocal output for the entire phrase.

   Song sheets were written so that the lyrics that were to be sung on one breath were written on one line. The patriotic classic, *America the Beautiful* (by Samuel Ward, with lyrics by Katherine Lee Bates), is a good example of this concept. The song sheet was initially presented as:

   > *Oh, beautiful*
   > *For spacious skies*
   > *For amber waves of grain* ---→

   A more "advanced" version was:

   > *Oh, beautiful, for spacious skies*
   > *For amber waves of grain* --→

   As breath control and vital capacity improve, the patient can logically transition into singing the entire phrase in one breath. We found that the use of phrase markings or breath markings was less effective than presenting the song sheet in the manner illustrated here. Again, the ending words of phrases that were to be extended had arrows drawn to the far right-hand side of the page to emphasize the expectation of sustained vocalization.

   We also used songs with repetitious lyrics that could be easily structured to facilitate increased volume and vocal output.

   An example of this concept is the African American spiritual, *I've Got Peace Like A River.* The lyric repeats throughout the song, providing the opportunity to crescendo on each consecutive line, requiring more and more breath control. To reinforce the concept, we utilized changing font size to emphasize the increase in volume (Azekawa, 2011). Crescendo and decrescendo markings did not have any meaning for the non-musician patients, but the increasing font size of the lyrics emphasized the desired increase in volume:

   I've got Peace like a river

   ## I've got Peace like a river

   ## I've got Peace like a river

   In my soul --→

3 *To increase intelligibility.* Songs that contained targeted phonemes for the patients were chosen. Not all of the patients had the same articulation difficulties, so the song sheets were customized to fit each patient's most challenging sounds. For example,

one patient had more difficulty with ending consonants, so these were highlighted on his song sheet, whereas another patient had difficulty with initial sounds, and her song sheet was highlighted accordingly. Each group member had a song that was more specifically tailored to their unique goals, but all of the patients sang all of the songs with their individualized highlighted versions of the song sheets. While the neurologic music therapist facilitated the singing with an autoharp, the speech therapist would move from patient to patient, specifically listening for successful articulation or cueing for improvement in the targeted sounds. After singing the song, the patients would then take turns to read the lines of the song out loud. Each line would be read by an individual, progressing around the table. In this manner we emphasized the transferring of the singing back into functional speech. By reading the lyrics line by line, the patients retained the rhythmic character of the song, which in turn provided a temporal structure with which they could pace themselves. This also reinforced the emphasis on the targeted sounds. As they read "solo" they worked very hard to make sure that they were loud enough and clear enough to be heard by the group.

An untargeted but significant result of the TS group was the camaraderie that developed among these patients. They would verbally encourage one another within the sessions (e.g. noting when someone was more intelligible during the follow-up reading of the lyrics). Overall, these patients showed increased interaction with one another, both during and outside of the sessions, thus highlighting the fact that patients can benefit from the extra motivation provided by therapeutic singing "because of the emotional (and possibly social) context music may provide" (Thaut, 2005, p. 176).

16.5.3 Clinical scenario for TS focused on respiratory rehabilitation

Patient diagnosis: cardiac arrest during surgery with emergent intubation, multiple systems failure resulting in an extended ICU stay.

Targeted area to be addressed through therapeutic singing:

1 decreased respiratory support and coordination of breath (volume).

Because of this patient's extensive debilitation from her medical course, she had great difficulty coordinating her breathing and voice production when her Passy–Muir speaking valve was capped.

Therapeutic singing was utilized in the following ways:

1 *To increase breath control and vocal output.* There was no specific neurological reason for the patient to be aphonic, and various attempts at utilizing OMREX techniques and VIT to structure opportunities for voice production were relatively unsuccessful. However, when the patient was asked to attempt to sing a well-loved song, even if it was only to complete the final words of the familiar lyrics, she was finally able to consistently vocalize. Although the neurologic music therapist and speech therapist continued to engage the patient in more specific exercises to build respiratory support, therapeutic singing was the most effective way for this patient to "find her voice" again and sustain her participation in therapy.

16.5.4 **Clinical scenario for TS with a 6-year-old patient with CVA**

Patient diagnosis: hemorrhagic CVA.

Targeted area to be addressed through TS:

1 decreased communication and engagement in therapy

2 normalizing ongoing speech and language development.

This otherwise healthy child had an unexplained sudden onset of CVA with resulting right-sided hemiplegia, visual disturbances, and decreased language skills and verbal communication.

Therapeutic singing was utilized in the following ways:

1 *To increase vocal output.* To engage a young child with mild expressive aphasia, singing familiar children's songs proved to be much more effective than attempting to address this goal area more "formally" with modified MIT. Initially the structure of *musical speech stimulation (MUSTIM)* was utilized by asking the child to complete a familiar lyric (e.g. "Twinkle, twinkle, little _____"). This quickly transitioned into singing the entire song as the child became more self-confident and comfortable with the neurologic music therapist.

   Therapeutic singing was an intervention employed on a regular basis throughout the period of several years for which this child was seen by a neurologic music therapist. Often the sessions would begin with the choosing of a song, followed by the child strumming the autoharp with the neurologic music therapist, and the therapist and child singing together. Since the therapeutic goal was to increase vocalization, as opposed to the motor task of strumming, the child strummed with her unaffected hand. In this way the direct focus of singing and vocalizing was diminished by engaging the child with the instrumental playing, in *combination* with singing.

2 *To enhance vision therapy goals.* Vision therapy goals required the repetition of visual scanning and tracking challenges, which we often addressed through modified versions of *musical neglect training (MNT)*. However, therapeutic singing also assisted in addressing this goal. Again using familiar songs, the patient would be encouraged to sing with the neurologic music therapist while locating pictures that matched key lyrics of the song, picking them out of a selection of pictures that required visual acuity and scanning. Once the pictures had been chosen and organized on a Velcro board, the therapist and child then sang the song together, focusing on singing with a "big voice." The final step of the intervention was to sing the song once more and remove the pictures in the correct order, which again required visual scanning and tracking. The judicious use of a song structured the rather boring task of visually scanning back and forth into something that was more motivating and pleasurable for the child, while continuing to engage her vocally.

   As the child learned to read at a higher level, the sessions also utilized song sheets for therapeutic singing, which obviously required her to practice her visual scanning during a more functional task.

16.6 **Conclusions**

It goes without saying that the level of success achieved with therapeutic singing interventions is dependent on the choice of song. Although patient preference is certainly a vital element to consider, an effective song choice involves consideration of a wide range of factors. The therapist must address the *musical logic* and the *therapeutic logic* of their song choice in order to foster meaningful success in therapy. It is important that songs have temporal flexibility—that is, they can be slowed down or speeded up and still maintain their temporal logic. Because rhythm is the driving force for the facilitation of speech motor movements within the lyrics, rhythmic anticipation and rhythmic complexity are also important elements to consider (Azekawa, 2011). If a song has temporal flexibility, the therapist can tailor the cueing to facilitate maximal response, yet still have a viable musical end product.

Simply singing a song with a patient at random and calling this "therapeutic singing" is not best practice. Combining and reinforcing the speech and language, respiratory, and other possible goal areas of a session into a natural opportunity for functional use in song can provide a powerful therapeutic experience. However, it is *perceptive* musical choices, implemented with *esthetic facilitation* of the singing opportunity, that elevate therapeutic singing above the "sing-along" and into an extremely effective therapeutic technique.

References

Azekawa, M. (2011). *The effect of group vocal and singing exercises for vocal and speech deficits in individuals with Parkinson's disease: a pilot study.* Master's thesis. Retrieved from Dissertations and Theses database (UMI No. 1492358).

Baker, F. and Tamplin, J. (2006). *Music Therapy in Neurorehabilitation: a clinician's manual.* London: Jessica Kingsley Publishers.

Baker, F. and Uhlig, S. (eds) (2011). *Voicework in Music Therapy.* London: Jessica Kingsley Publishers.

Baker, F., Wigram, T., and Gold, C. (2005). The effects of a song-singing programme on the affective speaking intonation of people with traumatic brain injury. *Brain Injury, 19,* 519–28.

Bonilha, A. G. et al. (2009). Effects of singing classes on pulmonary function and quality of life of COPD patients. *International Journal of Chronic Obstructive Pulmonary Disease, 4,* 1–8.

Brown, S., Martinez, M. J., and Parsons, L. M. (2006). Music and language side by side in the brain: a PET study of the generation of melodies and sentences. *European Journal of Neuroscience, 23,* 2791–803.

Cohen, N. S. (1992). The effect of singing instruction on the speech production of neurologically impaired persons. *Journal of Music Therapy, 29,* 87–102.

Cohen, N. S. (1994). Speech and song: implications for music therapy. *Music Therapy Perspectives, 12,* 8–14.

Conklyn, D. et al. (2012). The effects of modified melodic intonation therapy on non-fluent aphasia – a pilot study. *Journal of Speech, Language, and Hearing Research, 55,* 1463–71.

Darrow, A. A. and Starmer, G. J. (1986). The effect of vocal training on the intonation and rate of hearing impaired children's speech: a pilot study. *Journal of Music Therapy, 23,* 194–201.

Davis, W. B., Gfeller, K. E., and Thaut, M. H. (2008). *An Introduction to Music Therapy,* 3rd edition. Silver Springs, MD: American Music Therapy Association.

Di Benedetto, P. et al. (2009). Voice and choral singing treatment: a new approach for speech and voice disorders in Parkinson's disease. *European Journal of Physical and Rehabilitation Medicine, 45,* 13–19.

Ferriero, G. et al. (2013). Speech disorders from Parkinson's disease: try to sing it! A case report. *Movement Disorders, 28,* 686–7.

Hairston, M. (1990). Analyses of responses of mentally retarded autistic and mentally retarded nonautistic children to art therapy and music therapy. *Journal of Music Therapy, 27,* 137–50.

Haneishi, E. (2001). Effects of a music therapy voice protocol on speech intelligibility, vocal acoustic measures, and mood of individuals with Parkinson's disease. *Journal of Music Therapy, 38,* 273–90.

Kenny, D. T. and Faunce, G. (2004). The impact of group singing on mood, coping, and perceived pain in chronic pain patients attending a multidisciplinary pain clinic. *Journal of Music Therapy, 41,* 241–58.

LaGasse, A. B. (2009). *Oromotor kinematics of speech in children and the effect of an external rhythmic auditory stimulus.* Doctoral dissertation. Retrieved from ProQuest Digital Dissertations (AAT 3358724).

Lim, H. A. (2010). Effect of "developmental speech and language training through music" on speech production in children with autism spectrum disorders. *Journal of Music Therapy, 47,* 2–26.

Lord, V. M. et al. (2010). Singing teaching as a therapy for chronic respiratory disease – a randomized controlled trial and qualitative evaluation. *BMC Pulmonary Medicine, 10,* 41.

Miller, S. B. and Toca, J. M. (1979). Adapted melodic intonation therapy: a case study of an experimental language program for an autistic child. *Journal of Clinical Psychiatry, 40,* 201–3.

Ozdemir, E., Norton, A., and Schlaug, G. (2006). Shared and distinct neural correlates of singing and speaking. *NeuroImage, 33,* 628–35.

Pilon, M. A., McIntosh, K. W., and Thaut, M. H. (1998). Auditory vs visual speech timing cues as external rate control to enhance verbal intelligibility in mixed spastic-ataxic dysarthric speakers: a pilot study. *Brain Injury, 12,* 793–803.

Schlaug, G., Marchina, S., and Norton, A. (2008). From singing to speaking: why singing may lead to recovery of expressive language function in patients with Broca's aphasia. *Music Perception, 25,* 315–23.

Tamplin, J. (2008a). A music therapy treatment protocol for acquired dysarthria rehabilitation. *Music Therapy Perspectives, 26,* 23–6.

Tamplin, J. (2008b). A pilot study into the effect of vocal exercises and singing on dysarthric speech. *NeuroRehabilitation, 23,* 207–16.

Tamplin, J. and Grocke, D. (2008). A music therapy treatment protocol for acquired dysarthric rehabilitation. *Music Therapy Perspectives, 26,* 23–30.

Tamplin, J. et al. (2011). The impact of quadriplegia on muscle recruitment for singing and speech. *Archives of Physical Medicine and Rehabilitation, 92,* 250–56.

Thaut, M. H. (2005). *Rhythm, Music, and the Brain: scientific foundations and clinical applications.* New York: Routledge.

Thaut, M. H., McIntosh, K. W., McIntosh, G. C., and Hoemberg, V. (2001). Auditory rhythmicity enhances movement and speech motor control in patients with Parkinson's disease. *Functional Neurology, 16,* 163–72.

Wan, C. Y., Ruber, T., Hohmann, A., and Schlaug, G. (2010). The therapeutic effects of singing in neurological disorders. *Music Perception, 27,* 287–95.

Wiens, M. E., Reimer, M. A., and Guyn, H. L. (1999). Music therapy as treatment method for improving respiratory muscle strength in patients with advanced multiple sclerosis. *Rehabilitation Nursing, 24,* 74–80.

Wilson, S. J., Parsons, K., and Reutens, D. C. (2006). Preserved singing in aphasia: a case study of the efficacy of melodic intonation therapy. *Music Perception, 24,* 23–6.

Chapter 17

Developmental Speech and Language Training Through Music (DSLM)

A. Blythe LaGasse

17.1 Definition

Developmental speech and language training through music (DSLM) is the specific use of developmentally appropriate musical materials and experiences to enhance speech and language development through singing, chanting, playing musical instruments, and combining music, speech, and movement. This technique targets children who are developing speech and language skills for the first time. However, it may also be used with adolescents, teenagers, and adults with severely protracted language skills. DSLM can be used to target speech production (i.e. articulation and intelligibility), language development (i.e. vocabulary, grammar, and syntax), or both simultaneously. One key element of DSLM is that all efforts at improving speech and language are directed toward the functional use of communication.

17.2 Target populations

The DSLM technique can be utilized with a number of child populations that demonstrate speech and language delays. There are several populations in which the motor aspects of speech control would be targeted by DSLM. This includes children with developmental apraxia of speech, cerebral palsy, and Down syndrome. The language components of DSLM may be used to target children with learning disabilities, autism spectrum disorders, and intellectual disabilities. We shall now discuss the key characteristics of speech and language for each of these populations.

1 *Developmental apraxia of speech (DAS)* is a neurological disorder of unknown etiology that affects speech communication abilities (American Speech-Language-Hearing Association, 2007). Although the criteria for DAS are debated, the American Speech-Language-Hearing Association (ASHA) has proposed three key features of DAS, namely inconsistent errors in sound production, disrupted transitions between sounds and syllables, and inappropriate prosody. Children with DAS may also exhibit difficulties with motor speech function, prosody, structure of speech sounds, and literacy (American Speech-Language-Hearing Association, 2007). These characteristics can

have an impact on the child's ability to develop expressive language, and will require intensive treatment (American Speech-Language-Hearing Association, 2007).

2 *Autism spectrum disorder (ASD)* is a neurodevelopmental disorder that affects social, communicative, and cognitive functioning. As this is a spectrum disorder, a wide variety of speech and language abilities can be observed in children with ASD. Children with ASD may demonstrate difficulties with joint attention, speech prosody, verbal communication, abstract language, receptive language, and expressive language (Gerenser and Forman, 2007). It is estimated that up to 25% of children who have ASD lack speech communication skills altogether (Koegel et al., 2009). Furthermore, children with ASD may exhibit unique challenges, such as echolalia or perseverative language.

3 *Cerebral palsy* is a neurodevelopmental lifelong disorder that affects the motor system (Winter, 2007). Children with cerebral palsy will often exhibit both speech and language delays. Some children will demonstrate a high level of receptive language and a low level of expressive language, indicating difficulties in oromotor control. Other children may exhibit deficits in receptive and expressive language due to cognitive impairment (Winter, 2007). Children with cerebral palsy will often use assistive technology for communication purposes.

4 *Intellectual disabilities* are a range of cognitive limitations due to disease or disability, including fragile X syndrome, Williams syndrome, Angelman syndrome, Down syndrome, and Prader–Willi syndrome. Children with intellectual disabilities may exhibit both speech and language delays. The characteristics of individual deficits will be dependent on cognitive factors and individual disability characteristics. For example, children with Down syndrome will often have physical characteristics that can limit or affect speech production, such as abnormal dentition, tongue size, and mandible size. Therefore the music therapist must consider the individual characteristics along with cognitive delay when addressing speech and language needs.

5 *Specific language impairment (SLI)* is a language disorder in which children demonstrate deficits in language skills without the presence of any other intellectual, motor, or hearing disability. There is no known cause of SLI. However, research indicates a genetic link for the disorder (National Institute on Deafness and Other Communication Disorders, 2013). Children with SLI may exhibit severely protracted development of communication milestones, including difficulty with vocabulary acquisition, grammar/syntax, word usage, and receptive language (Paul, 2007).

17.3 Research summary

Research on the use of music to enhance speech and language skills in children is emerging. Initial studies have demonstrated that music can be beneficial to the development of speech and language. However, there is a need for more research with a variety of populations. For the purpose of this chapter we shall consider the literature on music neuroscience, education, and music therapy.

The literature on music neuroscience and education has demonstrated a relationship between music aptitude and language skills (Jentschke and Koelsch, 2009; Jentschke et al., 2008; Marin, 2009; Moreno et al., 2009; Strait et al., 2011), with the suggestion that strengthening one skill could influence the other (Moreno et al., 2009). Music training has been shown to enhance verbal intelligence (Moreno et al., 2011a), speech pitch perception (Moreno et al., 2009), phonemic learning (Corradino, 2009), phonological awareness (Lathroum, 2011), phonological memory (Grosz et al., 2010), reading comprehension (Corrigall and Trainor, 2011), reading ability (Moreno et al., 2009), and pre-literacy skills (Moreno et al., 2011b). This relationship between music and language may be due to the shared cortical activations observed in language and music engagement (Brown et al., 2006; Koelsch et al., 2002; Schon et al., 2010). Shared activations may enable therapeutic outcomes to be met in children who have disabilities that have an impact on language.

When applied in a systematic manner, music therapy has been shown to improve word recognition, logo identification, and pre-writing skills in children in early intervention programs (Register, 2001). Similarly, significant gains in word decoding, word knowledge, and reading comprehension have been demonstrated in children with a specific learning disability in reading (Register et al., 2007). In a study of second graders, when reading was paired with music this resulted in significantly higher comprehension scores and on-task behaviors (Azan, 2010). These initial studies indicate that music could be a powerful tool for enhancing the learning of language and literacy in young children.

A few studies have investigated the use of music for vocabulary acquisition. Kouri and Winn (2006) investigated the use of piggybacked sung scripts for *quick incidental learning (QUIL)* in children with speech and language delays. The results indicated that children produced more unsolicited target words following music intervention. Cooley (2012) replicated this study, with the change from piggybacked to original songs for QUIL. The replication study focused on children with ASD, and failed to demonstrate any significant difference between the sung and spoken conditions. Both of these studies had small sample sizes, which could have contributed to the results.

Much of the current research has focused on the use of music for communication in children with ASD. The emphasis on this area is probably due to the prevalence of ASD, and to findings that children with autism appear to have a unique attraction to musical stimuli (Emanuele et al., 2010). Furthermore, children with ASD show an increased cortical response to music compared with speech in the left inferior frontal gyrus and left superior temporal gyrus, areas known to be involved in speech and auditory processing in the brain (Lai et al., 2012). Increased activation when responding to music could be utilized as a unique approach to facilitate functional improvements in communication. Initial studies using music for verbal communication in autism have shown promising results, with improvements in verbal production in children who are "low functioning" or low verbal (Lim, 2010; Wan et al., 2011).

Wan et al. (2011) utilized an exercise approach which they called *auditory motor mapping training* with six children with autism who were low verbal or non-verbal. The children demonstrated significant gains in speech output after 8 weeks of intensive therapy.

The principles as well as the specific use of musical elements in auditory motor mapping fit the paradigm of the DSLM technique. There is one study that has specifically targeted DSLM for children with ASD. Lim (2010) used recorded speech or music training to determine whether music would affect verbal production. Although there were no statistically significant differences between the groups, children with ASD who were lower functioning demonstrated greater gains in the music condition.

Lim and Draper (2011) added music to an applied behavioral analysis verbal behavioral approach. Their results indicated that children in speech and music groups showed significant improvements. However, there were no differences between the groups. The music condition was found to be most effective for promoting echoic production of speech. Although the literature in this area is limited, these initial studies indicate that music may be useful in speech and language training of children.

17.4 **Therapeutic mechanisms**

The music used in the DSLM technique should be appealing to the child while at the same time targeting the functional objective. Therefore the music stimuli should be motivating, exploratory, esthetically pleasing, and goal-oriented. Additionally, the transformational design model (TDM) should be used to ensure that the music is an isomorphic translation of a non-musical functional exercise. The TDM will assist the neurologic music therapist in developing music that facilitates the goal, which will prevent the use of activity-based music that may not easily generalize back to the functional skill. Although goal-oriented music should be used at all times, this music should not lack creative child-like elements. Rather, the music should meet the child's musical preferences, while promoting function. The music therapist can systematically apply rhythm, melody, structure, and novelty in order to create an exciting and therapeutic DSLM experience.

Rhythm can be extremely useful for promoting speech production and anticipation of response. Although rhythm is naturally present in all music experiences, the music therapist should consider rhythm as a primary facilitator of speech responses. Therefore rhythm should be clear and strong in the experience, and should be used to promote the actual production of speech. For example, rhythm can be used when the child is hearing the phrase and when they are attempting the phrase. Since the rhythmic stimulus is helping to promote speech, the music therapist must have the necessary knowledge to choose a functional tempo for production and maintaining rhythmic stability.

Additional properties of music that should be considered are melodic elements and structure. Melody can be used to mimic the natural intonation of phrases, to develop music exercises that are engaging, and to help with response anticipation. The music therapist's creativity in melodic elements can help to make functional exercises motivating. For example, melodic/structural elements can create an "anchor" in the exercises, something that "pulls" the child in and captures their attention. Once the child is engaged, the functional component can be embedded in the musical stimuli. Therefore, rather than having a child simply produce initial phonemes, an engaging age-appropriate song about an animal can be created to target initial phonemes. As the child is motivated by the musical experience, they will probably not realize that they are completing the target repetitions, but rather they will complete them in order to be a part of the experience.

Music structure can further enhance the experience, as a simple ABA form can allow for multiple repetitions of the "anchor" in the A section and the target response in the B section. So long as the A section remains motivating for the child, the B section can be used to promote multiple opportunities for the desired speech or language behavior. This requires age-appropriate music, engaging music, preferential music, and the correct balance between novelty and repetition.

When working with children, there is a balance to be struck between novelty and support for mastery of skills. Initially the child will need more support (musically and through prompting), and this is where repetition of exercises can be useful. Although the exercise may be repeated, musical elements can be altered to promote engagement. The goal is not to teach the child how to have a particular response within a particular song, but rather to provide them with opportunities to practice communicating or to enhance their language skills. Therefore the experiences should involve a gradual decrease in therapist support, and an increase in novelty to allow the child to practice the skill in multiple experiences.

17.5 **Clinical protocols**

The range of possibilities in DSLM is vast. Speech and language is not an area where a few protocols will do justice to the intricacies of the scope of treatment. For this reason, we shall explore the clinical application of music to speech and language goals using the *transformational design model (TDM)*. Although the full range of possibilities cannot be covered, an understanding of how to appropriately use the TDM to systematically apply music can be generalized to any exercise in the realm of speech and language. This approach is being used for a number of reasons. First, the music therapist will probably be working in a setting that uses a specific approach to language and speech acquisition (e.g. the PROMPT system, verbal behavior approach, whole language approach, milieu training, TEACCH, etc.), and it is impossible to cover each and every approach or methodology within the scope of one chapter. Secondly, there is no one "protocol" within DSLM. This is a flexible technique whereby music is used to enhance and promote speech and language production and learning.

However, this does not affect the music therapist's ability to apply the TDM in order to become an integral member of the child's therapy team. Therefore the following exercises will begin with a population that is known to demonstrate the particular speech or language difficulty (note that this does not mean that these interventions are exclusive to these populations). Non-musical exercises will be presented from the current literature on speech and language. The highlighted non-musical exercise will then be isomorphically transformed using the TDM. This will provide readers with a map of logical transformation from non-musical to musical exercises, which could be replicated within any area of speech and language treatment.

17.5.1 **Speech sequencing**

17.5.1.1 Example population: developmental apraxia of speech (DAS)

17.5.1.1.1 Assessment and goal information

Children with DAS will demonstrate poor sequencing of speech phonemes, difficulty producing speech, and multiple articulation errors within productions. The goal of speech-sequencing exercises is to improve the correct and ordered production of phonemes in age-appropriate phrases.

17.5.1.1.2 Common non-musical exercises

The treatment guidelines by Wambaugh et al. (2006) listed articulatory kinematic approaches as "probably effective" and rate-controlled techniques as "possibly effective." According to these researchers, most of the interventions studied in articulatory kinematic methods involve modeling and repetition of the phrase, with emphasis on correct articulation production. Some methods involve motor cues, including the *prompts for restructuring oral muscular phonetic targets (PROMPT)* method (Square et al., 2001) and the *sound production treatment (SPT)* method (Wambaugh and Mauszycki, 2010).

Rate-controlled methods employ the use of an external cueing device, such as a metronome, to pace speech production (Mauszycki and Wambaugh, 2011). The literature focuses on adults with apraxia (Brendel and Ziegler, 2008; Wambaugh and Martinez, 2000), with the emphasis on slowing speech and bringing awareness to correct production (Dworkin et al., 1988; Dworkin and Abkarian, 1996; Wambaugh and Martinez, 2000). Computer-generated rate cues that conform to the natural prosody of the speech phrase have also been used in practice (Brendel and Ziegler, 2008).

Since most music therapists are not trained in PROMPT or SPT, the following example will focus on the basic model-repetition articulatory kinesthetic method. In this exercise, the therapist would choose an age-appropriate phrase or word that is of the right level of difficulty. For some children this may be on the level of a one consonant (C)-vowel (V)-consonant (CVC) word, such as "mom." Difficulty will often increase with the addition of more C-V combinations, such as the CVCVCV word "banana." The treatment team often establishes appropriate word lists and target phonemes. There are also texts that can be used, such as *Becoming Verbal and Intelligible* by Dauer et al. (1996). Once appropriate words or phrases have been identified, the therapist would model the word or phrase, the child would watch the therapist produce the word or phrase, and then the child would attempt production of the word or phrase. This would be repeated with feedback from the therapist about the success of the production.

17.5.1.1.3 Musical transformation

An isomorphic translation of phrase and word repetitions would involve the systematic addition of an external cueing device for these repetitions. The music therapist would utilize a metronome as an external cueing device, and would cue the child to pronounce words after listening to and watching the model. In order to help with sequencing, the child should first be shown how to produce one syllable per metronome beat. As children have perceptual motor differences, the music therapist should expect that the precise moment of speech production might not appear to synchronize with the external cueing device. The tempo should be within a functional range and should be subdivided if the child's rate is too slow, so that there is an anticipatory cue between production of each syllable. For example, anything below 1 Hz could have an anticipatory cue added to further promote production.

There is no doubt that this is hard work for children, and therefore the music therapist should consider a few elements to help the child with engagement. First, the therapist can provide these opportunities within a larger experience. For instance, the child could be engaged in a creative musical experience that involves a child-appropriate song about animals using an A-B-A structure. They could manipulate animal dolls in the song for the A section of the song. In the B section of the song, the child could practice contextually appropriate phrases using the external cue to pace the speech production (see Figure 17.1a). After a number of productions, the A section of the song could be repeated. This provides the child with opportunities to be creative and become engaged with the "anchors." The song utilized could change in future sessions while maintaining practice of the target words (see Figure 17.1b). Older children will often be able to complete speech production to external rhythmic cueing without extra activity.

If the child has no presenting motor disabilities, then motor movement may be added in order to further aid speech sequencing. This could include a range of movement from whole body movement with speech, to arm movement, to simply taping the rhythm on their leg. The music therapist should be aware that extra movements may enhance speech production, but may also deter production if the perceptual motor differences are too great.

17.5.1.1.4 Outcomes/assessments

According to Wambaugh et al. (2006), common assessments include phonemic transcriptions and ratings of phonemic accuracy. The music therapist could record the speech production of a child after treatment and have this recording transcribed by an unfamiliar but trained listener. Phonemic accuracy could be determined by the music therapist at a superficial level, and trained individuals could complete formal assessments at regular intervals to determine improvements. Diadochokinetic rate tests (e.g. quick repetitions of puh-tuh-kah), oromotor assessments, and prosodic assessments are also often used to determine improvements in coordination, intonation, and functional skill (American Speech-Language-Hearing Association, 2007).

17.5.2 Acquisition of phonemes and intelligibility

17.5.2.1 Population: Down syndrome

17.5.2.1.1 Assessment/goals

Articulatory issues arise when "motor skills are insufficient to produce the sounds for speech" (Farrell, 2012, p. 12). In children with Down syndrome, the size of the mandible

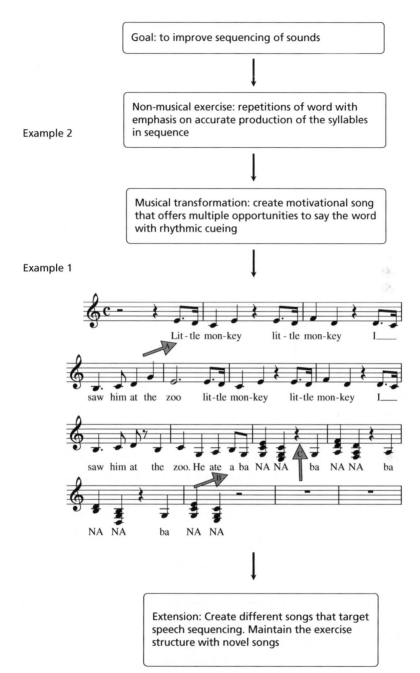

Fig. 17.1a Sequencing CV sounds or acquisition of phonemes.

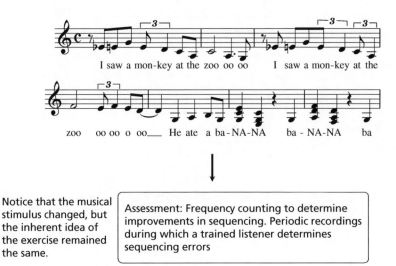

Notice that the musical stimulus changed, but the inherent idea of the exercise remained the same.

Assessment: Frequency counting to determine improvements in sequencing. Periodic recordings during which a trained listener determines sequencing errors

Fig. 17.1b Acquisition of phonemes and intelligibility.

in relation to the tongue, tongue protrusion, low tone, and motor difficulties contribute to poor intelligibility and phoneme production. The goal of speech intervention is to improve phoneme production and intelligibility. Differences from the speech-sequencing example in Section 17.5.1.1 would be the nature of the disability, as with Down syndrome the therapist must consider cognitive differences and anatomical differences that would affect communication.

17.5.2.1.2 **Common non-musical exercises**

As with the speech-sequencing example in Section 17.5.1.1, systems such as modeling repetition and PROMPT may be used for intelligibility and articulatory exercises. According to Kumin (2003), one way to work on articulation would be to have the child practice using different words with target phonemes. Depending on the skill level of the child, these can be practiced as sounds, isolated words, or target words in phrases. A pacing board can be used to help with phrases. An example is a strip with four circles on it that the child touches as they say each component of the phrase. Kumin also suggests using books as a way to target particular phonemes, and provides a list of appropriate books (Kumin, 2003, p. 153).

17.5.2.1.3 **Music translation**

Articulation of phonemes can be first practiced in isolation and then immediately followed with functional words. For example, if a child has difficulty with the phoneme /b/ then they could practice saying "ba, ba, ba, ba, ball." Since engagement is important in learning, the music therapist could complete these phoneme repetitions within a larger, more engaging experience. For example, they might create an experience using the TDM where a song is crafted to help the child to produce the syllable repetitions and then practice using words in context. In the above example, that could involve rolling a ball, bouncing a ball, or playing with different colored balls (see Figure 17.2). The exercise would not need to be

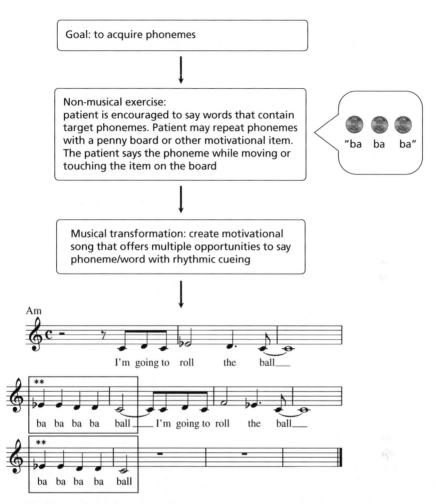

In this song example, the child is saying the repetitions while manipulating (rolling) a ball. The part where the child responds (marked with **) uses the same structure, promoting anticipation of the response. Engagement can be maintained by extending to different actions with the ball. The music therapist can choose different modes and feels for each action with the ball to further promote engagement.

Fig. 17.2 Acquisition of phonemes.

limited to one object, but could bring in different items with different consonant–vowel combinations in order to promote use of the phoneme with different vowels. This could also be easily placed within a phrase in order to practice communication of needs and wants (e.g. "I want [the] ball").

Musical creativity can also be added to children's books, using music as a way to promote further engagement, create structure and anticipation, and provide a stimulus for aiding in target productions. Within this area, the music therapist should be cognizant of musical form and choose books that have a natural flow that will work well in song (e.g. books with repeating themes that can be used as a musical anchor, then a variation with text that changes throughout).

Since the goal for many children is communication rather than isolated phoneme production, the music therapist should consider using experiences that are concrete, provide opportunities to practice real-world communication skills, and work on a variety of age-appropriate words or phrases. With a variety of language-rich experiences, the child will have more opportunities to practice using words and communication.

17.5.2.1.4 Outcomes/assessment

There are a couple of strategies that can be used to determine whether children are acquiring a greater level of motor speech ability. First, the child's speech can be recorded and transcribed by a trained but unfamiliar listener (such as a speech language pathologist or another music therapist). For instance, the music therapist could ask the child to tell them about a child-appropriate picture in order to have the child produce spontaneous speech. An unfamiliar listener would then dictate what the child said. This can be repeated following a course of treatment to determine whether the listener can better understand the child's speech. There are also some standardized speech assessments (such as the Goldman–Fristoe Test of Articulation, or the Kahn–Lewis Phonological Analysis) that can be completed by a trained individual.

17.5.3 **Pre-linguistic language**

17.5.3.1 Population: fragile X syndrome and autism spectrum disorder

17.5.3.1.1 **Assessment/goals**

Children with fragile X syndrome and autism may demonstrate protracted communication milestones. Early intervention can be utilized to establish pre-linguistic behaviors, including engagement, imitative skills, and reciprocation. These skills are important because they are used in later communication efforts and provide the building blocks for social communication exchanges. For the purpose of this example, we shall focus on gaining imitative play skills in pre-linguistic children. Note that the pre-linguistic phase in typical children is from around 9 months to 24 months; however, this may be protracted in children with disability.

17.5.3.1.2 **Common non-musical exercises**

Pre-linguistic interventions will often include opportunities for the child to engage in motor and vocal imitation. Sundberg and Partington (1998) have outlined various activities for imitative play with children. These include games such as peek-a-boo, making funny faces, making funny noises, or the simple command "Do this" followed by an action or vocal sound (Sundberg and Partington, 1998, pp. 95–7). The authors comment that these exercises must be motivating and fun for the child in order to engage and facilitate the behavior.

17.5.3.1.3 **Music transformation**

The music therapist can isomorphically translate the above exercises by using simple song structures in imitative games, in order to help with anticipation and engagement. Music is naturally engaging, and therefore the music therapist has an excellent tool for pre-linguistic imitative play. This may include common children's songs paired with movements or self-composed songs that allow for imitative opportunities. These musical games can be taught to parents and caregivers to provide them with concrete exercises that can be practiced in the home environment (see Figure 17.3). It is important to remember that musical games are a natural part of child development. The music therapist would bring in a variety of exercises that capture the core functional skill (in this case imitation).

17.5.3.1.4 **Assessment/outcomes**

The number of imitative responses can be measured by observation, to see whether their frequency increases. A trained individual may utilize early language assessments to determine improvements in the child's receptive and expressive abilities (including imitation), such as the Sequenced Inventory of Communication Development or the Symbolic Play Test.

17.5.4 Alternative/assisted expressive communication

17.5.4.1 Population: Angelman syndrome

17.5.4.1.1 **Assessment/goals**

Although children with Angelman syndrome will commonly demonstrate pro-social behaviors, they will often also have cognitive delays and severe language impairment (Williams, 2010). These children often exhibit little or no speech and will demonstrate stronger receptive than expressive skills (Gentile et al., 2010). Due to the lack of speech, *alternative and augmentative communication (AAC)* is often used as the primary method of communication. According to Calculator and Black (2010), one of the highest areas of need is the ability to express wants and needs. For the purpose of this example, we shall focus on the use of the *Picture Exchange Communication System (PECS)* to meet the goal of expressing wants.

17.5.4.1.2 **Non-musical exercise**

The child would be provided with an opportunity to express their wants using the AAC device. For example, if the child was attracted to an art program on the computer or iPad, the therapist would provide an opportunity to choose different aspects of the activity, such as the color of a virtual paintbrush, using the picture communication system. Communication pictures would be attached to a board and the child would be instructed to make a choice by pulling one of the pictures off the board and handing it to the therapist. In the case of an electronic picture system, the child would touch the picture, and would sometimes have to touch "speak" to make the device speak the words aloud. They would then have the opportunity to follow through with the choice that was indicated. This process would then be repeated for subsequent choices.

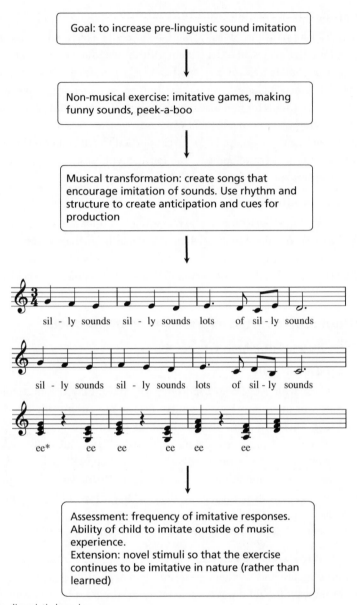

Fig. 17.3 Pre-linguistic learning.

17.5.4.1.3 **Music transformation**

The music therapist would use the same premise of having the child choose between different music items, preferred items, songs, etc. The translation is not in the item that the child chooses (any preferred item will suffice), but rather it is in using the music to help the child to anticipate a response, respond, and then be motivated by their choice. For example, an age-appropriate music structure could indicate the options available, present a

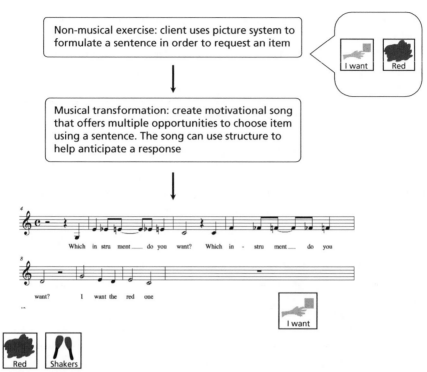

In this song example, the child is either handing the symbols to the music therapist or putting them on a Velcro board. The music therapist maintains the rhythm and musical cues for each word (providing music support as needed), singing the words in response to the child handing/placing them. Depending on the child's language abilities, the music therapist can adapt to include or exclude adjectives and/or instrument names.

Fig. 17.4 Alternative and augmentative communication.

question asking which one the child wants, and then prompt the child's response using an "I want . . ." phrase (see Figure 17.4). The musical stimuli should be engaging and motivating to the child, as should be the potential items that the child could choose. This can be repeated with different items. The musical structure can then indicate a new opportunity to express a want.

17.5.4.1.4 Assessment/outcomes

The focus of this exercise is not on decision making, but rather on the child picking up the picture symbol and giving it to the therapist (or touching the electronic symbol). There is a basic cause-and-effect paradigm where the child expresses their want using communication and then receives the item. Favorable outcomes are the child taking more initiative to communicate using the symbols, independently picking them and giving them to individuals in the environment. As their competence increases, the goal will probably progress to the child seeking out the communication device or individuals in the environment. Initial data can include the frequency of indicating choice. Some treatment teams might use distractor items (e.g. blank pictures) or non-preferred items in order to determine whether the child is truly communicating their wants. In this case, the team would be measuring the frequency of communicating non-distractor items.

17.5.5 Semantics

17.5.5.1 Population: intellectual disability

17.5.5.1.1 Assessment/goals

Children with intellectual disability may demonstrate difficulty with semantics, including the meaning of words, labeling, classification, and expression through words. Goals may include identifying items, grouping items, discriminating words with multiple meaning in context, or verbal expression through words. For the purpose of this example we shall focus on increasing expressive vocabulary through item labeling.

17.5.5.1.2 Common non-musical exercise

Exercises often target functional items from the child's environment. Several identification activities have been outlined by Kumin (2003, pp. 100–103) and Hilsen (2012, pp. 71–81). The child may be asked to identify actual items in the environment. This is often completed by the therapist holding up the item or picture and asking "What is this?" Engaging in the child's environment can also complete this exercise. For example, the adult may work with the child in a natural play environment, perhaps with a toy kitchen set. The child would be asked to identify the many items in the set through a play-like interaction. For example, the therapist might say "Look, I have a _____" and allow the child to expressively identify the item. The therapist may need to provide a model, initially identifying the different objects—for example, "Look, I have an apple." The therapist can also follow the child's gaze and prompt them to speak about what they are currently attracted to—for example, "Wow, that's a _____" or "What do you have?"

17.5.5.1.3 Musical transformation

Expressive communication is another area where music interventions can be isomorphically translated in order to help with anticipation, structured responses, and engagement. In the example with the toy kitchen set, the music therapist could use the same materials and create an interactive song about the subject at hand, where the child is periodically cued to respond and identify the different kitchen items. The musical experience can go beyond asking "What is this?", but use music as a way to create a situation for appropriately identifying items and engaging in play with the items (see Figure 17.5).

17.5.5.1.4 Assessment/outcomes

The child's correct identification of items can be tracked, using common vocabulary lists as a basis for learning. Careful communication with the treatment team should be maintained in order to reinforce words that are being emphasized in other environments.

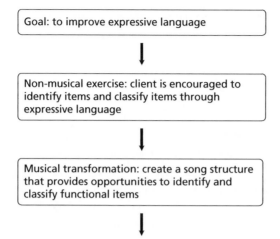

In the following song example, the child is working on identification and classification of food items. The A section of the song is the part where the child dances, signs, or seeks out new manipulatives. The B section is structured for classification and identification of items. In this example the items of focus are two types of apple. The child would be provided with pictures/cards/plastic manipulatives for this portion of the exercise. The desired response of the child is shown inside a box.

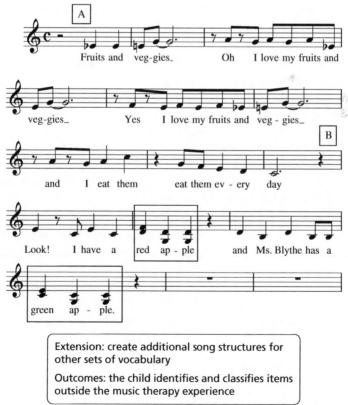

Fig. 17.5 Semantics.

Vocabulary is also assessed by individuals trained to administer tests including the Peabody Picture Vocabulary Test, the Expressive Vocabulary Test, or the One-Word Picture Vocabulary Test.

17.5.6 Receptive language skills

17.5.6.1 Population: specific language impairment (SLI)

17.5.6.1.1 Assessment/goals

The child with SLI may be able to comply with standard receptive tasks (e.g. "Touch the truck"), but demonstrate difficulties with tasks that involve function, feature, and class (e.g. "Touch the truck your dad drives"), or that omit the particular item (e.g. "Touch the one your dad drives") (Sundberg and Partington, 1998). Children with SLI may also demonstrate difficulty in complex or multi-step verbal stimuli (e.g. "Go to the table, get the cup, and give it to your mother").

17.5.6.1.2 Common non-musical exercises

Exercises would include having the child respond to a verbal command. The complexity of these commands would be based on the child's receptive language ability. For the purpose of this example, we shall focus on a child who demonstrates difficulty with function, feature, and class receptive language. As in the previous examples, the non-musical exercise will often be completed using stimuli in which the child is interested, for engagement purposes. For example, if the child and the therapist were playing with farm animals, the therapist might ask "Where is the cow?" Upon the child identifying a cow, the therapist could ask a question that requires classification, such as "Where is the spotted one?" This could be repeated in different situations that the child would encounter in their normal environment, including play and non-play situations (e.g. food items, clothing).

17.5.6.1.3 Musical transformation

In order to help with receptive language, music can be used to promote structure, anticipation, and further engagement. This will often require the music therapist to generate musical material quickly, in order to follow the child's interest. For example, if the child comes to the session and is naturally drawn to scarves, these could be utilized for the receptive language experience, so long as there are different scarves that would require classification, function, or features (e.g. moving a scarf with butterflies, particular colors, moving in different patterns, sizes of scarves, etc.). Musical material should be structured, allowing the child to anticipate responses, and can even be used to help the child to use self-language to complete the task (see Figure 17.6). For instance, if a prompt is presented with a certain musical structure, that structure can be replicated while the child is to complete the task to help with internal generation of the language in order to complete the task.

17.5.6.1.4 Assessment/outcomes

Receptive language tasks can be calculated through frequency calculations and the need for prompts to complete the task. The goal is to have the child generalize and be able to

Goal: to improve receptive language skills

Non-musical exercise: client is encouraged to touch specific items, as requested by facilitator. For example "touch the big truck"

Musical transformation: create a song that offers opportunities to practice receptive language skills by manipulating specific items

In the following song example, the child is asked to wave scarves that have different features including different sizes and patterns. The music is changed in accordance with the item, using smaller intervals for "little" and larger intervals for "big." Note that the child may or may not be singing since the goal is receptive language.

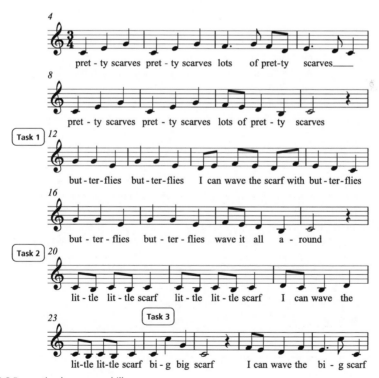

Fig. 17.6 Receptive language skills.

complete tasks of class, function, or feature outside of the music therapy session. This means that the use of non-musical items should be integrated into the session. Qualified individuals can assess receptive language with the Receptive-Expressive Emergent Language Test or the Expressive One-Word Picture Vocabulary Test.

17.6 Conclusion

The systematic application of music to enhance speech and language goals is a cornerstone of the DSLM technique. The neurologic music therapist can utilize known diagnostic, objective, and non-musical exercise information to inform their direction in treating children with speech and language difficulties. They can then explore music creativity in their isomorphic translation of the non-musical exercise to the application of music in therapy. Following the TDM when creating music experiences for DSLM will help to avoid activity-based therapy, and will maintain the therapeutic focus on motivating and creative musical experiences.

References

American Speech-Language-Hearing Association (2007). *Childhood Apraxia of Speech.* www.asha.org/policy/TR2007-00278 (accessed December 2013).

Azan, A. M. (2010). *The comparison of three selected music/reading activities on second-grade students' story comprehension, on-task/off-task behaviors, and preferences for the three selected activities.* Florida State University. ProQuest Dissertations and Theses.

Brendel, B. and Ziegler, W. (2008). Effectiveness of metrical pacing in the treatment of apraxia of speech. *Aphasiology, 22,* 77–102.

Brown, S., Martinez, M. J., and Parsons L. M. (2006). Music and language side by side in the brain: a PET study of the generation of melodies and sentences. *European Journal of Neuroscience, 23,* 2791–803.

Calculator, S. N. and Black, T. (2010). Parents' priorities for AAC and related instruction for their children with Angelman syndrome. *Augmentative and Alternative Communication, 26,* 30–40.

Cooley, J. (2012). *The use of developmental speech and language training through music to enhance quick incidental learning in children with autism spectrum disorders.* Unpublished thesis. Fort Collins, CO: Colorado State University.

Corradino, G. (2009). *Improving letter recognition and beginning sound identification through the use of songs with special education kindergarten students.* Unpublished thesis. Caldwell, NJ: Caldwell College.

Corrigall, K. A. and Trainor, L. J. (2011). Associations between length of music training and reading skills in children. *Music Perception, 29,* 147–55.

Dauer, K. E., Irwin, S. S., and Schippits, S. R. (1996). *Becoming Verbal and Intelligible: a functional motor programming approach for children with developmental verbal apraxia.* San Diego, CA: Harcourt Publishers Ltd.

Dworkin, J. P. and Abkarian, G. G. (1996). Treatment of phonation in a patient with apraxia and dysarthria secondary to severe closed head injury. *Journal of Medical Speech-Language Pathology, 2,* 105–115.

Dworkin, J. P., Abkarian, G. G., and Johns, D. F. (1988). Apraxia of speech: the effectiveness of a treatment regime. *Journal of Speech and Hearing Disorders, 53,* 280–94.

Emanuele, E. et al. (2010). Increased dopamine DRD4 receptor mRNA expression in lymphocytes of musicians and autistic individuals: bridging the music–autism connection. *Neuroendocrinology Letters*, 31, 122–5.

Farrell, M. (2012). *The Effective Teacher's Guide to Autism and Communication Difficulties*. New York: Routledge.

Gentile, J. K. et al. (2010). A neurodevelopmental survey of Angelman syndrome with genotype–phenotype correlations. *Journal of Developmental and Behavioral Pediatrics*, 31, 592–601.

Gerenser, J. and Forman, B. (2007). Speech and language deficits in children with developmental disabilities. In: J. H. Jacobson, J. A. Mulick, and J. Rojahm (eds) *Handbook of Intellectual and Developmental Disabilities*. New York: Springer. pp. 563–79.

Grosz W, Linden U, and Ostermann T (2010). Effects of music therapy in the treatment of children with delayed speech development – results of a pilot study. *BMC Complementary and Alternative Medicine*, 10, 39.

Hilsen, L. (2012). *Early Learners with Autism Spectrum Disorders*. Philadelphia, PA: Jessica Kingsley Publishers.

Jentschke S and Koelsch S (2009). Musical training modulates the development of syntax processing in children. *NeuroImage*, 47, 735–44.

Jentschke S, Koelsch S, Sallat S, and Friederici A (2008). Children with specific language impairment also show impairment of music-syntactic processing. *Journal of Cognitive Neuroscience*, 20, 1940–51.

Koegel, R. L., Shirotova, L., and Koegel, L. K. (2009). Brief report: using individualized orienting cues to facilitate first-word acquisition in non-responders with autism. *Journal of Autism and Developmental Disorders*, 39, 1587–92.

Koelsch, S. et al. (2002). Bach speaks: a cortical "language-network" serves the processing of music. *NeuroImage*, 17, 956–66.

Kouri, T. and Winn, J. (2006). Lexical learning in sung and spoken story script texts. *Child Language Teaching & Therapy*, 22, 293–313.

Kumin, L. (2003). *Early Communication Skills for Children with Down Syndrome: a guide for parents and professionals*. Bethesda, MD: Woodbine House.

Lai, G., Pantazatos, S. P., Schneider, H., and Hirsch, J. (2012). Neural systems for speech and song in autism. *Brain*, 135, 961–75.

Lathroum, L. M. (2011). *The role of music perception in predicting phonological awareness in five- and six-year-old children*. Doctoral dissertation. Coral Gables, FL: University of Miami.

Lim, H. A. (2010). Effect of "developmental speech and language training through music" on speech production in children with autism spectrum disorders. *Journal of Music Therapy*, 47, 2–26.

Lim, H. A. and Draper, E. (2011). The effects of music therapy incorporated with applied behavior analysis verbal behavior approach for children with autism spectrum disorders. *Journal of Music Therapy*, 48, 532–50.

Marin, M. (2009). Effects of early musical training on musical and linguistic syntactic abilities. *Annals of the New York Academy of Sciences*, 1169, 187–90.

Mauszycki, S. C. and Wambaugh, J. (2011). *Acquired Apraxia of Speech: a treatment overview*. www.asha.org/Publications/leader/2011/110426/Acquired-Apraxia-of-Speech--A-Treatment-Overview (accessed May 2014).

Moreno, S. et al. (2009). Musical training influences linguistic abilities in 8-year-old children: more evidence for brain plasticity. *Cerebral Cortex*, 19, 712–23.

Moreno, S. et al. (2011 a). Short-term music training enhances verbal intelligence and executive function. *Psychological Science*, 22, 1425–33.

Moreno, S., Friesen, D., and Bialystok, E. (2011 b). Effect of music training on promoting preliteracy skills: preliminary causal evidence. *Music Perception*, 29, 165–72.

National Institute on Deafness and Other Communication Disorders. (2013). *Specific Language Impairment Across Languages.* www.nidcd.nih.gov/news/meetings/01/developmental/pages/leonard.aspx (accessed December 2013).

Paul, R. (2007). *Language Disorders from Infancy through Adolescence: assessment and intervention*, 3rd edition. St Louis, MO: Mosby.

Register, D. (2001). The effects of an early intervention music curriculum on prereading/writing. *Journal of Music Therapy, 38,* 239–48.

Register, D., Darrow, A., Standley, J., and Swedberg, O. (2007). The use of music to enhance reading skills in second grade students and students with reading disabilities. *Journal of Music Therapy, 44,* 23–37.

Schon, D. et al. (2010). Similar cerebral networks in language, music and song perception. *NeuroImage, 51,* 450–61.

Square, P. A., Martin, R. E., and Bose, A. (2001). Nature and treatment of neuromotor speech disorders in aphasia. In: R.H. Chapey (ed.) *Language Intervention Strategies in Adult Aphasia*, 4th edition. Philadelphia, PA: Lippincott Williams & Wilkins. pp. 847–84.

Strait, D., Hornickel, J., and Kraus, N. (2011). Subcortical processing of speech regularities underlies reading and music aptitude in children. *Behavioral and Brain Functions, 7,* 44.

Sundberg, M. and Partington, J. (1998). *Teaching Language to Children with Autism or Other Developmental Disabilities.* Concord, CA: AVB Press.

Wambaugh, J. L. and Martinez, A. L. (2000). Effects of rate and rhythm control treatment on consonant production accuracy in apraxia of speech. *Aphasiology, 14,* 851–71.

Wambaugh, J. L. and Mauszycki, S. C. (2010). Sound production treatment: application with severe apraxia of speech. *Aphasiology, 24,* 814–25.

Wambaugh, J. L. et al. (2006). Treatment guidelines for acquired apraxia of speech: a synthesis and evaluation of the evidence. *Journal of Medical Speech-Language Pathology, 14,* 35–65.

Wan, C.Y. et al. (2011) Auditory-motor mapping training as an intervention to facilitate speech output in non-verbal children with autism: a proof of concept study. *PLoS ONE, 6,* e25505.

Williams, C.A. (2010). The behavioral phenotype of the Angelman syndrome. *American Journal of Medical Genetics. Part C, Seminars in Medical Genetics, 154C,* 432–7.

Winter, S. (2007). Cerebral palsy. In: J. H. Jacobson, J. A. Mulick, and J. Rojahm (eds) *Handbook of Intellectual and Developmental Disabilities.* New York: Springer. pp. 61–80.

Chapter 18

Symbolic Communication Training Through Music (SYCOM)

Corene P. Thaut

18.1 Definition

Symbolic communication training through music (SYCOM) is a technique in neurologic music therapy (NMT) that utilizes music performance exercises to simulate and train appropriate communication behaviors, language pragmatics, speech gestures, and emotional expression through a non-verbal "language" system. SYCOM exercises are designed for patients with a severe loss of expressive language (e.g. after a brain injury or stroke), or for patients with dysfunctional language or a complete lack of development of functional language. SYCOM exercises simulate and practice rules of communication through musical exercises such as structured instrumental or vocal improvisation. These exercises can effectively be used to train structural communication behavior such as dialoguing, asking questions and creating answers, listening and responding, appropriate speech gestures, appropriate timing of initiation and responding, initiating and terminating communication, appropriate recognition of a message being communicated, and other communication structures in social interaction patterns in real time (Thaut, 2005).

18.2 Target population

SYCOM was designed specifically for patients who either have a complete loss of language related to a stroke, brain injury, or neurologic disease, or have an absence of development of functional expressive language. Although it is rarely the case that speech and language skills are completely lost after a stroke or brain injury, the absence of the ability to use expressive language due to severe expressive aphasia and/or cognitive impairment can leave a patient frustrated and isolated, due to lack of ability to verbally communicate with their environment. Using symbolic communication patterns through musical improvisation exercises can provide an opportunity for emotional expression and non-verbal communication of thoughts and ideas.

In some cases, a therapist may see a patient in whom the development of functional language skills is absent due to a disorder such as pervasive developmental disorder, autism, Asperger's syndrome, Rhett's syndrome, or cerebral palsy. In these populations, SYCOM can play an important role by using musical exercises to simulate and train appropriate communication behaviors, language pragmatics, speech gestures, and emotional expression.

18.3 **Research summary**

Composers, performers, estheticians, and music critics from a variety of backgrounds and cultures do not dispute the fact that music has meaning that is communicated to both the participants and the listener. Whether the meaning arises from the abstract intellectual context of the musical work itself, or from the extra-musical world of concepts, actions, emotional states, and character, depends on the "absolutist" or "referentialist" perspective (Berlyne, 1971). However, all meaning in both musical language and verbal language is shaped and defined by the social and cultural context as well as by the intent and expectations of the situation in which the communication takes place (Kraut, 1992; Merriam, 1964).

Deutsch (2013) has described the auditory system groups in relation to various simple rules, which have been referred to as gestalt principles (Wertheimer, 1923). This ability to group in conformity with such principles enables us to interpret and communicate with our environment more accurately. Because of the natural groupings of sound elements through gestalt patterns of proximity, similarity, and good continuation that are inherently built into music, it can be an effective non-verbal tool for creating coherent communication patterns.

18.4 **Therapeutic mechanisms**

Language pragmatics refers to the rules for social language, such as using language for different purposes (e.g. to communicate a question, statement, or demand), changing the tone of language based on the listener or the situation, or following the rules for conversation and interaction. Although music does not have specific semantic meaning, through its rule structure and associated extra-musical ideas it can incorporate language pragmatics using the auditory modality in a similar way to speech. Musical exercises can create opportunities for dialoguing, asking questions and creating answers, listening and responding, initiating responses, and appropriately reflecting on a discussion. In addition to practicing the verbal components of communication, non-verbal language patterns and gestures such as turn taking and listening can be addressed through SYCOM exercises. Additional parallels between musical language and spoken language can be seen in phonology, prosody, morphology, and syntax.

18.5 **Clinical protocols**

SYCOM can be implemented through a variety of improvisational musical exercises that are used to train verbal and non-verbal structural communication behaviors, such as turn taking, gesturing, dialoguing, asking questions and creating answers, listening and responding, appropriate timing of initiation and responding, initiating and terminating communication, and appropriately recognizing a message that is being communicated. A patient can participate in a SYCOM exercise at any level of musical ability. However, in order to ensure a successful and therapeutic musical experience, the therapist needs to be sensitive to the patient's cognitive and physical abilities. The level of musical complexity may need to be adjusted through the use of adaptive equipment, visual cues, and modal music. The following examples involve typical clinical scenarios using SYCOM to address various aspects of verbal and non-verbal communication behaviors.

18.5.1 Turn taking and gesturing

In a therapy setting in which the patient has an absence of development of speech, SYCOM may begin with very simple exercises to practice the appropriate gesturing and non-verbal rules and structures that accompany functional communication. For example, the therapist and the patient may sit facing each other with a xylophone between them. The therapist plays 8 beats on the xylophone and then makes eye contact with the patient and passes them the mallets. The patient is then expected to play a few bars on the xylophone, make eye contact with the therapist, and pass the mallets back. After several repetitions, this example may progress to the patient having their own instrument and mallets, and simply stopping and gesturing when it is the therapist's turn to play. This level of SYCOM may take several sessions or several months for the patient to master, depending on their level of impairment.

18.5.2 Listening before responding

One aspect of pragmatics when communicating involves following the rules for conversation and interaction. If everyone is talking at the same time, it will be difficult to hear what other people are saying, and therefore difficult to respond in an appropriate manner. Creating musical exercises that require the patient to listen to a musical statement before creating a response can be an effective way to practice appropriate listening and responding in context at the appropriate times.

18.5.3 Dialoguing and responding to musical context

Once the patient is able to musically implement appropriate gestures of communication, and has established the ability to listen before responding through the previous exercises, the next step in SYCOM would involve implementing some level of dialoguing between the therapist and the patient. For example, the therapist may ask the patient to play a few short phrases on the xylophone. The therapist then plays something that reflects what the patient has just played. This process may be repeated several times. The therapist and patient should then switch roles. The therapist should play something on the xylophone, after which the patient should play something that reflects what the therapist has just played. This interaction could symbolize the way that communication between two people should reflect the fact that they are listening to each other and responding in context to the interaction.

18.5.4 **Asking questions and creating answers**

During this stage of SYCOM, the therapist can begin to introduce the concept of asking a question as opposed to making a statement. The therapist should explore with the patient what a musical question might sound like (e.g. an upward scale to imitate the upward inflection of the voice when a question is asked). Next the therapist and patient would explore a musical statement or answer to a question. The therapist and patient would then take turns to ask each other a question and respond with a musically appropriate answer.

18.6 **Summary**

SYCOM is a technique that uses structured musical improvisation exercises to train and practice appropriate communication behaviors, language pragmatics, speech gestures, and emotional expression through a non-verbal "language" system. Because music is sensorily structured, requires social awareness, has strong affective saliency, and evolves in real time, it can be an effective tool for simulating communication structures and social interaction patterns in a therapeutic setting (Thaut, 2005).

References

Berlyne D E (1971). *Aesthetics and Psychobiology*. New York: Appleton-Century-Crofts.

Deutsch D (2013). Grouping mechanisms in music. In: D Deutsch (ed.) *The Psychology of Music*, 3rd edition. San Diego, CA: Elsevier. pp. 183–248.

Kraut R (1992). On the possibility of a determinate semantics for music. In: M Riess Jones and S Holleran (eds) *Cognitive Bases of Musical Communication*. Washington, DC: American Psychological Association. pp. 11–22.

Merriam A P (1964). *The Anthropology of Music*. Evanston, IL: Northwestern University Press.

Thaut M H(2005). *Rhythm, Music, and the Brain: scientific foundations and clinical applications*. New York: Routledge.

Wertheimer M (1923). Untersuchung zur Lehre von der Gestalt II. *Psychologishce Forschung, 4*, 301–50.

Useful websites

American Speech-Language-Hearing Association. www.asha.org

Chapter 19

Musical Sensory Orientation Training (MSOT)

Audun Myskja

19.1 Definition

Musical sensory orientation training (MSOT) is an application of neurologic music therapy (NMT) that has been found particularly useful in patients with clinical conditions that affect attention, arousal, and sensory response. According to Michael Thaut:

> This technique uses live or recorded music to stimulate arousal and recovery of wake states and to facilitate meaningful responsiveness and orientation to time, place, and person. In more advanced recovery or developmental stages, active engagement in simple musical exercises increases vigilance and trains basic attention maintenance with emphasis on quantity rather than quality of response (Ogata, 1995). It includes sensory stimulation, arousal, orientation, and vigilance and attention maintenance.

> (Thaut, 2005, p. 196)

19.2 Target populations

MSOT has shown promise and has a particular clinical application in the following conditions:

- *dementia*: Alzheimer's disease, vascular dementia, Lewy body dementia, frontal lobe dementia
- *developmental disabilities*: traumatic brain injury (TBI), birth defects, learning disorders, chromosomal disorders (e.g. Down syndrome)
- *disorders of consciousness*: coma, vegetative states, stages of post-trauma recovery.

There have also been reports of the use of MSOT in patients with autism spectrum disorder, and it has potential applications in patients with attention deficit hyperactivity disorder (ADHD), attention deficit disorder (ADD), and related states.

19.3 Research

Several reviews encourage the use of music for patients with dementia symptoms (Sherratt et al., 2004), emphasizing the need for specific techniques that address the core symptoms of dementia (Myskja, 2005). The use of music in dementia care is increasingly becoming part of established supportive treatment, and is being implemented systematically in the health services (Hara, 2011). The main research challenges are documenting the most effective methods tailored to specific symptoms, and optimal modes of implementation (Myskja, 2006). The application of song techniques to aid sensory orientation and cooperation in washing and other procedures is one example of the promising areas of clinical application (Gotell et al., 2009). Music therapy for developmental disorders has a growing evidence base (Wigram and De Backer, 1999). The use of music for patients with autism spectrum disorder (ASD) has shown efficacy according to a Cochrane review (Gold et al., 2006). There is an increasing research base for the use of music therapy in disorders of consciousness (O'Kelly and Magee, 2013a), and improved assessment methods may enable a more precise use of musical elements to facilitate attention and arousal (O'Kelly and Magee, 2013b). Randomized controlled trials (RCTs) indicate a specific effect of music on the after-effects of stroke and post-traumatic injury (Sarkamo, 2011).

19.4 **Therapeutic mechanisms**

Therapeutic mechanisms for the effect of music in cognitive and sensory rehabilitation of dementia, developmental disabilities, and consciousness disorders include the following (Myskja, 2012):

- Direct interaction between auditory signals and motor activation may enhance executive function and motor skills.
- Auditory cortical plasticity acts as a substrate for retraining functions even in a damaged brain.
- Auditory stimulation can increase autobiographical recall in cognitive problems by recruiting alternative pathways.
- Specific music therapy methods such as the spaced retrieval technique can improve face/name recognition in memory loss.
- The differential cognitive load embedded in music perception can provide a range of stimuli, from basal pleasant auditory stimulation to more complex sensory stimulation.
- Familiar musical stimuli can create a template that serves as an aid to retain the patterning implied in memory functions, thereby recruiting working memory circuits.

Neuroscientific research on the effects of music on cognition, memory, and attention is progressing rapidly (Koelsch, 2009). One research strand is moving toward the implication of the mirror neuron system in mediation of the link between perception and action (Molnar-Szakacs and Overy, 2006). Although still putative, the application of basic research to successful clinical strategies is being presented (Wan et al., 2010). This research may aid the development of basic principles for successful psychosocial strategies in dementia. For instance, it has been shown that sentences which describe actions activate frontal lobe motor circuits (Tettamanti et al., 2005). Thus the emphasis on giving clear simple instructions and ascertaining that these instructions are understood before proceeding may have a sound foundation in a learning system in the brain (Avanzini et al., 2005). The mood-arousal hypothesis synthesizes research to state that the reciprocal influence of level of arousal and mood states can give access to untapped resources in cognition and attention (Thompson et al., 2001).

19.5 **Clinical protocols**

MSOT can be applied in a number of ways, ranging from simplified therapeutic procedures to techniques that require specific advanced skills in NMT. MSOT techniques are applied at three hierarchically ordered levels of increasing complexity and cognitive demand, each of which will now be described in turn.

19.5.1 **Sensory stimulation**

At this level, MSOT uses basal stimulation techniques with sound—possibly combined with other sensory modalities—to achieve some level of basic response to the sound and to induce physiological arousal. Sensory stimulation is most commonly used in patients with low levels of disorders of consciousness or recovery states, severe developmental disorders, or advanced states of dementia. Playing familiar recorded music, playing instruments of different timbres with sustained sounds, using the human singing voice, and asking the patient to touch "musical" surfaces that create sounds are all intended to create structured auditory sensory input, the goal being for the patient to show a psychomotor response to the stimulation in some "cause-and-effect" way.

19.5.2 **Arousal and orientation**

This level includes therapeutic music exercises to help the patient to achieve or maintain basic levels of cognitive processing. Arousal and orientation exercises are important for improving recovery states in disorders of consciousness, for building basic cognitive processing skills in developmental disorders, and for maintaining orientation and alertness in dementia. Exercises may be built around familiar songs and music, helping the patient to orient to time, place, and person. Music may be used to reduce anxiety and agitation. Musical instruments may be played in different space positions to help the patient to track and orient to the sound source. Simple cognitive demands may be built around arousal and orientation exercises such as "Nod your head if you like the song", "Turn your chair/ raise a hand when the music starts", or "Try to sing along if you know the song."

19.5.3 **Vigilance and attention maintenance (VAM)**

VAM exercises constitute the highest level of MSOT techniques. Frequently they serve as a gateway for more specific cognitive rehabilitation techniques, such as *musical attention control training (MACT)* or *auditory perception training (APT)*. The emphasis in VAM exercises is on sustained (quantitative) participation in musical activities without the specific (qualitative) response requirements that are introduced in MACT. The therapist must provide accessible yet musically meaningful resources for the patient to participate. Criteria for success are duration of engagement and sustained attention to the activity without qualitative criteria on how to respond or participate. The therapist may sing a familiar song and offer the patient accessible instruments —that are easily manipulated to create sounds—with which to play along. The electronic touch surfaces of cue or omnichords are good examples of musical accessibility. The therapist may program sustained sound patterns such as arpeggios or glissandi, and change chords on the chord buttons while the patient moves their hand on the surface for as long as the therapist sings. Useful acoustic options may include wind chimes, bells, or large tone bars. Touch boards or wands with digital interfaces are also appropriate options. In addition, sustained instrumental improvisations may be used for sustained VAM involvement. The patient plays freely on pitched percussion instruments (e.g. marimba, xylophone, metallophone) that have been prepared by the therapist in a modal scale set-up, such as one of the five diatonic pentatonic modes (do, re, mi, so, la modes), one of the four pentachordic modes (major, minor, Phrygian, or Lydian within the interval space of a fifth), or one of the seven heptatonic modes (Ionian, Dorian, Phrygian, Lydian, Mixolydian, Aeolian, or Locrian), which offer the widest melodic range for improvisation. The therapist responds to or frames, directs, guides, or anchors the patient's playing with patterns of modal harmonies at a slow pace without emphasizing metric rhythmicity. In modal music—since scale notes have no use in "vertical" functional harmony—polyphony can be easily created by simultaneous layers of melodic lines or intervals without the effect of "wrong" notes and chords.

19.5.4 **Other protocols**

19.5.4.1 Care singing for washing and other procedures in dementia and disorders of consciousness

Patients are assessed for preference with the assessment approaches of individualized music (Myskja, 2012), with a specific focus on finding at least two familiar songs that yield a strong positive response on repeated assessments by at least two independent raters. All staff and family members are instructed to sing these songs when they initiate procedures, to give the subject a recognizable sensory input with optimal arousal state, to facilitate attention and thus improve cooperation. Participants must take care to create and maintain a safe, supportive environment (Whall et al., 1997). For staff who are insecure about their own singing ability, care singing is taught and trained through role plays. Lyrics for the chosen songs are posted above the bed for bed-ridden patients, and in the bathroom for residents who are able to walk. The singing is continued intermittently as needed throughout the procedures, to monitor optimal levels of stimulation, arousal, and attention. Care singing is normally used as an intervention at the sensory stimulation or arousal and orientation level of MSOT.

19.5.4.2 Individualized music (pre-recorded and live) to regulate sensory stimulation, arousal, and attention

Subjects are assessed for preference with regard to the assessment approaches of individualized music (Gerdner, 2005). A selection of at least six recorded selections that have given a maximum positive response on direct rating (Myskja, 2005) are played to the subject, monitoring the volume and distance according to the response. The therapist sings above the pre-recorded selections, augmenting and modulating the output to monitor the responses to the music cadences, as gauged by facial action, gestures, and body movement. The singing is varied as needed throughout the session, to monitor optimal levels of stimulation, arousal, and attention. Individualized music presentations are part of sensory stimulation or arousal and orientation exercises in MSOT.

19.5.4.3 Group exercises in individualized music

Participants are assessed for preference with regard to the assessment approaches of individualized music (Myskja, 2012). Familiar songs are selected in accordance with optimum stages of sensory stimulation, by selecting familiar rhythmic songs that provide active stimulation and induce a response to initiate the musical dialogue. Examples of musical phrases that are found to give high response rates include songs which acknowledge the participant, such as *Skip to my Lou*.

For stimulating arousal (sensory stimulation and arousal and orientation level), it is important to regulate rhythm and volume in order to avoid both hypo- and hyperarousal. Examples of options that give strong therapeutic responses include changing between rhythmic songs that induce motor response, and slower ballads.

For orientation (arousal and orientation level), use familiar songs that refer to known structures, such as the patient's own name, their home town, the season, or nursery rhymes (but be careful not to introduce these in a way that may be perceived as childish).

For attention maintenance (VAM level), build up the program with careful monitoring of the correct blend of stability/predictability and variation/novelty. Pay particular attention to rhythmic phrasing, subtle changes in volume, and physical distance from the participants. Ensure that there is proper closure of the session.

References

Avanzini, G., Lopez, L., Koelsch, S., and Majno, M. (eds) (2005). *The Neurosciences and Music II: From perception to performance*. New York: New York Academy of Sciences.

Gerdner, L. A. (2005). Use of individualized music by trained staff and family: translating research into practice. *Journal of Gerontological Nursing, 31*, 22–30.

Gold C, Wigram T, and Elefant C (2006). Music therapy for autistic spectrum disorder. *Cochrane Database of Systematic Reviews, 2*, CD 004381.

Gotell, E., Brown, S., and Ekman, S.-L. (2009). The influence of caregiver singing and background music on vocally expressed emotions and moods in dementia care: a qualitative analysis. *International Journal of Nursing Studies, 46*, 422–30.

Hara, M. (2011). Music in dementia care: increased understanding through mixed research methods. *Music and Arts in Action, 3*, 15–33.

Koelsch, S. (2009). A neuroscientific perspective on music therapy. *Annals of the New York Academy of Sciences, 1169*, 374–84.

Molnar-Szakacs, I. and Overy, K. (2006). Music and mirror neurons: from motion to 'e'motion. *Social Cognitive and Affective Neuroscience, 1*, 235–41.

Myskja A (2005). Musikk som terapeutisk hjelpemiddel i sykehjemsmedisin. *Tidsskrift for den norske Lægeforening, 120*, 1186–90.

Myskja A (2006). *Den Siste Song.* Bergen: Fagbokforlaget.

Myskja A (2012). *Integrated music in nursing homes – an approach to dementia care.* Doctoral thesis. Bergen: University of Bergen.

Ogata S (1995). Human EEG responses to classical music and simulated white noise: effects of a musical loudness component on consciousness. *Perceptual and Motor Skills, 80,* 779–90.

O'Kelly, J. and Magee, W. L. (2013a). Music therapy with disorders of consciousness and neuroscience: the need for dialogue. *Nordic Journal of Music Therapy, 22,* 93–106.

O'Kelly, J. and Magee, W. L. (2013b). The complementary role of music therapy in the detection of awareness in disorders of consciousness: an audit of concurrent SMART and MATADOC assessments. *Neuropsychological Rehabilitation, 23,* 287–98.

Sarkamo T (2011). *Music in the recovering brain.* Doctoral dissertation. Helsinki: University of Helsinki.

Sherratt, K., Thornton, A., and Hatton, C. (2004). Music interventions for people with dementia: a review of the literature. *Aging & Mental Health, 8,* 3–12.

Tettamanti M et al. (2005). Listening to action-related sentences activates fronto-parietal motor circuits. *Journal of Cognitive Neuroscience, 17,* 273–81.

Thaut M H (2005). *Rhythm, Music, and the Brain: scientific foundations and clinical applications.* New York: Routledge.

Thompson, W. F., Schellenberg, E. G., and Husain, G. (2001). Arousal, mood, and the Mozart effect. *Psychological Science, 12,* 248–51.

Wan CY et al. (2010). From music making to speaking: engaging the mirror neuron system in autism. *Brain Research Bulletin, 82,* 161–8.

Whall A et al. (1997) The effect of natural environments upon agitation and aggression in late stage dementia patients. *American Journal of Alzheimer's Disease and Other Dementias, 12,* 216–20.

Wigram T and De Backer J (1999). *Clinical Applications of Music Therapy in Developmental Disability, Paediatrics and Neurology.* London: Jessica Kingsley Publishers.

Chapter 20

Auditory Perception Training (APT)

Kathrin Mertel

20.1 Definition

Auditory perception training (APT) focuses on auditory perception and sensory integration. It is composed of musical exercises that help one to identify and discriminate between different components of sound, such as time, tempo, duration, pitch, rhythmic patterns, and speech. APT integrates different sensory modalities (visual, tactile, and kinesthetic) during active musical exercises, such as playing from symbolic or graphic notation using tactile sound transmission or integrating movement and music.

The area of cognition training includes both auditory perception and sensory integration.

20.2 Target populations

Auditory discrimination is crucial for sharpening cognitive function and for regaining or developing speech and language. Auditory perception disturbances occur in different forms, and can stem from neural impairment, genetic causes, or a variety of developmental delays.

Examples of target populations for the application of APT include the following:

- Patients with *developmental disorders*, including delays in or problems with sensory faculties.

- Patients with *intellectually disabling conditions* of various etiologies, such as inadequate prenatal care during pregnancy, perinatal insults, or complications occurring shortly after birth.

- Individuals of any age with various types and degrees of *hearing disorders and/or hearing loss*. Congenital or acquired hearing disorders and/or hearing loss during early childhood can have a severe impact on communication throughout life. Auditory training enables the individual to improve their ability to understand speech and environmental sounds. Another typical goal of auditory training is the improvement of speech comprehension.

- Patients with *central auditory processing disorder (CAPD)* or *auditory processing disorder (APD)*. CAPD is an auditory-based receptive communication or language learning dysfunction. The symptoms are probably caused by delayed maturation of the central auditory system, and can be triggered by certain neurological disorders or developmental abnormalities. Children or adults with this disorder have a structurally intact ear and auditory apparatus, but the brain has abnormal difficulty processing or interpreting aural stimuli, especially when these are presented in unfavorable acoustic conditions.

Other disorders that affect auditory perception and cognitive functioning include the following:

◆ *Down syndrome* is the most common chromosomal disorder and inherited cause of mental retardation. There are multiple ways to develop Down syndrome, but around 95% of cases are known as *trisomy 21,* when the condition results from the presence of all or part of an extra copy of chromosome 21. Down syndrome is associated with a substantial decrease in cognitive ability as well as a particular set of facial characteristics, and associations with heart defects, leukemia, and early-onset Alzheimer's disease. Among affected individuals, language and communication skills tend to vary widely. Surveys suggest that as many as 80% of people with Down syndrome will have some problem with hearing (Shott, 2000), which may be difficult to detect. Competencies such as speech and language as well as socialization and general intellectual development are primarily acquired by hearing, so the importance of hearing and auditory processing cannot be overemphasized. The early detection and treatment of hearing deficits is therefore essential for the child with Down syndrome (Kirk et al., 2005; Sacks and Wood, 2003).

◆ *Autism spectrum disorders* are a group of disorders linked by difficulties in communication, social interaction, and/or cognitive functioning as a result of uneven or delayed development, while sensory abilities remain intact. In many cases, hearing or vision problems are overlooked or overshadowed during the diagnostic process. Behaviors caused by hearing and vision problems can be misattributed to the classic signs of autism, such as lack of attention, problems with speech, clumsiness, and lack of eye contact, or shading of the eyes.

Impairments in basic cognitive functioning and sensory deficits (e.g. auditory perception and discrimination, central hearing loss) can occur following various types of neurological damage, including the following:

◆ *Traumatic brain injury (TBI)* is a major cause of death and lifelong disability that presents with a broad spectrum of severity. Head injuries can cause widespread damage to the brain which may result in many complex physical, linguistic, cognitive, social, and behavioral changes for the individual.

◆ *Strokes* are broadly classified as being ischemic or hemorrhagic. Ischemic strokes are caused by blockage within the arterial system of the brain, resulting in an interruption of blood supply, leading to tissue death. This type of stroke is more common and is thought to account for around 80% of strokes. Hemorrhagic strokes (which account for about 20% of strokes) result from the rupture of a blood vessel within the brain that leads to local tissue destruction. Strokes are typically followed by persistent impairments of movement (paresis or frank paralysis), and/or of speech and cognitive abilities, which vary depending on the location and severity of the stroke.

20.3 **Research summary**

The beneficial effects of specific auditory perception training have been shown by a variety of studies comparing musicians with non-musicians. In general, musicians show stronger and faster neurophysiological reactions to musical stimuli compared with non-musicians, whether measured in conscious or unconscious conditions.

Musicians are able to more accurately discriminate differences in pitch, estimate the duration of tone or sound, recognize breaks between notes, identify timbres, assess sound intensity, and accurately localize the origin of a sound in three dimensions. The perception and production of music are powerfully modified by deliberate training. Such training results in modifications of the auditory system. For example, several research groups have documented a higher density of gray matter in areas of the auditory system of musicians compared with non-musicians. Musicians were found to have a density of gray matter in Heschl's gyrus double that of non-musicians. Furthermore, the tempo of nerve cell activity during the presentation of tones and sounds is four times faster in musicians than in non-musicians. This phenomenon can even be demonstrated when comparing professional musicians with music students; the auditory nerve activity of professional musicians has been found to be twice as fast as it is in music students. Such results support the neurological changes that occur after deliberate musical training. Effects like these can be replicated when working with non-musicians. For example, 14 hours of pitch discrimination training led to a significant improvement in auditory discrimination, nearly reaching the level found in professional musicians (Koelsch et al., 1999; Tervaniemi et al., 2006). Similar results were seen in a group of non-musicians after a short training period of 2 hours. Following this brief training, participants were able to detect minute differences within a sequence of 10 sounds (Watson, 1980).

Pantev et al. (2001) revealed that long-term practicing of one instrument led to stronger neural reactions in the auditory cortex when hearing the same instrument being played. Musicians showed significantly stronger nerve activity when identifying the sounds of their own instrument among other instruments.

Anvari et al. (2002) demonstrated that there is a link between phonological awareness, working memory, and musical ability, especially for the perception of sound, pitch, rhythm, and melody. Compared with non-musicians, musicians showed a more robust frequency following response (FFR) during EEG measures while listening to musical sounds (Musacchia et al., 2007). The same effect was shown when comparing tonal (Mandarin) and non-tonal (English) speakers (Song et al., 2008). Results like these provide evidence for neurological modification at the level of the brainstem following musical training for sound processing in music and language.

Similar effects were indicated by elevated P2 values after auditory perception training in both language and music training. The participants in the study by Reinke et al. (2003) showed more distinct P2 values after a short training sequence in which they distinguished vowels compared with individuals who did not undergo this training sequence. In the same year, Shahin et al. (2003) documented a similar effect with musicians. In their experiment, musicians were found to be superior to non-musicians in differentiating pitches. Receiving a higher P2 amplitude after focused musical and speech-based training serves as an indicator that there are shared neural networks for spectral and temporal analysis of music and speech. On the basis of these findings it can be concluded that musical training has a high benefit for neural speech analysis. Marie et al. (2011) demonstrated that musicians are better at detecting metric structures within speech compared with non-musicians. This difference was also shown by higher P2 values in the musician group. Higher P2 amplitudes seem to be a consequence of musical training, which leads to a better perception of metric speech elements and thus has a positive effect on analyzing metric language structure.

20.4 **Therapeutic mechanisms**

As described earlier, shaping of the auditory system is largely accomplished through long-term musical training. A musician's expertise comes at the cost of countless hours spent learning, analyzing, and rehearsing music. This has been demonstrated in various studies throughout the last 15 years comparing musicians with non-musicians.

Music is primarily an auditory art form, and can be an enjoyable and excellent tool for therapy so long as the auditory and communicative characteristics of the individual are accommodated. Auditory discrimination is crucial for sharpening cognitive functions and for developing or regaining speech and language. In APT, musical exercises are designed to aid the identification and discrimination of different sound components, such as time, tempo, duration, pitch, timbre, rhythmic patterns, and speech sounds.

Gaab et al. (2005) were able to demonstrate a positive effect of musical training on reading and writing skills. They concluded that the detection of prosodic characteristics is crucial when listening to spoken language and acquiring new information. Moreno et al. (2009) confirmed the transfer of musical abilities to linguistic abilities. In their study, 8-year-old children received either music or art lessons for a period of 6 months. In the post-tests, only the children who had received music lessons showed improvements in reading abilities. Musical training improves basic auditory analysis and the ability to distinguish subtle differences in sound and pitch. Skills like these support the development of phonological representations, which are in turn important for reading skills. These results support the evidence for an increase in brain plasticity after musical training.

Listening to instruments being played helps to define the parameters of sound and other musical qualities, while playing instruments provides consistent auditory feedback to patients. The act of playing music is a highly motivating tool for encouraging participation in rehabilitation therapy, and has a high rate of spontaneous transfer to real-world auditory discrimination.

For individuals with hearing loss, auditory training is an intervention that enables the individual to make maximum use of residual hearing, or aids the development of new hearing skills after the implantation of a cochlear implant. The ultimate goal of auditory training for these patients is typically to improve their ability to understand speech and distinguish environmental sounds. Because music and speech share common structural characteristics, such as pitch and duration of sounds, music can effectively contribute to an auditory training program by motivating the use of residual hearing (Amir and Schuchman, 1985; Bang, 1980; Darrow and Gfeller, 1996; Fisher and Parker, 1994; Gfeller, 2000).

In most people the auditory system is trained through normal environmental exposure during childhood. Individuals who suffer from brain injury or various sensory dysfunctions must in many respects relearn these abilities and execute them volitionally. Playing an instrument allows the individual to see a cause–effect relationship between an action (striking the instrument) and the reaction (the resulting sound). For many patients, playing an instrument is also a positive and motivating experience during which they actively create and perceive sounds.

20.4.1 **Using APT with children**

The application of APT exercises in children with various impairments is similar to their application in adults. Children with autism or hearing difficulties tend to show deficits in expressive and receptive communication skills. Music therapy can encourage basic cognitive functions as well as receptive language (listening, and understanding signs and gestures) and expressive language (singing and speaking).

Nearly all children enjoy playing musical instruments, and the use of therapeutic music exercises encourages prolonged listening and attention. Playing different-sounding instruments can help to improve auditory discrimination of sounds and tones.

20.5 **Clinical protocols**

Auditory discrimination is crucial for sharpening cognitive functions and for developing or regaining speech and language. In APT, musical exercises consist of the discrimination and identification of different sound components, namely time, tempo, duration, pitch, timbre, rhythmic patterns, and speech sounds. APT can also be organized through active musical exercises such as playing from symbolic or graphic notion, using tactile sound transmission, or integrating one's movement to music. In this way, different sensory modalities (e.g. visual, tactile, kinesthetic) are integrated during active musical exercises.

Percussion instruments and low-pitched mallet instruments (e.g. xylophone, glockenspiel) can be used effectively to work on the following goals: *sound detection* (the presence or absence of sound), *sound discrimination* (sounds that are the same or different), *sound identification* (recognizing the sound source), and *comprehension* (understanding) *of sound* (Darrow and Gfeller, 1996).

Music therapy sessions using APT may be held in an individual setting or among small groups of patients who are working toward similar goals.

It is important to remember that the primary goal in auditory perception exercises is to improve basic cognitive function and awareness of sufficient sound distinction, rather than to correct voice or instrumental playing quality.

20.5.1 **Sound**

Box 20.1 Sound detection: sound versus silence

Specific target of exercise:	Sound detection
NMT technique:	APT
Outcome goal:	Introduce or practice the concept of sound versus silence
Clientele description:	Children with hearing loss
	Rehabilitation of adults with cochlear implants
	Patients with neurological injury or illness
Session type:	Group (3–4 participants)
	Single setting
Equipment needed:	Tomtom on a stand

Step-by-step procedure:

Sound–silence with visual control:

♦ All of the participants sit in a circle. The tomtom is placed on a stand in the middle of the circle so that all of the participants can see the instrument.

♦ The therapist starts to play the tomtom and shows a sign like "I hear sound" for as long as the instrument is being played.

♦ The therapist stops playing the instrument and shows a sign for "stop–silence."

♦ Each participant repeats this procedure.

Sound–silence without visual control:

♦ All of the participants can move around the room. The tomtom is placed on a stand at the edge of the room and should be played from behind the instrument.

♦ The therapist plays the instrument, and for as long as the instrument sounds the participants walk round the room.

♦ As soon as the therapist stops playing, all of the participants freeze until they hear the sound of the instrument again.

♦ Each of the participants will take it in turn to play the tomtom.

Box 20.2 Sound detection: directional hearing

Specific target of exercise:	Sound detection
	Directional hearing
NMT technique:	APT
Outcome goal:	Introduce or practice spatial orientation
Clientele description:	Children with hearing loss
	Rehabilitation of adults with cochlear implants
	Patients with neurological injury or illness
Session type:	Group (3–4 participants)
	Single setting
Equipment needed:	Four tone bars
	Four drums
	A variety of different rhythm instruments

Step-by-step procedure:

Sound detection with visual control: front and back

◆ Four chairs are placed so that there is one in each corner of the room, and a tone bar, a drum, and one of the rhythm instruments are placed on each chair.

◆ One chair is placed in the middle of the room.

◆ One of the participants sits on the middle chair, while the rest of the group members and the therapist take the other chairs.

◆ The two players *in front of* the participant sitting in the center play the drums or the tone bars together, so that the participant in the center can listen to the sound in front of him or her.

◆ Then the two players *behind* the participant sitting in the center play the drums or the tone bars together, so that the participant in the center can listen to the sound behind him or her.

◆ Finally, the participant in the center will hear the sound *alternating from front to back* played by the other group members.

◆ Each of the participants will take it in turn to sit in the center of the room and listen to sound coming from in front of them and from behind them.

Sound detection with visual control: left and right

◆ The same room set-up and sound presentation procedure as before will be used.

◆ The two players on the *right-hand side* of the participant sitting in the center play the drums or the tone bars together, so that the participant in the center can listen to the sound coming from his or her right side.

Box 20.2 Sound detection: directional hearing *(continued)*

- Then the two players on the *left-hand side* of the participant sitting in the center play the drums or the tone bars together, so that the participant in the center can listen to the sound coming from his or her left side.
- Finally, the participant in the center will hear the sound *alternating from right to left* played by the other group members.
- Each of the participants will take it in turn to sit in the center of the room and listen to sound coming from their right or left side.

Sound detection without visual control:

- The same room set-up will be used, but the participant seated in the center is blindfolded.
- The same procedure as described previously can be repeated, and the participant has to point to the direction from which he or she hears the sound (left, right, front, or back).
- Each corner of the room can be identified with a different instrument (e.g. front right, drum; front left, tone bar c1; back right, rattle; back left, tone bar g2), so that the direction is easier to identify.
- Then the position of these instruments is changed and the participant seated in the center has to point to the direction from which he or she hears the sound.
- As a variation, all of the instruments can be played in turn, and the participant in the center has to work out whether the sound is going around him or her in a clockwise or anticlockwise direction.
- Each of the participants will take it in turn to sit in the center

20.5.2 Tempo

Box 20.3 Distinguishing tempi: I

Specific target of exercise:	Distinguishing tempi: I
NMT technique:	APT
Outcome goal:	Introduce and practice the concept of slow and fast tempo
Clientele description:	Children with hearing loss
	Rehabilitation of adults with cochlear implants
	Patients with neurological injury or illness
Session type:	Group (3–4 participants)
	Single setting

Box 20.3 Distinguishing tempi: I *(continued)*

Equipment needed: One pair of claves per participant

One conga per participant

Step-by-step procedure:

- The group is seated in a circle, and each participant has a conga or a pair of claves.
- The therapist introduces a *slow* rhythm pattern on their conga/claves and the participants repeat this together.
- Then the therapist plays a *fast* rhythm pattern on their conga/claves and the participants repeat this together.
- After the two rhythm patterns have been set, the therapist chooses one of the patterns and plays it to the participants.
- The participants listen to it and only repeat the pattern when they have identified the *fast* rhythm pattern. If they hear the *slow* pattern, they do not repeat it.
- After some repetitions the therapist gives other group members the opportunity to present one of the two rhythms to the group.

Variation:

- The therapist plays randomly either a *slow* or a *fast* rhythm pattern to the participants.
- The participants listen and only repeat the *fast* rhythm.
- The participants listen and only repeat the *slow* rhythm.

Box 20.4 Distinguishing tempi: II

Specific target of exercise:	Distinguishing tempi: II
NMT technique:	APT
Outcome goal:	Introduce and practice the concept of slow and fast tempo
Clientele description:	Children with hearing loss
	Rehabilitation of adults with cochlear implants
	Patients with neurological injury or illness
Session type:	Group (3–4 participants)
	Single setting
Equipment needed:	One pair of claves per participant or one conga per participant
	Piano

Step-by-step procedure:

- The group is seated in a circle, and each participant has a conga or a pair of claves.
- The therapist introduces a steady *slow* beat on the piano by playing a cadence scheme.

Box 20.4 Distinguishing tempi: II *(continued)*

- While playing, the therapist invites the group to join in with the slow pattern on their congas or claves.
- Then the therapist plays a steady *fast* beat on the piano using the same cadence scheme.
- While playing, the therapist invites the group to join in with the fast pattern on their instruments.
- Finally, the therapist and the participants play together. The participants have to listen to the tempo of the therapist and synchronize their own playing to it as it changes from slow to fast, and vice versa.

Variation:

- For a more subtle change of tempo, the therapist uses *accelerando* and *ritardando* in his or her performance, so that the participants have to listen more carefully in order to synchronize their action.

20.5.3 **Duration**

Box 20.5 **Distinguishing the duration of sounds: I**

Specific target of exercise:	Distinguishing the duration of sounds: I
NMT technique:	APT
Outcome goal:	Differentiate between and produce short and long sounds
Clientele description:	Children with hearing loss
	Rehabilitation of adults with cochlear implants
	Patients with neurological injury or illness
Session type:	Group (3–4 participants)
	Single setting
Equipment needed:	*Long-sounding instruments*:
	Cymbals, tomtom, tone bars, rainmaker
	Short-sounding instruments:
	Snare drum, hand drum, wood blocks
	Instruments that produce both long and short sounds:
	Piano, vibraphone, flute
Step-by-step procedure:	

- The group is seated in a circle, with all of the instruments in the center of the circle.

Box 20.5 Distinguishing the duration of sounds: I *(continued)*

♦ The therapist introduces all of the *short-sounding* instruments by playing them to the participants.

♦ The participants are invited to try out these instruments for themselves.

♦ Then the therapist introduces all of the *long-sounding* instruments by playing them to the participants.

♦ The participants are invited to try out these instruments for themselves.

♦ Finally, the therapist introduces all of the available instruments, which can produce *both short and long sounds*:

  – piano: playing notes with (*long*) and without (*short*) pedal

  – vibraphone: playing notes with (*long*) and without (*short*) pedal

  – for more subtle changes, the therapist demonstrates how the sound changes when using different kinds of mallets on the vibraphone

  – flute: blow for 4 beats (*long*) or for only 1 beat (*short*).

♦ The participants are invited to try out these instruments for themselves and demonstrate the *difference between long and short sounds*.

Box 20.6 Distinguishing the duration of sounds: II

Specific target of exercise:	Distinguishing the duration of sounds: II
NMT technique:	APT
Outcome goal:	Differentiate between and produce short and long sounds
Clientele description:	Children with hearing loss
	Rehabilitation of adults with cochlear implants
	Patients with neurological injury or illness
Session type:	Group (3–4 participants)
	Single setting
Equipment needed:	A variety of tone bars or a vibraphone
	A variety of drums and mallets
	Synthesizer or piano
	Paper and pencils for the participants

Step-by-step procedure:

♦ All of the participants are seated in a semicircle, each holding a piece of paper and a pencil. The therapist has the piano or synthesizer, and all of the other instruments are in front of the group.

Box 20.6 Distinguishing the duration of sounds: II *(continued)*

- The therapist gives an example of *long* sounds by playing chords on the piano, tone bars, or vibraphone and letting them sound for 4 beats by holding down the pedal and then stopping the sound by muting the instrument.
- Then the therapist gives an example of *short* sounds by hitting the drum once for a duration of a quarter note (1 beat) or playing the same chords on the piano or vibraphone without using the pedal (also only for 1 beat).
- This procedure can be repeated several times.
- Finally, the therapist plays *either a long or a short variation of the chord*, and the participants have to decide after each pattern whether they heard the long or the short version of the chord.
- Each of the participants in turn should then try to play the *difference between long and short* on the piano or vibraphone while the others listen and give feedback.
- As a next step, drums are distributed among the participants.
- Then the therapist and the group play together, with the therapist *switching randomly between the long and short version* and the participants only playing with the therapist when they hear the short notes (1 beat per note). (It is important to make sure that the participant cannot see the therapist playing!)
- Next the therapist plays a sequence of three sounds and the participants have to note down what they heard (e.g. short—long—long) and discuss their results together.

Variations (for adult participants):

- The participants receive sheets on which there is a template of short and fast sequences.

  Example: ▬ refers to *long,* - refers to *short*

  1. ▬ ▬ - -

  2. - - - ▬

  3. ▬ - ▬ -

  4. ▬ - - ▬

- The participants have to listen and check whether the presented line is correctly played by the therapist.
- Then the participants have to work out which line was played

20.5.4 Rhythm

Box 20.7 Distinguishing rhythms

Specific target of exercise:	Distinguishing rhythms
NMT technique:	APT
Outcome goal:	Identify and recognize whether two rhythmic patterns sound equal or not
Clientele description:	Children with hearing loss
	Rehabilitation of adults with cochlear implants
	Patients with neurological injury or illness
Session type:	Group (3–4 participants)
	Single session
Equipment needed:	A conga or other rhythm instrument for the therapist
	Paper and pencils for the participants

Step-by-step procedure:

♦ All of the participants are seated in a circle, each holding a piece of paper and a pencil. The therapist has a conga in front of him or her.

♦ The therapist gives an example of *two consonant-sounding rhythmic patterns*. He or she plays a short rhythm pattern on the conga, and then after a short break he she plays *the same rhythmic pattern* again.

♦ Then the therapist gives an example of *two different-sounding rhythmic patterns*. He or she plays a short rhythm pattern on the conga, and then after a short break he or she plays *a different rhythmic pattern*.

♦ Finally, the therapist plays two rhythmic patterns in sequence and the participants have to decide after each pair whether the rhythms were equal or different.

♦ This procedure can be repeated several times.

♦ As a next step, the therapist plays five pairs one after the other and the participants have to note down whether the pairs were equal or different.

♦ The group then discusses their results with the therapist.

♦ This procedure is repeated several times.

♦ The rhythmic pairs could also be presented in a pre-recorded format on an audio file

Box 20.8 Recognizing rhythms

Specific target of exercise:	Recognizing rhythms
NMT technique:	APT
Outcome goal:	Recognize and identify different rhythmic patterns
Clientele description:	Children with hearing loss
	Rehabilitation of adults with cochlear implants
	Patients with neurological injury or illness
Session type:	Group (3–4 participants)
	Single session
Equipment needed:	One conga for each participant
	One agogo bell

Step-by-step procedure:

◆ All of the participants are seated in a circle, with the therapist within the group, and each person has a conga.

◆ The therapist introduces three different rhythmic patterns (in a 4/4 meter) and the participants learn to play them together.

◆ Then the therapist plays one of the three rhythms and the participants repeat it together. This continues for several repetitions.

◆ Finally, all of the participants play together while the therapist leads and chooses between the three rhythms and the group pays attention to the changes and synchronizes their playing to the rhythm (there is a change of rhythm after all of the participants have played the current rhythmic pattern together).

◆ If it is too hard to distinguish between the conga sounds made by the group and the therapist, the therapist can use an agogo bell to play the rhythmic patterns.

◆ For more challenging listening conditions the group can be seated in a line and the therapist then plays the rhythms in random order *behind* the participants (again, if the conga sound of the therapist is too hard to identify, an agogo bell can be used).

20.5.5 **Pitch**

Box 20.9 Distinguishing pitch: high versus low

Specific target of exercise:	Distinguishing pitch: high versus low
NMT technique:	APT
Outcome goal:	Experience and identify high- and low-pitched sound
Clientele description:	Children with hearing loss
	Rehabilitation of adults with cochlear implants

Box 20.9 Distinguishing pitch: high versus low *(continued)*

	Patients with neurological injury or illness
Session type:	Group (3–4 participants)
	Single session
Equipment needed:	A piano or synthesizer
	One pair of claves per participant
	Three bass tone bars in a major triad (g-h-d)
	Three tone bars in a major triad (g2-h2-d2)
	One mallet

Step-by-step procedure:

+ The participants are seated in a semicircle, each holding a pair of claves, with the therapist at the piano or synthesizer in front of the group.

+ The therapist gives an example of *high-pitched* notes by playing a short melody pattern (within a fifth) on the high-pitched keys of the piano or synthesizer.

+ Then the therapist gives an example of *low-pitched* notes by playing a short melody pattern (within a fifth) on the low-pitched keys of the piano or synthesizer.

+ This procedure can be repeated several times.

+ Finally, the therapist plays the short melody pattern on *either the low- or the high-pitched* keys, and the participants have to decide after each pattern has been played whether they heard the low- or the high-pitched version of the melody

+ Next the therapist and the group play together, with the therapist switching randomly between the high- and low-pitched version and the participants only playing with the therapist when they hear the melody in the high-pitched version. (It is important to ensure that the participants cannot see the therapist playing!)

+ This procedure can also be carried out using tone bars.

Variation:

+ The group can be divided into two subgroups, one group playing to the high-pitched version of the melody, and the other group playing to the low-pitched version.

Variation (for adult participants):

+ The participants are given sheets on which there is a template of high- and low-pitched sequences.

  For example, "H" refers to high pitch and "L" refers to low pitch (the pitch is now presented in only one note, e.g. c4 and C):

  1. H H L H L L H 2. L L H H L H L 3. H H H L L H L 4. L L H H H L H

+ The participants have to decide while listening whether the presented line is being correctly played by the therapist.

+ The participants have to work out which line was played.

Box 20.10 Distinguishing pitch: equal versus unequal

Specific target of exercise:	Distinguishing pitch: equal versus unequal
NMT technique:	APT
Outcome goal:	Identify and recognize whether or not two notes sound equal
Clientele description:	Children with hearing loss Rehabilitation of adults with cochlear implants Patients with neurological injury or illness
Session type:	Group (3–4 participants) Single session
Equipment needed:	A piano or synthesizer for the therapist Paper and pencils for the participants

Step-by-step procedure:

◆ All of the participants are seated in a semicircle, each holding a piece of paper and a pencil, with the therapist at the piano or synthesizer in front of the group.

◆ The therapist gives an example of *two consonant-sounding pitches*.

◆ Then the therapist plays a note on the piano, and after a short break he or she plays the *same* note again.

◆ Next the therapist gives an example of two *different-sounding pitches*. The therapist plays a note on the piano, and after a short break he or she plays a *higher- or lower-pitched* note.

◆ This procedure can be repeated several times.

◆ Finally, the therapist plays two notes in sequence and the participants have to decide after each pair of notes have been played whether the pitches were the same or different.

For adult participants:

◆ The therapist plays five tone pairs one after the other, and the participants have to note down whether the pairs were the same or different.

◆ The participants discuss their results with the therapist.

◆ The procedure is repeated several times.

◆ The tone pairs could also be presented in a pre-recorded format on an audio file.

Box 20.10 Distinguishing pitch: equal versus unequal *(continued)*

Variation:

◆ The participants are given sheets on which there is a template of tone-pair sequences. For example: "=" refers to equal tones and "+" refers to different tones.

1. = = += + + = 2. + + = = + = + 3. = = = + + = + 4. + + = = = + =

◆ The participants have to decide while listening whether the presented line is being correctly played by the therapist

Box 20.11 Pitch identification

Specific target of exercise:	Pitch identification
NMT technique:	APT
Outcome goal:	Learn, identify, and distinguish between different pitches
Clientele description:	Children with hearing loss
	Rehabilitation of adults with cochlear implants
	Patients with neurological injury or illness
Session type:	Group (3–4 participants)
	Single setting
Equipment needed:	Seven tone bars (c1, e1, g1, c2, e2, g2, and c3)
	One mallet for each participant

Step-by-step procedure:

◆ The group and the therapist are seated around a table with the tone bars in a random set-up placed on the table.

◆ To begin with, all of the participants play in a clockwise sequence one of the tone bars, and are asked to silently pay attention to the pitch changes.

◆ Then one participant plays a tone bar and points to the next participant to indicate that they should play the next tone bar.

◆ After this all of the group members discuss whether the second tone was *lower or higher* in pitch compared with the first one.

◆ This playing procedure and pitch identification continues for a while.

◆ The therapist then plays all of the tone bars successively in the random set-up, and asks the participants whether they can identify the *lowest-pitched* tone bar.

◆ After the lowest-pitched tone bar has been identified, the therapist removes it from the set-up and places it on another part of the table.

Box 20.11 Pitch identification (continued)

- Next the therapist plays all of the remaining tone bars in succession, and asks the participants whether they can identify the *highest-pitched* tone bar.

- After the highest-pitched tone bar has been identified, the therapist removes it from the set-up and places it next to the lowest-pitched tone bar.

- This procedure continues with identification of the *lowest- or highest-pitched* tone bar out of the remaining set-up.

- In this way, the first random set-up will disappear piece by piece, and a new set-up will be built up, in which all of the tone bars are arranged in a row from *the lowest to the highest pitch*.

- When this has been achieved, each of the participants can play the tone bars from lowest to highest pitch, and vice versa.

Box 20.12 Distinguishing pitch: direction of melodic lines

Specific target of exercise:	Distinguishing pitch: direction of melodic lines
NMT technique:	APT
Outcome goal:	Identify and recognize the direction of a melodic line
Clientele description:	Children with hearing loss Rehabilitation of adults with cochlear implants Patients with neurological injury or illness
Session type:	Group (3–4 participants) Single session
Equipment needed:	A piano or synthesizer for the therapist Paper and pencils for the participants

Step-by-step procedure:

- All of the participants are seated in a semicircle, each holding a piece of paper and a pencil, with the therapist at the piano or synthesizer in front of the group.

- The therapist gives examples of *ascending melodic lines*, by playing several sequences of five ascending notes on the piano, on low-, high-, and middle-pitched keys and in different rhythms, tempi, and intervals (e.g. octaves, fifths, thirds, seconds, and mixed).

Box 20.12 Distinguishing pitch: direction of melodic lines *(continued)*

- Then the therapist gives examples of *unchanging melodic lines*, by playing several sequences of the same five notes on the piano, on low-, high-, and middle-pitched keys and in different rhythms and tempi.

- Finally, the therapist gives examples of *descending melodic lines*, by playing several sequences of five descending notes on the piano, on low-, high-, and middle-pitched keys and in different rhythms, tempi, and intervals (e.g. octaves, fifths, thirds, seconds, and mixed).

- This procedure can be repeated several times.

- After a while, the therapist plays a sequence and the participants have to decide whether it was an ascending, descending, or unchanged melodic line.

For adult participants:

- As a next step, the therapist plays five sequences in a row and the participants have to note down the kinds of sequences that are being played, where:
  - "A" refers to ascending
  - "D" refers to descending
  - "U" refers to unchanging.

- The group discusses their results together with the therapist.

- This procedure is repeated several times.

- The melodic sequences could also be presented in a pre-recorded format on an audio file.

Variation:

- The participants receive sheets showing six templates of sequence combinations, where each melodic direction is represented in each example.

For example:

   " ⁄ " refers to an *ascending melodic line*

   " ＼" refers to a *descending melodic line*

   " ___ " refers to an *unchanging melodic line*

   1. ⌃ ___   2. ⌄ ⁄ ‾   3. ⁄ ⌃
   4. ⌄ ⁄   5. ⁄ ⌃ ＼   6. ＼ ⁄ ___

- The participants have to work out which pattern was played by the therapist.

20.5.6 **Timbre**

Box 20.13 Identifying timbre: I

Specific target of exercise:	Identifying timbre: I
NMT technique:	APT
Outcome goal:	Learn, identify, and distinguish between different instruments
Clientele description:	Children with hearing loss Rehabilitation of adults with cochlear implants Patients with neurological injury or illness
Session type:	Group (3–4 participants) Single setting
Equipment needed:	One hand drum, one tone bar, and one rattle for each participant and for the therapist Mallets

Step-by-step procedure:

- The group is seated in a circle without instruments.
- The therapist hands out a hand drum with a mallet to each participant, and introduces the name "drum."
- Each member of the group beats their drum in turn after saying "Listen to my drum", so that the participants can listen to the sound of a drum.
- Then the therapist hands out a rattle to each participant and introduces the name "rattle."
- Each member of the group shakes their rattle in turn after saying "Listen to my rattle", so that the participants can listen to the sound of a rattle.
- Next the therapist plays either the drum or the rattle and the participants have to repeat the correct sound.
- Each of the group members in turn take the part of the sound creator.
- As a next step, the therapist hands out a tone bar to each participant and introduces the name "tone bar."
- Each member of the group plays their tone bar in turn after saying "Listen to my tone bar" so that the participants can listen to the sound of a tone bar.
- The exercise continues with the therapist playing one of the three different instruments and the group repeating the correct sound.
- Each of the group members in turn take the part of the sound creator.

Box 20.13 Identifying timbre: I *(continued)*

More challenging versions with the therapist placed behind the group:

- The therapist plays one of the instruments and the participants repeat the correct sound together.
- The therapist plays one of the instruments and the participants take it in turn to repeat the correct sound, while the others give feedback as to whether the sound was correctly identified.
- The therapist chooses one of the instruments and the participants synchronize to the sound and react to the changes in the instruments played.
- The role of the sound creator can also be given to the group members, with the sound creator and the group sitting back to back, and the sound creator has to confirm that the group has correctly identified the presented sound.

Box 20.14 Identifying timbre: II

Specific target of exercise:	Identifying timbre: II
NMT technique:	Auditory perception training (APT)
Outcome goal:	Identify and experience different timbres
Clientele description:	Children with hearing loss
	Rehabilitation of adults with cochlear implants
	Patients with neurological injury or illness
Session type:	Group (3–4 participants)
	Single session
Equipment needed:	Three distinctly different-sounding instruments (e.g. piano or synthesizer, xylophone, flute)

Step-by-step procedure:

- All of the participants are seated in a circle, with all of the instruments in the center of the circle.
- The therapist introduces all of the instruments by playing them in turn, mentioning their name and providing some background information (e.g. the history and origin of the instrument, and how and in which musical style it is most commonly used).
- All of the instruments should be played at all pitches and at the end with the same melody.
- The participants are invited to try out these instruments for themselves.
- Next the participants are seated in a line and the therapist plays the melody to them again on each instrument.

Box 20.14 Identifying timbre: II *(continued)*

- Then the participants turn round, the therapist plays the melody randomly on one of the instruments, and the participants have to identify which instrument was selected.
- At the end of the session, the therapist plays a pre-recorded piece on each instrument in its typical musical style of playing.

Variations (for adult participants):

- This procedure can also be used with very similar sounding instruments (e.g. flute, recorder, and organ, or snare drum, conga, and stand tom).
- For this version, a synthesizer would be a good choice, because one melody can be easily played with different timbres.
- In this case, the therapist should use pictures of the instruments when they are introduced as described earlier.
- When using a synthesizer, the therapist could pre-record a musical piece using short ascending and descending melodic lines (e.g. six melody parts). Between each line there should be one or two measures' break (e.g. ascending line/*break*/descending line/*break*/descending line in different pitch/*break*, etc.).
- Two or three different instruments are selected (e.g. trumpet, piano, cello), with pictures, and the piece is presented with each timbre (which here also can be selected from very different or very similar timbres).
- Then the therapist plays the melody randomly using one of the timbres and the participants have to identify which instrument was selected.
- To make it more challenging for the participants, the therapist can change the timbre during the breaks of the piece.
- First, the therapist tells the participants in which order they will hear the different instruments, and plays the piece to them.

    Then the participants are given paper and pencils and have to note down the order of the presented timbres. The participants receive sheets with a template of timbre sequences. For example,

    "T" refers to trumpet "P" refers to piano "C" refers to cello

    1. T T C P P C T   2. C C P P T T   3. P T C C T P   4. C C T P T P
- The participants have to work out while listening whether the presented line is being correctly played by the therapist.
- Then the participants have to find out which line was played

20.5.7 **Sensory integration**

In this way, in addition to the acoustic stimulus, different sensory modalities (e.g. visual, tactile, kinesthetic) are integrated during active musical exercises.

Box 20.15 Sound detection on strong vibrating instruments: sound versus silence

Specific target of exercise:	Sound detection on strong vibrating instruments: sound versus silence
NMT technique:	APT
	Sensory integration
Outcome goal:	Introduce or practice the concept of sound versus silence
Clientele description:	Rehabilitation of children with cochlear implants
	Low-awareness patients
Session type:	Single session
Equipment needed:	Strong vibrating instruments (e.g. Big Bom, kalimba, tomtom, large cymbals, grand piano, bass drum)

For low-functioning patients with a short attention span (e.g. after neurological dam-age) or for non-verbal individuals (e.g. infants after implantation of cochlear implants), the vibrotactile element of music may foster alerting responses (e.g. blinking, smiling, making eye contact, crying). For individuals who are not able to respond at a verbal level, the auditory and tactile stimulation of music can be a valuable tool for eliciting initial or more adaptive responses (Gfeller, 2002a). The vibrotactile aspect of music then serves as a valuable form of sensory input for individuals who are profoundly deaf or receive little input though the sense of hearing.

Step-by-step procedure:

Sound versus silence

- The instruments should be positioned so that the participants can have physical contact with them.

- For the tomtom, large cymbals, kalimba, and bass drum, the therapist places the hands or other body parts of the participant on the instrument and makes a sign to indicate "silence."

- The therapist then starts to play the instrument and makes a sign for "I hear sound" for as long as the instrument is being played and therefore being felt by the participant.

- The therapist stops playing, mutes the instrument, and shows the sign for "silence" again.

- This procedure is repeated several times.

Box 20.15 Sound detection on strong vibrating instruments: sound versus silence *(continued)*

- For the grand piano or Big Bom, if body size, weight, and other factors allow this, the participant can be positioned so that they are lying on top of the grand piano or Big Bom, or in a sound cradle.

- The therapist starts to play the instrument and shows a sign like "I hear sound" for as long as the instrument is being played and therefore being felt by the participant

- The therapist stops playing, mutes the instrument, and shows the sign for "silence" again.

- This procedure is repeated several times.

Box 20.16 Distinguishing sound patterns and movement

Specific target of exercise:	Distinguishing sound patterns and movement
NMT technique:	APT
	Sensory integration
Outcome goal:	Recognize sound patterns and match gross motor skills
Clientele description:	Children with hearing loss
	Rehabilitation of children with cochlear implants
	Children with various disabilities
Session type:	Group (3–6 participants)
	Single session
Equipment needed:	Bass drum
	Piano

Step-by-step procedure:

- A group of children is seated around a bass drum which is lying on the floor.

- The therapist introduces a special tune on the piano and the children drum to it ("drum music").

- While playing the children have to listen out for a special signal to stop the drumming and stand up ("stand-up signal").

- Next the therapist plays a playful tune on the higher-pitched keys and the children have to dance on tiptoe around the drum while listening carefully to the tempo at which the tune is played ("tiptoe dance").

- The faster the tempo, the faster the children have to dance on tiptoe. During the task the children have to listen carefully for when the therapist stops playing.

- After the therapist has stopped playing, the children sit down again around the drum and play to the "drum music" until the "stand-up signal" sounds again for them to stand up.

Box 20.16 Distinguishing sound patterns and movement *(continued)*

- Next the therapist plays heavy chords on the lower part of the keyboard and the children have to stamp their feet to the tempo of the tune ("stamp dance") until the therapist stops playing.

- The game will then start over again with the therapist playing the drum until the sound of the "stand-up signal" to stand up and identify whether the "tiptoe dance" or the "stamp dance" signal is being made.

Box 20.17 Combination of different tactile stimuli with different sound patterns

Specific target of exercise:	Combination of different tactile stimuli with different sound patterns
NMT technique:	APT Sensory integration
Outcome goal:	Experiencing three different kinds of tactile stimulation in combination with three matching sound patterns
Clientele description:	Children with hearing loss Rehabilitation of children with cochlear implants Children with various disabilities Patients with TBI
Session type:	Group (3–6 participants) Single session
Equipment needed:	One conga per participant Piano

Step-by-step procedure:

- First, the therapist uses the flat of their hand to pat the drum, and lets the children listen to the sound that this movement creates. Then the children are encouraged to produce the same movement.

- The therapist and children try to describe the sound and name it (e.g. "wind gusting").

- The therapist introduces a suitable sound pattern on the high-pitched keys of the piano. The children have to listen to this pattern while stroking the drum. At the same time they have to pay attention to the beginning and ending of the "wind tune."

- Then the therapist shows the children how it may sound when they are drumming the congas with their fingers. Again the children first have to listen and then have to try to perform the same movement pattern. This sound can be referred as "raindrops."

Box 20.17 Combination of different tactile stimuli with different sound pattern *(continued)*

- The therapist again translates this movement into a piano pattern on the middle keys. As in the first step, the "raindrop tune" should be played while additional attention is also being paid to the start and stop of the "raindrop tune."

- Finally, the therapist drums on the congas with the flat of their hands, lets the children listen to this new sound and then encourage them to make the sound for themselves. The new movement pattern can be referred to as "thunder."

- "Thunder" is also translated into a piano pattern, using the lower-pitched keys. The procedure continues as in the previous two steps.

- After all three movement patterns and their matching sound patterns have been introduced, the children have to listen after every stop for which movement will come next. They then have to identify the tune and match it with the corresponding movement pattern.

Box 20.18 Combination of visual and auditory stimuli

Specific target of exercise:	Combination of visual and auditory stimuli
NMT technique:	APT
	Sensory integration
Outcome goal:	React to a visual cue and combine it with an auditory response
Clientele description:	Children with hearing loss
	Rehabilitation of children with cochlear implants
	Children with various disabilities
Session type:	Group (3 participants)
	Single session
Equipment needed:	Four rattles
	Four tone bars
	Four drums
	Four triangles
	Mallets
	Six large colored sheets of paper (e.g. two red, two blue, and two yellow sheets)

Step-by-step procedure:
Version 1:

- The group is seated in a circle with the therapist in the center.

- The therapist hands out a rattle to the first participant, a tone bar to the second participant, and a triangle to the third participant.

Box 20.18 Combination of visual and auditory stimuli *(continued)*

- The therapist places the three colored sheets in the center of the circle.
- The children are asked to name the colors and decide together on which color which instrument has to be placed (e.g. rattle on red, tone bar on blue, triangle on yellow).
- Then the children have to work out which color is referring to their own instrument, after which they will receive the second colored sheet, on which they should place their own instrument.
- Next the therapist goes to the red sheet with the rattle and introduces the child with the rattle to play with him or her.
- This procedure continues with the yellow sheet (triangle) and blue sheet (tone bar).
- The therapist now steps from color to color, and the children react to their colors by playing the corresponding instrument.
- After a while, the children change places so that they are each sitting in front of a different color, and the game starts all over again.
- Alternatively, instead of changing positions, the instruments on the colors can be switched round and the game started all over again.

Variation 1:

- The group is seated in a circle with the therapist in the center.
- The therapist hands out a rattle, a tone bar, and a triangle to each participant.
- The therapist places the three colored sheets in the center of the circle.
- The children have to name the colors and decide together on which color each instrument has to be placed (e.g. rattle on red, tone bar on blue, triangle on yellow).
- Next the therapist goes to the red sheet with the rattle and introduces the children to play the rattle with him or her.
- This procedure continues with the yellow sheet (triangle) and blue sheet (tone bar).
- The therapist then steps from one colored sheet to the next, and the children play the instrument corresponding to the selected color.
- After a while, the instruments are placed on different colors and the game starts all over again.
- One of the children will be on the therapist's position and steps between the colors while the rest are playing the instruments that correspond to those colors.

Variation 2:

- The therapist plays the guitar and sings a song while one child is selecting colors and the rest are playing the instruments that correspond to those colors.

20.5.8 **Voice/speech sounds**

Box 20.19 Speech and sound identification: I

Specific target of exercise:	Speech and sound identification: I
NMT technique:	APT
Outcome goal:	Identify voice or instrumental sounds
Clientele description:	Rehabilitation of adults with cochlear implants
	Patients with neurological injury or illness
Session type:	Group (3–4 participants)
	Single session
Equipment needed:	Various pre-recorded songs and instrumental pieces
	CD player

Step-by-step procedure:

- The group is seated in a horseshoe-shaped arrangement, and the therapist places a CD player in front of the group.
- The therapist plays either a song or an instrumental piece on the CD player.
- The participants have to identify whether they heard a voice singing or instruments playing.

Variation:

- The group members also have to identify whether the voice was male or female.

Box 20.20 Speech and sound identification: II

Specific target of exercise:	Speech and sound identification: II
NMT technique:	APT
Outcome goal:	Identify voice or speech sounds
Clientele description:	Children with hearing loss
	Rehabilitation of adults with cochlear implants
	Patients with neurological injury or illness
Session type:	Group (3–4 participants)
	Single session
Equipment needed:	Piano for the therapist
	One pair of claves for each participant
	Music sheet of a popular song that is known by all of the participants

Box 20.20 Speech and sound identification: II *(continued)*

Step-by-step procedure:

- The group is seated in a line, and the therapist is positioned at the piano in front of the group.

- First the participants sing the song together with the therapist *a capella*.

- Then the group listens to the therapist playing the melody of the song *on the piano* with an easy accompaniment pattern.

- Next the group alternately sings the song together and listens to the instrumental version.

- The participants now turn around so that the therapist is sitting behind the group.

- The therapist then either sings or plays the melody of the song to the participants.

- The participants have to identify the singing version and join in with the singing.

- Finally, the participants have to identify the instrumental version and join by playing the claves to the beat of the song.

References

Amir, D. and Schuchmann, G. (1985). Auditory training through music with hearing-impaired preschool children. *Volta Review, 87*, 333–43.

Anvari, S. H., Trainor, L. J., Woodside, J., and Levy, B. A. (2002). Relations among musical skills, phonological processing, and early reading ability in preschool children. *Journal of Experimental Child Psychology, 83*, 111–30.

Bang, C. (1980). A work of sound and music. *Journal of the British Association for Teachers of the Deaf, 4*, 1–10.

Darrow, A. A. and Gfeller, K. E. (1996). Music therapy with children who are deaf and hard of hearing. In: C. E. Furman (ed.) *Effectiveness of Music Therapy Procedures: documentation of research and clinical practice*, 2nd edition. Washington, DC: National Association for Music Therapy. pp. 230–66.

Fisher, K. V. and Parker, B. J. (1994). A multisensory system for the development of sound awareness and speech production. *Journal of the Academy of Rehabilitative Audiology, 25*, 13–24.

Gaab, N. et al. (2005). Neural correlates of rapid spectrotemporal processing in musicians and nonmusicians. *Annals of the New York Academy of Sciences, 1060*, 82–8.

Gfeller, K. (2000). Accommodating children who use cochlear implants in the music therapy or educational setting. *Music Therapy Perspectives, 18*, 122–30.

Kirk, J. W., Mazzocco, M. M., and Kover, S. T. (2005). Assessing executive dysfunction in girls with fragile X or Turner syndrome using the Contingency Naming Test (CNT). *Developmental Neuropsychology, 28*, 755–77.

Koelsch, S., Schröger, E., and Tervaniemi, M. (1999). Superior pre-attentive auditory processing in musicians. *Neuroreport, 10*, 1309–13.

Marie, C., Magne, C., and Besson, M. (2011). Musicians and the metric structure of words. *Journal of Cognitive Neuroscience, 23*, 294–305.

Moreno, S. et al. (2009). Musical training influences linguistic abilities in 8-year-old children: more evidence for brain plasticity. *Cerebral Cortex, 19*, 712–23.

Musacchia, G., Sams, M., Skoe, E., and Kraus, N. (2007). Musicians have enhanced subcortical auditory and audiovisual processing of speech and music. *Proceedings of the National Academy of Sciences of the USA, 104*, 15894–8.

Pantev, C. et al. (2001). Timbre-specific enhancement of auditory cortical representations in musicians. *Neuroreport, 12*, 169–74.

Reinke, K. S., He, Y., Wang, C., and Alain, C. (2003). Perceptual learning modulates sensory evoked response during vowel segregation. *Brain Research: Cognitive Brain Research, 17*, 781–91.

Sacks, B. and Wood, A. (2003). Hearing disorders in children with Down syndrome. *Down Syndrome News and Update, 3*, 38–41.

Shahin, A. J., Bosnyak, D. J., Trainor, L. J., and Roberts, L. E. (2003). Enhancement of neuroplastic P2 and N1c auditory evoked potentials in musicians. *Journal of Neuroscience, 23*, 5545–52.

Shott, S. R. (2000). Down syndrome: common paediatric ear, nose and throat problems. *Down Syndrome Quarterly, 5*, 1–6.

Song, J. H., Skoe, E., Wong, P. C., and Kraus, N. (2008). Plasticity in the adult human auditory brainstem following short-term linguistic training. *Journal of Cognitive Neuroscience, 20*, 1892–902.

Tervaniemi, M., Castaneda, A., Knoll, M., and Uther, M. (2006). Sound processing in amateur musicians and nonmusicians: event-related potential and behavioral indices. *Neuroreport, 17*, 1225–8.

Watson, C. S. (1980). Time course of auditory perceptual learning. *Annals of Otology, Rhinology and Laryngology Supplement, 89*, 96–102.

Chapter 21

Musical Attention Control Training

Michael H. Thaut and James C. Gardiner

21.1 **Definition**

Musical attention control training (MACT) provides "structured active or receptive musical exercises involving precomposed performance or improvisation in which musical elements cue different musical responses to practice . . . attention functions" (Thaut, 2005, p. 196). When linked with non-musical information, music adds structure and organization, emotion, and appeal to the information in order to increase the probability that attention will be focused, maintained, and/or switched.

Attention is the ability of an individual to select and focus on a mental or behavioral task, concentrate on that task for as long as necessary, and shift their attention, when needed, between several tasks. Attention is the foundation skill for good cognitive functioning. Without attention, it would not be possible to think, learn, remember, communicate, or take action to solve problems. For more information on the neuroscientific foundation for attention, see Posner (2011).

There are three essential ways in which the brain controls attention. The first is to *select and focus*. In order to accomplish a mental task, you first must tune out the millions of things that are competing for your attention and focus your attention fully on the task at hand. When your attention system is working well, you will tune out all the competing stimuli and focus only on what you wish to accomplish. Secondly, you need to be able to *sustain* attention for as long as is necessary to complete the job. Thirdly, your brain has the ability to use your executive ability to control and *switch* attention. This skill is sometimes called alternating or shift of attention, and it involves focusing on different processes in sequence. Finally, some tasks may require paying attention to two or more events or stimuli simultaneously. This process is called divided attention. The brain achieves this by rapid switching of the focus of attention, so that it is perceived as if we are tracking stimuli simultaneously. However, physiologically divided attention is a sub-form of extremely fast alternating attention operations.

Another framework for studying attention functioning, developed and refined by Klein and Lawrence (2011), presents two modes of attention. The *exogenous* mode seeks your attention from outside of you, through your senses. For example, you hear a fire alarm in the building and your attention is drawn to investigating the cause of the alarm. The *endogenous* attention mode, which originates from within you, is a result of your goals and intentions. Along with the modes of attention, Klein and Lawrence propose four domains in which attention operates:

1 Attention to *space* involves (a) overtly searching the environment with your senses to gain useful information about the space and objects around you, and (b) covertly analyzing spatial information in order to help you to better understand and use the newly acquired knowledge.

2 Attention to *time* allows you to be aware of the passing of time, and to organize time schedules in order to accomplish tasks and goals.

3 The *sensory* domain enables you to pay attention to the information that is arriving through your senses, and to effectively switch your attention between your senses in order to examine and compare the incoming information in its various forms.

4 Attention to *task* allows you to focus on a behavioral goal and to switch your attention between the various behaviors that you need to perform in order to achieve your goal.

When attention skills are damaged in the brain after a neurological injury or illness, it is often necessary to provide rehabilitation to improve those abilities. Fortunately, attention skills are often amenable to successful rehabilitation (Cicerone et al., 2011; Mateer, 2000), and are normally one of the first cognitive areas to be targeted for improvement by rehabilitation specialists. Therapeutic music exercises provide powerful and complex sensory stimulation to the attention system in our brain, assisting in the rehabilitation process. In fact, rhythm is considered to be vital for training attention (Klein and Riess Jones, 1996; Miller et al., 2013; Sohlberg and Mateer, 1989; Thaut, 2005).

21.2 **Target populations**

Neurologic music therapy (NMT) has been demonstrated to be useful for improving attention functioning in a variety of populations, including patients who have experienced traumatic brain injury, stroke, autism, or dementia. It is also likely to be helpful in the management of cognitive difficulties associated with brain tumor, multiple sclerosis, Parkinson's disease, and other neurological diseases or injuries. Musical treatment is also useful for strengthening attention skills in wellness training, when individuals wish to improve their ability to concentrate.

21.3 **Research summary**

There have been several reviews of the literature on the rehabilitation of attention and other cognitive skills. Manly et al. (2002) reported that rehabilitation efforts have been effective in improving scanning. Functional, goal-directed approaches that encourage clients to focus on real-world outcomes have been shown to be effective in training attention. Spatial attention has been successfully improved by teaching scanning and training clients in response readiness and alertness. The need for careful assessment of attention deficits, so that rehabilitation can target the specific needs of the clients, was emphasized. The Society for Cognitive Rehabilitation recommends that "Attention skills should be seen as the underlying foundation of all other cognitive skills" (Malia et al., 2004, p. 27). Gordon et al. (2006) reported that the use of attention process training and compensatory strategies was useful for improving attention. Cicerone et al. (2011) recommended that attention training should be included in treatment after brain injury. O'Connell and Robertson (2011) summarized the studies on the effectiveness of cognitive training on attention, and concluded that such training is a "promising avenue for cognitive rehabilitation" (p. 470). They also emphasized the need to help clients to generalize their improved skills to everyday tasks.

Sohlberg and Mateer (1987, 1989) have developed, clinically tested, and researched the effectiveness of attention process training, which includes hierarchical attention tasks that target specific aspects of attention. They include sustained, selective, alternating, and divided attention. Numerous studies have demonstrated that attention process training has improved attention skills in clinical populations (Bennett at al., 1998; Mateer, 2000; Palmese and Raskin, 2000; Pero et al., 2006; Sohlberg et al., 2000). They emphasize the need for assessment of attention skills, individualized planning of attention skill training, and generalization of the attention tasks to everyday situations. Attention process training exercises also include tracking auditory rhythms via finger tapping.

Studies have been conducted that demonstrate the effectiveness of attention training in a variety of rehabilitation settings (Barrow et al., 2006; Ben-Pazi et al., 2003). In a study of cognitive outcomes in brain-injured patients who engaged in systematic cognitive rehabilitation, Bennett et al. (1998) found that systematic training of attention deficits improved attention skills, as measured by neuropsychological tests and ratings of everyday functioning skills. Another study, by McAvinue et al. (2005), showed that patients with brain injuries are likely to have attention deficits, and that giving them feedback on their cognitive errors improves sustained attention.

Adults with cognitive deficits in the age range 70–95 years participated in two group music therapy sessions which involved listening to and identifying the title of the song that they heard. The results indicated that elderly adults with cognitive deficits could sustain attention to music for 3.5 minutes (Gregory, 2002). In another study of elderly people with dementia, group singing sessions influenced attention in a positive direction (Groene, 2001).

Attentive behavior among preschool children with visual impairments was found to be significantly improved during music sessions as compared with play sessions (Robb, 2003). Children with autism who engaged in improvisational music therapy improved significantly more in attention behaviors than autistic children who engaged in formal play therapy (Kim et al., 2008).

A total of 60 patients who were recovering from middle cerebral artery stroke were randomly assigned to daily music listening, listening to audio books, or control conditions, and underwent neuropsychological assessment 1 week, 3 months, and 6 months after the stroke. They participated in standard medical and rehabilitation care. The music condition produced significantly greater improvement in focused attention than the audio book or control conditions (Sarkamo et al., 2008).

In a single subject design, the alternating attention skills of a brain-injured subject were improved with the Musical Attention Training Program, which required the client to switch their concentration between a melodic line and a drum track (Knox et al., 2003).

A cognitive rehabilitation group featuring NMT showed improvement in both visual and verbal attention. Gardiner and Horwitz (2012) studied the outcomes of 22 patients with traumatic brain injuries who participated in an average of 53 sessions of NMT and psycho-educational group psychotherapy. The participants significantly improved in ability to concentrate on both verbal and visual materials.

21.4 **Therapeutic mechanisms**

Music adds new dimensions as an auditory sensory language to the rehabilitation process of attention.

1　Music "rhythmic patterns drive attention focus by interacting with attention oscillators via coupling mechanisms" (Thaut, 2005, p. 74). Thaut's research established that music can enhance the oscillation associated with ability to shift attention (Miller and Buschman, 2011). Research by Robertson et al. (1997) has shown that auditory stimuli, activating right-hemispheric dominant sustained attention systems, can have a modulatory (improvement) influence on spatial attention, including unilateral neglect.

2　Music can facilitate divided (alternating) attention by providing multidimensional stimuli, such as melody and rhythm.

3　Music brings timing, grouping, and organization, so that attention can be sustained.

4　Music recruits shared or parallel brain systems that assist the frontal lobes with alternating attention.

5　Music provides the additional dimensions of emotion and motivation to help to facilitate concentration and keep the person on task (Thaut, 2005).

21.5 **Clinical protocols**

21.5.1 **Attention: auditory perception**

NMT technique used: Musical attention control training (MACT): selective and sustained.

Cognitive area targeted: Attention.

Brain system and function targeted: The attention system (including the frontal lobes and brainstem) and the auditory perception system (including the right temporal and right parietal areas).

Goal of the exercise: Each participant will be able to continue to focus their attention on a given stimulus and will be able to correctly interpret the nature of the information that they perceive.

Clientele description: Anyone who wishes to improve their auditory attention and perception.

Setting: Individual or group.

Equipment needed: Recorded music player (CD, MP3, etc.), recorded songs with words, a band recording, a symphony recording, paper, pencils, and clipboards.

Step-by-step procedure:

1 If you are working in a group, assemble the participants where they can comfortably sit and hear the recorded music.

2 Carefully explain the purpose of the procedure you about to lead them through, so that they are at ease with what you wish to achieve.

3 Answer any questions that the participants may have before you begin.

4 Play a recorded song with words and ask the group to listen for and note every time a certain word is sung (e.g. "back" in *Back in the Saddle*). After the song has ended, ask the group to compare notes on how many times they heard the chosen word being sung.

5 Play another recorded song, and this time ask the group to listen for and record *two* words that occur in the song. Again the participants should compare notes after the song.

6 Play a band song (marching band, big band, or dance band), and ask the participants to write down every musical instrument they can hear playing on the recording. After the song has ended, ask the group members which instruments they heard. Then play the song again, asking the group members to identify the instruments as they join the song.

7 Repeated Step 6 with a symphony recording.

Application to everyday life: For a homework assignment, participants can be asked to listen to a variety of recorded songs with a friend or family member. They should then identify the instruments heard as well as the words sung in the vocal songs. After this they can compare their results with those of the other person, in order to receive feedback about the accuracy of their perceptions. This exercise will further enhance their skills in listening and concentrating on the meaning derived from listening to other people.

Possible methods for measuring changes:

1 Immediately after taking part in the exercise, participants can be asked to rate on a 10-point scale their confidence in their ability to listen accurately.

2 A few weeks after taking part in this exercise, the participants can be asked to describe, orally or in writing, situations in which they needed to accurately listen to auditory stimuli.

21.5.2 **Attention: living in the here and now**

NMT technique used: Musical attention control training (MACT): sustained.

Cognitive area targeted: Attention.

Brain system and function targeted: Attention system, bilateral frontal lobes, and brainstem.

Goal of the exercise: Participants will be able to continue focusing attention on a stimulus from the environment.

Clientele description: Anyone who wishes to improve their ability to sustain attention.

Setting: Individual or group.

Equipment needed: Music for relaxation, and a source of rhythm (e.g. drum, autoharp, guitar, piano).

Step-by-step procedure:

1 If you are working with a group, assemble the participants in a circle, where they can sit comfortably and have plenty of personal space.

2 Carefully explain the purpose of the procedure you are about to lead them through, so that they are at ease with what you wish to achieve.

3 Answer any questions that the participants may have before you begin.

4 Begin by explaining and demonstrating the concept of *living in the here and now (LITHAN)* to the group members. Do this by "thinking aloud" and describing every intention and move made over a short period of time. For example, "Now I am going to play a song for you. First I will place my feet correctly, stand up, and walk carefully to the table and pick up my guitar. Watching my moves carefully, I will walk back to the group, sit down where I can see all of you, and start playing the guitar." After the song has been played, the instructor can again describe aloud each move made as the guitar is put away.

5 LITHAN is then practiced by the group members in an exercise designed to keep track of keys, as follows:

6 With soft music playing in the background, guide the group in becoming comfortable, closing their eyes, and paying close attention to their breathing.

7 After each person has become relaxed, turn off the music and, using piano, guitar, autoharp, or drums, establish a rhythm that is suitable for chanting.

8 As the participants take their keys from their pocket or purse, they chant to the rhythm "I'm taking out my keys, I'm taking out my keys . . .".

9 Then everyone places their keys on an empty chair, chanting "My keys are on the chair, my keys are on the chair . . .".

10 While walking toward the door, they chant "I'm walking out the door, I'm walking out the door . . .".

11 They then go back for their keys, chanting "My keys are on the chair, I'm coming for my keys . . .".

12 As they pick up their keys, they chant "I'm picking up my keys, I'm picking up my keys . . .".

13 While putting the keys back in their pocket or purse, they chant "The keys are in my pocket (purse), the keys are in my pocket (purse) . . .".

14 The group then discusses the exercise. Each participant is asked how they will use this process in everyday life.

Possible methods for measuring changes:

1 Immediately after taking part in the exercise, the participants can be asked to rate on a 10-point scale their confidence in their ability to effectively sustain attention.

2 Participants can be administered a standardized measure of sustained attention skills after participating in the musical exercise.

21.5.3 Attention: select and focus

NMT technique used: Musical attention control training (MACT): select and focus.

Cognitive area targeted: Attention.

Brain system and function targeted: Attention system, bilateral frontal lobes.

Goal of the exercise: Participants will be able to successfully select a stimulus from the environment, remain focused on that stimulus, respond appropriately, and ignore input from competing stimuli.

Clientele description: Anyone who wishes to improve their ability to select and focus their attention.

Setting: Group (four or more participants).

Equipment needed: Drums, percussion instruments (e.g. maracas, bells, wood block).

Step-by-step procedure:

1 Assemble the participants in a circle, where they can sit comfortably and have plenty of personal space.

2 Carefully explain the purpose of the procedure that you are about to lead them through, so that they are at ease with what you wish to achieve.

3 Answer any questions that the participants may have before you begin.

4 Distribute the percussion instruments among the participants.

5 The group members are numbered alternately 1, 2,1, 2, etc.

6 Using drums or other rhythm instruments, the group leader plays a simple, sustained 4/4 rhythm with beats on 1, 2, 3, and 4.

7 The group members designated as 1s are invited to practice the rhythm with the leader.

8 The leader stops the 4/4 rhythm.

9 The group members designated as 2s are invited to practice a sustained 3/4 rhythm with beats on 1, 2, and 3.

10 The leader stops the 3/4 rhythm.

11 Next, the leader plays only on the first beat of each measure with a bell or clave, while all the 1s in the group play a 4/4 rhythm and all the 2s play a 3/4 rhythm. Everyone in the group plays beat 1 together, but they are at odds when the 1s play beats 2, 3, and 4, equally spaced through each measure, while the 2s are playing beats 2 and 3, equally spaced through each measure. Thus each person in the group experiences having

someone on either side of them playing a rhythm that is different from the one they are playing.

12 After practicing for a few minutes, the process is then switched so that the 2s play a 4/4 rhythm together, and the 1s play a 3/4 rhythm together.

13 After drumming for a few minutes, the leader stops the drumming and the group discusses the experience.

Application to everyday life: By practicing ignoring what is happening on either side of them and focusing only on the task at hand, the participants in this exercise will be able to stay better focused on everyday events that require full concentration in the face of distractions.

Possible methods for measuring changes: Immediately after participating in the exercise, group members can be asked to rate on a 10-point scale their confidence in their ability to effectively select and focus attention while tuning out unwanted input.

Note: Additional MACT exercises are available in *Rhythm, Music, and the Brain* (Thaut 2005), Appendices C, D, E, F, and G.

21.5.4 Sustained attention: therapeutic music exercise for attention improvement

NMT technique used: Musical attention control training (MACT): sustained.

Cognitive area targeted: Attention.

Brain system and function targeted: Attention system, bilateral frontal lobes, and brainstem.

Goal of the exercise: To maintain attention to and follow changes in a sustained auditory stimulus.

Clientele description: Anyone who wishes to improve their ability to sustain their attention to a stimulus.

Setting: This therapeutic music exercise is usually done in individual sessions because such a setting supports the client's ability to focus on sustained attention without other stimuli or people present. However, it can also be adapted to a group setting in which several participants track the therapist's musical cues.

Equipment needed: Pitched instruments (e.g. xylophones, metallophones, marimbas) and non-pitched instruments (e.g. drums, timpani, congas, bongos, roto toms, hand drums).

If pitched instruments are used—for example, if the therapist uses a keyboard and the client uses a xylophone —the added dimension of changes in pitch/register can also be used.

Procedure:

The basic structure is as follows. The therapist and client play together on musical instruments, with the client following as closely as possible the variation introduced by the therapist.

Elements of musical variation that the therapist can use include the following:

- changes between play and rest
- changes in tempo
- changes in rhythmic pattern
- changes in note duration
- changes in loudness
- changes in pitch/register.

If pitched instruments are used, the therapist should only use single pitches or melodic lines, and never use chord structures, so that the client can follow easily.

The task difficulty should be structured around two dimensions, namely the number of change elements and the duration of the exercise.

Depending on the client's attention level, the therapist may use only one change initially for a short period of time that is as long as the client can attend. The best baseline variation is "play vs. rest", because it focuses on the basic auditory attention function of "sound present" vs. "sound absent." The therapist may then add sequentially other variations one at a time with increasingly long exercise duration. At higher levels of attention function the therapist may eventually challenge the client's sustained attention capability by mixing all of the change elements.

Application to everyday life: This exercise applies to any daily activity that requires sustained attention. It helps to prepare the client, for example, to finish reading a passage in a book or to complete the preparation of a meal.

Possible methods for measuring changes:

1 Immediately after taking part in the exercise, participants can be asked to rate on a 10-point scale their confidence in their ability to effectively sustain their attention.
2 Participants can be administered a standardized measure of sustained attention skills, such as the Digit Span Test, after taking part in the musical exercise.

21.5.5 Selective attention: therapeutic music exercise for attention improvement

NMT technique used: Musical attention control training (MACT): selective.

Cognitive area targeted: Attention.

Brain system and function targeted: Attention system, bilateral frontal lobes, and brainstem.

Goal of the exercise: To select and respond to an auditory target stimulus from an array of continuous auditory stimuli.

Clientele description: Anyone who wishes to improve their selective attention.

Setting: This therapeutic music exercise is usually implemented in an individual setting to help to maximize patient focus on the attention task at hand. However, it can also be adapted to a group setting in which either all of the patients have to respond to the selective attention cue by the therapist, or only one patient responds while the others continue to play following the basic musical outline.

Equipment and procedure: The therapist and client play together following a basic improvisational scheme, and every so often in random sequence a specific musical cue appears to which the client has to respond musically. For example, the therapist and client play on two xylophones in Dorian mode in free heterophony. At random moments in the improvisation the therapist plays a distinct melodic motif of 3 or 4 notes which has been shown to the client before the start of the improvisation and which is never played during the basic improvisation. If the therapist plays on a keyboard or on a chromatic marimba, the motif could be using accidentals to highlight the distinction. The therapist could also have a second instrument (e.g. a triangle) ready that they strike at random moments during the improvisation. The task for the client is to give a specific musical response to the "signal." One of the more basic responses would be to stop playing when the signal sounds and resume playing when the signal occurs again.

The exercise structure provides selective attention training because the client has to "select" from a large array of signals—in this case musical events—one distinct auditory event and respond to it. Music contains many elements from which to create a range, from very simple to very complex auditory structures in multiple dimensions of pitch, loudness, timbre, and rhythm, and therefore lends itself very effectively to the creation of very diversified "task challenges" to train selective attention capabilities.

Application to everyday life: By practicing ignoring what is happening around them and focusing only on the task at hand, participants in this exercise will be able to stay better focused on everyday events that require full concentration in the face of distractions. For example, the participant should be better able to talk on the telephone while those around them are conversing.

Possible methods for measuring changes: Immediately after participating in the exercise, group members can be asked to rate on a 10-point scale their confidence in their ability to effectively select and focus attention while tuning out unwanted input.

21.5.6 **Alternating attention**

NMT technique used: Musical attention control training (MACT): alternating.

Cognitive area targeted: Attention.

Brain system and function targeted: Attention system, bilateral frontal lobes, and brainstem.

Goal of the exercise: To alternate attention between two or more auditory stimuli and follow each stimulus when it is presented.

Clientele description: Anyone who wishes to improve their alternating attention.

Setting: This therapeutic music exercise lends itself well to a group setting, but can also be adjusted to individual settings, most likely requiring some technology. The exercise can be implemented with simple hand percussion instruments or body percussion such as hand clapping.

Equipment and procedure:

The clients have to follow with their musical responses alternating musical cues that come from two or more different cue sources and are distinct in their musical patterns. Each cue must have a different response so that the alternating attention shift leads to a different "behavioral" response.

For example, in a group two "cue" leaders are placed at opposite ends of the room or group circle. Leader 1 claps a brief rhythmic pattern (e.g. "long-short-short-long") which the groups follows. When Leader 1 stops, Leader 2 starts seamlessly offering a different clapping pattern (e.g. "short-long-short-long"), which the group now has to follow. The leaders "play" the patterns back and forth at random durations so that the group members cannot anticipate when to shift attention to a new source.

If the group members close their eyes, the focus on the auditory attention challenge is strengthened. Furthermore, a clear spatial separation of the cue leaders helps to focus on "alternating." If the cues are closely spaced, the patient starts to perceive a single cue with variations similar to a sustained attention exercise.

If implemented in individual sessions, the therapist may set up two sound sources spaced apart, and use remote control to activate them alternately.

Application to everyday life: This exercise will help the participant with the essential daily challenge of changing their focus from one process to another and then back to the original process, if appropriate. For example, it will improve their ability, while participating in a conversation with several friends, to pay attention to what one person is saying, switch to what the second person is saying, then switch back to what the first one is saying, and so on.

Possible methods for measuring changes:

1 Immediately after taking part in the exercise, the participants can be administered a 10-point scale asking them to rate their confidence in their ability to effectively switch attention between two different things.

2 Participants can be administered Part B of the Trail Making Test to measure their alternating attention skills after participating in the musical exercise.

21.5.7 Divided attention: therapeutic music exercise for attention improvement

NMT technique used: Musical attention control training (MACT): divided.

Cognitive area targeted: Attention.

Brain system and function targeted: Attention system, bilateral frontal lobes, and brainstem.

Goal of the exercise: To track and respond to two or more auditory stimuli simultaneously.

Clientele description: Anyone who wishes to improve their divided attention.

Setting: This therapeutic music exercise is best implemented in a group session.

Equipment and procedure:

The basic structure is as follows. The client has to track two musical stimuli simultaneously and adjust their playing when a change in one of the musical stimuli occurs. Each musical stimulus "communicates" a different musical task to the client.

For example, in a group of three clients, the "target" client plays a low and high conga or a roto tom with a low and high drum head. The second client plays a marimba or xylophone, and the third client plays a standing tom or timpani. The marimba player plays in either the lower or the upper register. The registers are separated by colored dots. The marimba signals the "target" client to play on either the low or the high instrument. The third client changes between playing and resting, signaling to the "target" client to do the same.

The "cue clients" change their playing at random moments, requiring the "target client" to stay focused on both musical cues simultaneously in order to be able to respond accordingly.

In individual implementation the therapist would have to play two different instruments at the same time and change the playing of each instrument accordingly in order to engage the client's divided attention system.

Application to everyday life: This exercise will be of benefit in situations where the participant needs to carefully attend to more than one thing, such as a traffic signal, other automobiles, and the presence of children while driving.

Possible methods for measuring changes: Immediately after taking part in the exercise, the participants can be administered a 10-point scale asking them to rate their confidence in their ability to effectively divide their attention between two things.

References

Barrow, I. M., Collins, J. N., and Britt, L. D. (2006). The influence of an auditory distraction on rapid naming after mild traumatic brain injury: a longitudinal study. *Journal of Trauma, 61*, 1142–9.

Bennett, T. et al. (1998). Rehabilitation of attention and concentration deficits following brain injury. *Journal of Cognitive Rehabilitation, 16*, 8–13.

Ben-Pazi, H. et al. (2003). Abnormal rhythmic motor responses in children with attention-deficit-hyperactivity disorder. *Developmental Medicine and Child Neurology, 45*, 743–5.

Cicerone, K. D. et al. (2011). Evidence-based cognitive rehabilitation: updated review of the literature from 2003 through 2008. *Archives of Physical Medicine and Rehabilitation, 92*, 519–30.

Gardiner, J. C. and Horwitz, J. L. (2012). *Evaluation of a cognitive rehabilitation group featuring neurologic music therapy and group psychotherapy*. Unpublished manuscript.

Gordon, W. A. et al. (2006). Traumatic brain injury rehabilitation: state of the science. *American Journal of Physical Medicine and Rehabilitation, 85*, 343–82.

Gregory, D. (2002). Music listening for maintaining attention of older adults with cognitive impairments. *Journal of Music Therapy, 39*, 244–64.

Groene, R. (2001). The effect of presentation and accompaniment styles on attentional and responsive behaviors of participants with dementia diagnoses. *Journal of Music Therapy, 38*, 36–50.

Kim, J., Wigram, T., and Gold, C. (2008). The effects of improvisational music therapy on joint attention behaviors in autistic children: a randomized controlled study. *Journal of Autism and Developmental Disorders, 38*, 1758–66.

Klein, J. M. and Riess Jones, M. (1996). Effects of attentional set and rhythmic complexity on attending. *Perception and Psychophysics, 58*, 34–46.

Klein, R. M. and Lawrence, M. A. (2011). On the modes and domains of attention. In: M I Posner (ed.) *Cognitive Neuroscience of Attention,* 2nd edition. New York: Guilford. pp. 11–28.

Knox, R., Yokota-Adachi, H., Kershner, J., and Jutai, J. (2003). Musical attention training program and alternating attention in brain injury: an initial report. *Music Therapy Perspectives, 21*, 99–104.

McAvinue, L., O'Keeffe, F., McMackin, D., and Robinson, I. H. (2005). Impaired sustained attention and error awareness in traumatic brain injury: implications of insight. *Neuropsychological Rehabilitation, 15*, 569–87.

Malia, K. et al. (2004). *Recommendations for Best Practice in Cognitive Rehabilitation Therapy: acquired brain injury.* Exton, PA: Society for Cognitive Rehabilitation.

Manly, T., Ward, S., and Robertson, I. (2002). The rehabilitation of attention. In: P. J. Eslinger (ed.) *Neuropsychological Interventions: clinical research and practice.* New York: Guilford. pp. 105–36.

Mateer, C. A. (2000). Attention. In: S. A. Raskin and C. A. Mateer (eds) *Neuropsychological Management of Mild Traumatic Brain Injury.* New York: Oxford. pp. 73–92.

Miller, E. K. and Buschman, T. J. (2011). Top-down control of attention by rhythmic neural computations. In: M. I. Posner (ed.) *Cognitive Neuroscience of Attention,* 2nd edition. New York: Guilford. pp. 229–41.

Miller, J. E., Carlson, L. A., and McCauley, J. D. (2013). When what you hear influences when you see: listening to an auditory rhythm influences temporal allocation of visual attention. *Psychological Science, 24*, 11–18.

O'Connell, R. G. and Robertson, I. H. (2011). Training the brain: nonpharmacological approaches to stimulating cognitive plasticity. In: M. I. Posner (ed.) *Cognitive Neuroscience of Attention,* 2nd edition. New York: Guilford. pp. 454–74.

Palmese, C. A. and Raskin, S. A. (2000). The rehabilitation of attention in individuals with mild traumatic brain injury, using the APT-II programme. *Brain Injury, 14*, 535–48.

Pero, S. et al. (2006). Rehabilitation of attention in two patients with traumatic brain injury by means of 'attention process training'. *Brain Injury, 20*, 1207–19.

Posner, M. I. (ed.) (2011). *Cognitive Neuroscience of Attention,* 2nd edition. New York: Guilford.

Robb, S. L. (2003). Music interventions and group participation skills of preschoolers with visual impairments: raising questions about music, arousal, and attention. *Journal of Music Therapy, 40*, 266–82.

Robertson, I. H. et al. (1997). Auditory sustained attention is a marker of unilateral spatial neglect. *Neuropsychologia, 35*, 1527–32.

Sarkamo, T. et al. (2008). Music listening enhances cognitive recovery and mood after middle cerebral artery stroke. *Brain, 131*, 866–76.

Sohlberg, M. M. and Mateer, C. A. (1987). Effectiveness of an attention-training program. *Journal of Clinical and Experimental Neuropsychology, 9*, 117–30.

Sohlberg, M. M. and Mateer, C. A. (1989). *Attention Process Training.* Puyallup, WA: Association for Neuropsychological Research and Development.

Sohlberg, M. M. et al. (2000). Evaluation of attention process training and brain injury evaluation in persons with acquired brain injury. *Journal of Clinical and Experimental Neuropsychology, 22*, 656–76.

Thaut, M. H. (2005). *Rhythm, Music, and the Brain: scientific foundations and clinical applications.* New York: Routledge.

Chapter 22

Musical Neglect Training (MNT)

Mutsumi Abiru

22.1 Definition

Musical neglect training (MNT) includes active performance exercises on musical instruments that are structured in time, tempo, and rhythm, and use appropriate spatial configurations of the musical instruments to focus attention on a neglected or inattentively viewed visual field. A second application consists of receptive music listening to stimulate hemispheric brain arousal while engaging in exercises that address visual neglect or inattention (Frassinetti et al., 2002; Hommel et al., 1990; Thaut, 2005).

22.2 Target populations

Hemispatial neglect, also called spatial neglect, or unilateral visual neglect, is a neuropsychological condition in which, after damage to one hemisphere of the brain, a deficit in attention to and awareness of one side of space is observed. It is defined by the inability of an individual to process and perceive stimuli on one side of the body or environment that is not due to a lack of sensation (Unsworth, 2007). Most hemispatial neglect is commonly contralateral to the damaged hemisphere (Kim et al., 1999).

Hemispatial neglect most commonly results from brain injury or stroke to the right cerebral hemisphere (see Figure 22.1), causing neglect of the left visual field. Right-sided spatial neglect is rare. This disparity is thought to reflect the fact that the right hemisphere of the brain is specialized for spatial perception and memory, whereas the left hemisphere is specialized for language—there is redundant processing of the right visual fields by both hemispheres. Thus the right hemisphere is able to compensate for the loss of left hemisphere function, but not vice versa (Iachini et al., 2009).

A patient with neglect behaves as if the left side of sensory space is non-existent. For example, a patient with neglect might fail to eat the food on the left half of their plate, even though they complain of being hungry. If someone with neglect is asked to draw a clock, their drawing might show only numbers 12 to 6, or all 12 numbers on one half of the clock face, the other side being distorted or left blank. Neglect patients may also ignore the contra-lesional side of their body, shaving or applying make-up only to the non-neglected side. These patients may frequently collide with objects or structures such as door frames on the side that is being neglected.

Treatment consists of finding ways to bring the patient's attention toward the left. This is usually done incrementally, by going just a few degrees past the midline, and progressing

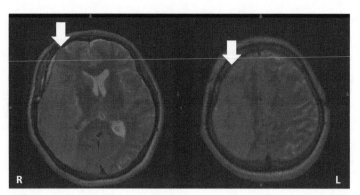

Fig. 22.1 Hemispatial neglect most commonly results from brain injury or stroke to the right cerebral hemisphere.

from there. Rehabilitation of neglect is often carried out by neuropsychologists, occupational therapists, speech-language pathologists, and neurologic music therapists, as well as by physical therapists.

Emerging treatment options include the use of prisms, visual scanning training, mental imagery training, video feedback training, and trunk rotation. Of these emerging treatment options, the most promising intervention is prism adaptation, given the growing evidence of relatively long-term functional gains from comparatively short-term usage. However, these treatment interventions are relatively new and the amount of evidence is still limited. Further research is mandatory in this field of research in order to provide more support in evidence-based practice (Luaute et al., 2006).

22.3 **Research**

Hommel and colleagues studied the variations in copying drawings induced by passive stimulation in patients with left-sided visual neglect. Experimental conditions of no sensory stimulation, tactile unilateral and bilateral, binaural auditory verbal, and non-verbal stimuli (music, white noise) were randomly applied to patients with right-hemisphere strokes. Only the non-verbal stimuli decreased the neglect (Hommel et al., 1990). In another music listening study, patients with neglect showed enhanced visual awareness associated with increased fMRI activation of regions related to emotion and attention while they listened to music they liked, but not while listening to music they did not like, or to silence (Soto et al., 2009). Frassinetti et al. (2002) reported that auditory tone presentation and auditory alerting can temporarily ameliorate visuospatial attention deficits in patients with unilateral neglect (Robertson et al., 1998).

Van Vleet and Robertson (2006) investigated the proposed mechanisms of cross-modal interaction in order to determine the conditions in which auditory stimulation affects spatial and non-spatially lateralized attention deficits in a patient with hemispatial neglect. Although the results suggest a beneficial effect of both general alerting and cross-modal spatial integration on visual search efficiency, the most significant improvement occurred when the target and a tone were both presented in contra-lesional space.

A research study in Japan by Noto et al. (1999) reported that a patient with left spatial neglect improved attention toward the left side on a cancellation test after having been trained to play a xylophone which was reversely placed with ascending keys from right to left. Using a similar training method, Kouya and Saito (2004) reported that patients with left spatial neglect extended their personal hygiene activities to the left side of the face after training with a xylophone again set in reverse, and by having the patients play melodies that emphasized ascending pitch patterns, thus moving attention and arm movement from the right side to the neglected left side.

Abiru et al. (2007) reported improvements in performance on a line cancellation test (see Figure 22.2) and a flower drawing test (see Figure 22.3), as well as reductions in left side collision during wheelchair movement, after exercises that involved playing tone bars in spatial arrangements adjusted to the severity of the patients' neglect. All of these studies are based on similar protocols with music-based exercises involving instrumental playing in various spatial arrangements to emphasize the neglect side, or arranging chord progressions or melodic patterns that move attention and movement, adjusted for the patients' severity of neglect. Unilateral spatial neglect is a major factor that can significantly interfere with a patient's activities of daily living. Research indicates that receptive and active forms of MNT can bring added functional value to the duration and effect of conventional neglect rehabilitation.

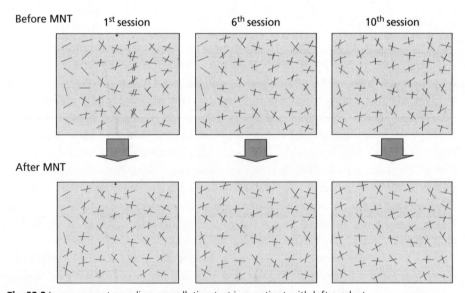

Fig. 22.2 Improvement on a line cancellation test in a patient with left neglect.

Before MNT
Session 1 Session 6 Session 10

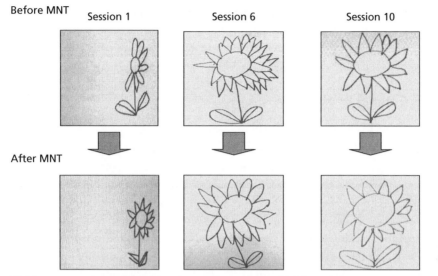

After MNT

Fig. 22.3 Improvement on a flower drawing test in a patient with left neglect.

22.4 **Therapeutic mechanisms**

It is important to take into consideration the fact that auditory pathways have bilateral projections which activate both hemispheres ipsi- and cross-laterally (Carpenter, 1978). Furthermore, auditory stimuli can be presented in both verbal and non-verbal forms. During verbal listening and processing, not only can increases in left-hemispheric cerebral blood flow be demonstrated (Knopman et al., 1982; Larsen et al., 1977), but also increases in cerebral blood flow in the right hemisphere are present. This is believed to be because the right hemisphere is more involved with high levels of attention and motivation (Heilman and van Den Abell, 1980), leading to the increases in cerebral blood flow or metabolism in the right hemisphere. However, an inter-hemispheric imbalance between right and left hemispheric activation has been suggested as a cause of neglect (Kinsbourne, 1970). Only verbal auditory stimuli may not modify inter-hemispheric imbalance due to the left hemispheric specialization in speech and language processing. Music processing, in contrast, involves bi-hemispheric activation with enhanced right hemispheric activation depending on the task and processing strategy. An increase in cerebral blood flow (Lassen et al., 1977; Roland et al., 1981) and metabolism (Mazziotta et al., 1982) has been shown to occur while listening to music, but the side and the extent of this increase depend on the strategy employed in the processing of the stimulus. If an analytic (syntactical) processing strategy is used, the metabolic increase is more marked in the left hemisphere. If a non-analytic (structural, holistic) approach is used, there is more activation in the right hemisphere (Alluri et al., 2012; Peretz and Zatorre, 2005). Thus the effect of music in neglect training may be based on enhanced recruitment of right hemispheric brain regions which are more involved in attentional mechanisms (Bhattacharya et al., 2001), and enhanced interconnectivity between hemispheres. In addition to mechanisms based on general music perception, emotional processing of music may also enhance recruitment of right hemispheric brain regions, at least during receptive musical neglect training (Soto et al., 2009).

22.5 **Clinical protocols**

22.5.1 **Receptive music listening exercises**

For patients with severe neglect, the music therapist could produce auditory, tactile, and/or vibratory stimulation through music to stimulate neglect side attention. For example, the therapist could provide live music by playing instruments on the neglect side. Alternatively, they could just play sustained and soothing sounds, such as tone chimes or energy chimes. When the patient hears the sound, they might try to localize it, and if they cannot localize it visually, the therapist could guide them to touch the instrument or feel the vibration, temperature, or texture of the instrument located in the neglect field (see Figure 22.4). Through these sensory-based exercises, the patient could become aware of the existence of objects in neglect space by the activation of visual, auditory, and tactile channels. Stimulation may be decreased gradually depending on the severity of neglect.

Another receptive technique—based on research data—involves playing familiar and preferred music for the patient(s) during activities of daily living that require full spatial awareness (e.g. eating, dressing).

22.5.2 **Active performance exercises on musical instruments**

For patients with severe neglect, simple music performance exercises on musical instruments would be preferred. In all protocols the therapist guides the patient's playing with

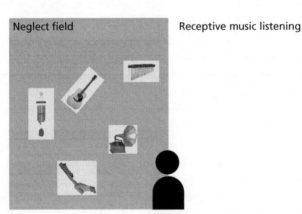

Neglect field

Receptive music listening

Fig. 22.4 For patients with severe neglect, just listening to some music being performed or even played on a CD from the neglect side could be effective. The music therapist could also play a relaxing sound, such as a tone chime, from the neglect side.

appropriate accompaniments that involve melodic, harmonic, and rhythmic patterns. To train appropriate sequencing skills, a metronome may added as an external time cue once the patient has understood the exercise pattern. For example, the therapist could set up some simple rhythmic pattern on instruments spaced from the non-neglect field into the neglect field, such as the Don(drum)-Shan(tambourine)-Twinkle (tree chime) pattern (see Figure 22.5a). Since this pattern is very simple, the patient could easily memorize "Don-Shan-Twinkle" after a few repetitions. Patients with neglect have a tendency to revert back quickly and without realizing it to the un-neglect field space. So they might play "Don-Shan-Don" even though they tried to play "Don-Shan-Twinkle." However, the auditory feedback may remind them of the missing sounds in the pattern and initiate a visual search within the neglect field.

Melodic patterns are more suitable for building longer spatial instrumental configurations (e.g. using tone bars) to play familiar patterns from the un-neglect field in the neglect field, such as a simple scale "C-B-A-G-F-E-D-C" (see Figure 22.5b). Since such tone progressions are very familiar even to a person with no musical experience, patients will seek to complete the pattern although they have run out of "playable" tone bars in the non-neglect field and are therefore being guided by the musical structure to search within the neglect space. Movable tone bars allow for precise spacing to adjust for the patient's neglect status. One may start with two or three bars centered in the patient's visual field, and then begin to add tone bars to the left. The starting tone bar should be in the midline or slightly to the right of the patient's field of vision.

The patient could also try some short chord with the pattern "C-E-G-Twinkle" (see Figure 22.5c). Even though this pattern involves a C chord, since the last sound is made by the tree chime, the sound and timbre of the progression are softer and have added tone color, motivating the patient to repeat the exercising of the pattern and moving their attention to the neglect side. Additional feedback for completing a musical pattern may come from the use of familiar songs so that the patient is guided to complete the musical pattern not only by playing the appropriate pitches, but also by following the lyrics. The patient may sing along, but such "dual-task" involvement may only be appropriate if it does not overload the patient's executive and attentional capabilities.

Finally, the therapist could challenge the patient by adding visual cues to the instruments. For example, the therapist could code by color different triads in tone bar arrangements that comprise an octave or more. For example, the C chord [C-E-G] could be coded with blue color, the F chord [F-A-C] with red color, and the G chord [G-B-D] with green color. This example would require nine tone bars, again spaced appropriately from the non-neglect field to the neglect field. In this set-up the patient would not only play adjacent tone bars in sequence, but would also have to search for "like" bars in a different location and play them in sequence, skipping over other "non-like" bars and resetting the starting pitch for each chord. Songs that use two, three, or more chords are the most appropriate musical materials. Song material could progress from easy (e.g. two chords alternating regularly, with single repetitions) to advanced (e.g. three chords changing asymmetrically, e.g. blues pattern) (see Figure 22.5d).

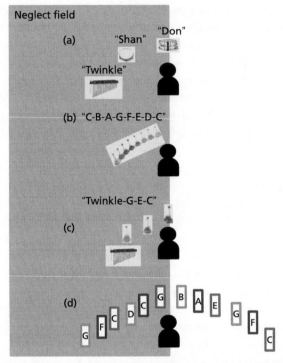

Fig. 22.5 For the patient with severe neglect, simple music performance exercises on the instruments would be preferred. (a) The therapist could set up some simple catchy rhythmic pattern from the non-neglect field to the neglect field, such as the "Don(drum)-Shan(tambourine)-Twinkle (tree-chime)" pattern. (b) During the sessions, the patient could try some longer but familiar pattern from the non-neglect field to the neglect field, such as [C-B-A-G-F-E-D-C]. Such tone progressions are very familiar even to people who have no musical experience. (c) The patient could also try some chord pattern. For example, if the chord is C, the composing sounds would be [C-E-G and tree-chime]. (d) The therapist could also present a greater challenge to the patient, from the neglect field to the non-neglect field, by using various different chords, such as I(C)-IV(F)-V(G). For example, the therapist could code the C-chord progress in [C-E-G] with blue color, the F chord in [F-A-C] with red color, and the G chord in [G-B-D] with green color, and move each tone from the non-neglect field to the neglect field one after the other. The patient could play some songs with these three chords, or even 12-bar blues.

It is important to use simple and familiar or easily recognizable musical patterns to enable these patients to recognize mistakes (e.g. omissions, missing pitches) and self-correct by adjusting their attentional focus and control of the visual and auditory field space.

22.5.3 **Points to keep in mind in clinical settings**
- Hemiparetic patients with spatial neglect should play with the arm on the non-neglect and non-paretic side (i.e. the right side) in order to focus their training on attention without interference from motor control problems.

◆ It is important for the patient to train in a comfortable sitting position with the therapist positioned on the non-neglect side of the patient.

22.6 **Assessment**

Well-researched and easy-to-use clinical assessment tools are the line cancellation test (see Figure 22.2) and the clock and/or flower drawing test (see Figure 22.3). If the patient is wheelchair bound, the therapist may also check the reduction in the number of neglect-side collisions during wheelchair movement before and after the MNT session. Observational logs for activities of daily living may also be useful, to check how the patient performs in the neglect-sided field or how they use compensatory strategies to attend to the *un*attended side.

References

Abiru M et al. (2007). The effects of neurologic music therapy on hemispatial neglect in a hemiparetic stroke patient. A case study. *Neurological Medicine, 67*, 88–94.

Alluri V et al. (2012). Large-scale brain networks emerge from dynamic processing of musical timbre, key and rhythm. *NeuroImage, 59*, 3677–89.

Bhattacharya J, Petsche H, and Pereda E (2001). Interdependencies in the spontaneous EEG in the brain during listening to music. *International Journal of Psychophysiology, 42*, 287–301.

Carpenter M B (1978). *Core Text of Neuroanatomy*. Baltimore, MD: Williams & Wilkins.

Frassinetti F, Pavani F, and Ladavas E (2002). Acoustical vision of neglected stimuli: interaction among spatially converging audiovisual inputs in neglect patients. *Journal of Cognitive Neuroscience, 14*, 62–9.

Heilman K M and Van Den Abell T (1980). Right hemisphere dominance for attention: the mechanism underlying hemispheric asymmetries of inattention (neglect). *Neurology, 30*, 327–30.

Hommel M et al. (1990). Effects of passive tactile and auditory stimuli on left visual neglect. *Archives of Neurology, 47*, 573–6.

Iachini T, Ruggiero G, Conson M, and Trojano L (2009). Lateralization of egocentric and allocentric spatial processing after parietal brain lesions. *Brain and Cognition, 69*, 514–20.

Kim M et al. (1999). Ipsilesional neglect: behavioural and anatomical features. *Journal of Neurology, Neurosurgery, & Psychiatry, 67*, 35–8.

Kinsbourne M (1970). A model for the mechanism of unilateral neglect of space. *Transactions of the American Neurological Association, 95*, 143–6.

Knopman D S, Rubens A B, Klassen A C, and Meyer M W (1982). Regional cerebral blood flow correlates of auditory processing. *Archives of Neurology, 39*, 487–93.

Kouya I and Saito Y (2004). A report with regard to the efficacy of the Japanese drum therapy carried out for the rehabilitation of a cerebral apoplexy patient: Part 2. *Japanese Journal of Music Therapy, 4*, 198–207.

Larsen B et al. (1977). The pattern of cortical activity provoked by listening and speech revealed by rCBF measurements. *Acta Neurologica Scandinavica Supplementum, 64*, 268–9, 280–1.

Lassen N A et al. (1977). Mapping of human cerebral functions: a study of the regional cerebral blood flow pattern during rest, its reproducibility and the activations seen during basic sensory and motor functions. *Acta Neurologica Scandinavica Supplementum, 64*, 262–3.

Luaute J et al. (2006). Prism adaptation first among equals in alleviating left neglect: a review. *Restorative Neurology and Neuroscience, 24*, 409–18.

Mazziotta J C, Pheips M E, Carson R E, and Kuhl D E (1982). Topographic mapping of human cerebral metabolism: auditory stimulation. *Neurology, 32*, 921–37.

Noto S et al. (1999). Effect of "xylophone therapy" for a patient of unilateral spatial neglect. *Journal of the Japanese Occupational Therapy Association, 18*, 126–33.

Peretz I and Zatorre R J (2005). Brain organization for music processing. *Annual Review of Psychology, 56*, 89–114.

Robertson I H, Mattingley J B, Rorden C, and Driver J (1998). Phasic alerting of neglect patients overcomes their spatial deficit in visual awareness. *Nature, 395*, 169–72.

Roland P E, Skinhoj E, and Lassen N A (1981). Focal activations of human cerebral cortex during auditory discrimination. *Journal of Neurophysiology, 45*, 1139–51.

Soto D et al. (2009). Pleasant music overcomes the loss of awareness in patients with visual neglect. *Proceedings of the National Academy of Sciences of the USA, 106*, 6011–16.

Thaut M H (2005). *Rhythm, Music, and the Brain: scientific foundations and clinical applications.* New York: Routledge.

Unsworth C A (2007). Cognitive and perceptual dysfunction. In: T J Schmitz and S B O'Sullivan (eds) *Physical Rehabilitation.* Philadelphia, PA: F.A. Davis Company. pp. 1149–85.

Van Vleet T M and Robertson L C (2006). Cross-modal interactions in time and space: auditory influence on visual attention in hemispatial neglect. *Journal of Cognitive Neuroscience, 18*, 1368–79.

Chapter 23

Musical Executive Function Training (MEFT)

James C. Gardiner and Michael H. Thaut

23.1 Definition

Executive function (EF) is the pinnacle of your brain's many impressive skills. Centered in the prefrontal area and extending into complex networks throughout your brain, EF facilitates your ability to create new aspirations, set goals, make plans to accomplish those goals, become motivated to act, organize your efforts, inhibit behaviors that are not compatible with your goals, initiate and execute your plans, monitor the outcomes of your efforts, and, when necessary, make adjustments in order to guide your plans to their completion. For more information on the nature of EF, the reader is referred to Goldberg (2001), Stuss and Knight (2002), and Miller and Cummings (2007).

After a neurological injury or illness, people with executive dysfunction often have serious difficulty integrating back into the community in which they may have previously thrived (Gordon al., 2006). Cognitive rehabilitation in EF is a highly important and delicate process. It needs to be approached with a knowledge of the theory of EF. People who suffer from executive dysfunction may do so because of a frontal lobe injury, a neurological illness that affects the frontal lobes, or difficulties with attention, memory, or other brain functions that are closely connected with EF. When working with someone who is struggling with executive difficulties, it is important to conduct a thorough assessment, so that you know exactly where the problem originates from. Then efforts to improve EF can be directed to the source of the problem and thus be more successful.

Musical executive function training (MEFT) includes "improvisation and composition exercises in a group or individually to practice executive function skills such as organization, problem solving, decision making, reasoning, and comprehension" (Thaut, 2005, p. 197).

23.2 Target populations

Neurologic music therapy (NMT) is useful for improving executive functioning with various populations. Research has demonstrated its effectiveness in patients with attention deficit disorder, traumatic brain injury, stroke, and in people with behavioral disorders. It is also likely to be useful in patients who are experiencing EF difficulties after brain tumor, multiple sclerosis, Parkinson's disease, anoxia, exposure to toxins, or other neurological diseases or injuries. It can also be useful for strengthening planning, organizational, and problem-solving skills in wellness training when healthy individuals wish to improve their executive functioning.

23.3 **Research summary**

After their exhaustive review of the literature on cognitive rehabilitation, Cicerone et al. (2000) reported that several studies had demonstrated improvement in EF after cognitive rehabilitation. They offered the following practice guideline. Rehabilitation of EF deficits should include "training of formal problem-solving strategies and their application to everyday situations and functional activities" (Cicerone et al., 2000, p. 1606). In addition, the Society for Cognitive Rehabilitation has recommended working on "executive skills and awareness at all stages of cognitive development" (Malia et al., 2004, p. 27).

Burgess and Robertson (2002) have offered six helpful principles for rehabilitation of EF, based on theory, research, and practice in cognitive rehabilitation of EF:

1 Use moment-to-moment feedback systems to remind the person of their goals and the appropriateness of their behaviors.

2 When clients are off task, use simple interrupts to prompt them to re-orient to their goal behaviors.

3 Instructions should be simple and clear.

4 Use reward and reinforcement, preferably actions plus verbal reward and reinforcement, rather than verbal alone.

5 Evaluation and treatment of EF need to consider competencies in a variety of settings, so that "rehabilitation efforts can then be targeted to the specific situation in which the patient has problems" (Burgess and Roberston, 2002, p. 566).

6 Rather than starting rehabilitation with the most troublesome behavior, begin training the lacking foundation skill (e.g. planning, awareness, attention) that may be causing the undesirable action.

There is evidence that music making activates the frontal executive area of the brain. In a study using near-infrared spectroscopy, piano performance produced a significantly greater total hemoglobin volume in the frontal area of the brain than did control conditions (Hashimoto et al., 2006).

Children with attention deficit hyperactivity disorder (ADHD) were administered either electroencephalography (EEG) neurofeedback, or EEG neurofeedback plus musical treatments. The results showed that children in the music group improved significantly on several EF measures. Miller (2007) concluded that the music added to neurofeedback could yield significantly better results for overcoming ADHD than non-musical feedback protocols.

Older normal adults (aged 60–85 years) showed significant improvement in EF after 6 months of *individualized piano instruction*, which was recommended as an intervention for age-related cognitive decline (Bugos et al., 2007).

Hitchen et al. (2010) studied the effects of music therapy on two patients with neurobehavioral disorders after head injuries. They found that music therapy improved functional abilities in everyday activities, increased independent behavior, and decreased behavioral episodes. They concluded that "music therapy may be effective in decreasing agitation and anxiety, overcoming initiation difficulties, and promoting positive behaviors in populations with neurobehavioral disorders" (Hitchen et al., 2010, p. 63).

In their review of the literature on non-pharmacological treatment for apathy after acquired brain injury, Lane-Brown and Tate (2009, p. 481) concluded that for individuals with severe impairments, "the strongest evidence suggested music therapy."

Thaut et al. (2009) demonstrated that one 30-minute session of NMT emphasizing ability to switch between two rhythms at unpredictable intervals significantly improved the participants' mental flexibility.

Gardiner and Horwitz (2012) evaluated the EF changes of 22 brain-injured patients who had participated in an average of 54 weekly sessions of NMT and group psychotherapy. They found that the patients significantly improved from low average to average in planning. They also improved from severely impaired to mildly impaired in mental flexibility.

Ceccato et al. (2006) have extended music applications to psychiatric rehabilitation in a pilot study. However, further research extending cognitive applications of NMT to psychiatric rehabilitation is needed.

23.4 **Therapeutic mechanisms**

Music adds many dimensions to the process of rehabilitation of EF:

1 Music stimulates the brain and raises the level of activity needed to accomplish the EF task.

2 It provides tangible cues and reminders when linked with specific tasks that need to be completed to accomplish a project.

3 It provides timing, grouping, and organization so that the person can stay on task.

4 It recruits shared or parallel brain systems that assist the frontal lobes in EF.

5 Therapeutic music exercises create a task process and task product in real time.

6 Music integrates affective and cognitive processes in EF training and, finally, adds emotion and motivation to keep the person on task (Thaut, 2005). The critical importance of extending EF training to include affective processes has been recently shown by Schweizer et al. (2011).

23.5 **Clinical protocols**

23.5.1 **Executive function**

NMT technique used: Musical executive function training (MEFT): organization, problem solving, decision making, reasoning, comprehension.

Brain system and function targeted: Frontal lobe executive control system.

Goal of the exercise: Participants will be able to improve all aspects of their executive skills by visualizing an outcome, setting an appropriate goal, deciding on a plan of action, organizing all the necessary materials, initiating action, inhibiting behaviors that would take them off course, monitoring the progress of the action, and adjusting their behaviors until the plan is successfully completed.

Clientele description: Anyone who wishes to improve their problem-solving abilities.

Setting: Individual or group.

Equipment needed: Drums, percussion instruments (e.g. maracas, bells, wood blocks).
Step-by-step procedure:

1 If a group setting is used, assemble the participants in a circle, where they can comfortably sit and have plenty of personal space.

2 Carefully explain the purpose of the procedure that you are about to lead them through, so that they understand and are at ease with what you wish to help them to achieve.

3 Answer any questions that the participants may have before you begin.

4 Have drums and percussion instruments available for the group members.

5 Start by asking the group members to picture the outcome of their efforts and the process they will go through to achieve the outcome.

6 Choose a group member, and instruct them to decide on a rhythm, choose the individuals with whom they want to perform the rhythm, choose an instrument for each person, and teach the chosen individuals the rhythm.

7 Build in obstacles to the group member's plan. For example, have another group member play the wrong rhythm, sit outside the circle, or at first refuse to participate.

8 Assist the leader in monitoring the obstacles and overcoming them.

9 Signal the leader to end the rhythm performance when they have successfully accomplished their goal.

10 Repeat Steps 6 to 9 until all of the group members have had an opportunity to accomplish their plans.

11 Discuss the process with the group, emphasizing how the skills that they have just learned can be used in everyday life.

Application to everyday life: Participants will be able to set a goal for a group activity, plan the activity, organize it, execute their plans, and make adjustments if necessary.

Possible methods for measuring changes:

1 Immediately after taking part in the exercise, participants can be asked to rate on a 10-point scale their confidence in their ability to think of an outcome, set a goal, and plan, organize, execute, monitor, and successfully accomplish their plans.

2 A few weeks after taking part in this exercise, participants can be asked to describe, orally or in writing, situations where they were able to set goals and to plan and execute their plans.

3 Participants can be administered an executive function test before and after taking part in the musical exercise.

23.5.2 Goal-setting support

NMT technique used: Musical executive function training (MEFT): problem solving, decision making.

Cognitive area targeted: Executive function, social.

Brain system and function targeted: Executive function, frontal lobe system.

Goal of the exercise: Each participant will be able to set and achieve a goal of their choice and receive social support for reaching the goal.

Clientele description: Anyone who wishes to improve their ability to set and reach goals.

Setting: Group.

Equipment needed: Drums, percussion instruments (e.g. maracas, bells, wood blocks).
Step-by-step procedure:

1 Assemble the participants in a circle, where they can comfortably sit and have plenty of personal space.

2 Carefully explain the purpose of the procedure that you are about to lead them through, so that they are fully informed and at ease with what you wish to help them to achieve.

3 Answer any questions that the participants may have before you begin.

4 Assist the participants in choosing specific behavioral goals.

5 Distribute drums or other percussion instruments to the group members.

6 Assist each group member in developing a rhythm that allows them to chant their goal to the group.

7 Help the group to join in the rhythm, chanting the goal with the person.

8 Process the reactions of the group members after the exercise is finished.

Application to everyday life: Participants will feel supported by the group members when they later focus on reaching their goals. They will also be more likely to support other people in their lives who have goals to accomplish.

Possible methods for measuring changes:

1 Immediately after taking part in the exercise, participants can be asked to rate on a 10-point scale their confidence in their ability to reach their goals, now that they have additional support.

2 A few weeks after taking part in this exercise, participants can be asked to describe, orally or in writing, situations where they made progress toward reaching their own goals, or supported other people who were attempting to achieve goals.

23.5.3 **External interactive motivation**

NMT technique used: Musical executive function training (MEFT).

Cognitive areas targeted: Executive function, psychosocial.

Brain system and function targeted: Frontal executive function system.

Goal of the exercise: The participants will be able to recognize an external source of motivation and decide how to react to it.

Clientele description: Anyone who wishes to improve their ability to recognize and appropriately react to external motivation sources.

Setting: Individual or group.

Equipment needed: Hand drums.

Step-by-step procedure:

1 Assemble the participants in a circle, where they can comfortably sit and have plenty of personal space.

2 Carefully explain the purpose of the procedures that you are about to lead them through, so that they are aware of and at ease with what you wish to help them to achieve.

3 Answer any questions that the participants may have before you begin.

4 Divide the group into pairs.

5 Within each pair, an initiator will present a motivating rhythm to the receiver.

6 The receiver will respond by copying that rhythm, and then initiating a motivating rhythm of their own, which they present to the initiator.

7 The initiator joins the receiver in presenting the new motivating rhythm.

8 After a few interchanges, the initiator performs a "good-bye" beat on the drum, and the interchange is over.

9 After each dialogue, the group discusses the rhythms, their observations, and their reactions to the motivating aspects of the rhythms.

Application to everyday life: Participants will be able to use music to motivate themselves and others. They will hopefully have increased awareness of the forces around them that are attempting to motivate or persuade them.

Possible methods for measuring changes: A few weeks after taking part in this exercise, participants can be asked to describe, orally or in writing, how they handled situations where they felt influenced or motivated by other people.

23.5.4 **Initiation**

NMT technique used: Musical executive function training (MEFT): organization, decision making, initiation.

Cognitive areas targeted: Executive function, social.

Brain system and function targeted: Frontal lobe executive function system involved with initiation.

Goal of the exercise: Participants will be able to effectively initiate and execute an action.

Clientele description: Anyone who wishes to improve their ability to initiate behavior.

Setting: Individual or group.

Equipment needed: Drums, percussion instruments (maracas, bells, wood blocks, etc.).

Step-by-step procedure:

1 Assemble the participants in a circle, where they can comfortably sit and have plenty of personal space.

2 Carefully explain the purpose of the procedure that you are about to lead them through, so that they are informed and at ease with what you wish to accomplish with them.

3 Answer any questions that the participants may have before you begin.

4 Hand out rhythm instruments to the group.

5 Ask for a volunteer to start a rhythm.

6 Instruct the volunteer to choose a rhythm, initiate it with the group, and stop the group when the rhythm is complete.

7 Repeat Step 6 until all the group members have participated.

Application to everyday life: Participants will be able to take initiative in a group setting, where they may have been hesitant to act in the past.

Possible methods for measuring changes:

1 Immediately after taking part in the exercise, participants can be asked to rate on a 10-point scale their confidence in their ability to take initiative.

2 A few weeks after taking part in this exercise, participants can be asked to describe, orally or in writing, situations where they were able to appropriately take initiative.

23.5.5 **Impulse control**

NMT technique used: Musical executive function training (MEFT): problem solving, decision making.

Cognitive area targeted: Executive function.

Brain system and function targeted: The orbital-frontal system that works to control impulses.

Goal of the exercise: Participants will be able to anticipate undesired behaviors and prevent them from occurring.

Clientele description: Anyone who wishes to improve their ability to control impulses.

Setting: Individual or group.

Equipment needed: Drums, percussion instruments (e.g. maracas, bells, wood blocks).

Step-by-step procedure:

1 If working in a group setting, assemble the participants in a circle, where they can comfortably sit and have plenty of personal space.

2 Carefully explain the purpose of the procedure, so that they are familiar with what you wish to achieve.

3 Answer any questions that the participants may have before you begin.

4 The group leader teaches the group members a simple rhythm pattern, such as "1-2-3-4", and the group learns to follow the pattern.

5 The leader then introduces an inhibition into the pattern by instructing the group members not to respond to the third beat. The group will beat "1-2-_-4" on this round.

6 The leader varies the inhibition by eliminating other beats (i.e. 1, 2, or 4).

7 Finally, the group members are given the opportunity to introduce a rhythm, decide which beat they want to eliminate from the rhythm, and then lead the group with their rhythm.

Application to everyday life: When faced with situations where they need to control their behaviors, participants will be able to hesitate, think, and stop their actions before behaving inappropriately.

Possible methods for measuring changes:

1 Immediately after taking part in the exercise, participants can be asked to rate on a 10-point scale their confidence in their ability to inhibit their behaviors.

2 A few weeks after taking part in this exercise, participants can be asked to describe, orally or in writing, situations where they felt, thought, or acted appropriately.

23.5.6 **Inhibition**

NMT technique used: Musical executive function training (MEFT): inhibition.

Cognitive area targeted: Executive function.

Brain system and function targeted: Frontal executive control system, orbital frontal area.

Goal of the exercise: Participants will be able to be aware when an urge for inappropriate behavior occurs, and will be able to stop the urge from being translated into action.

Clientele description: Anyone who wishes to improve their ability to appropriately inhibit behaviors.

Setting: Individual or group.

Equipment needed: Drums, percussion instruments (e.g. maracas, bells, wood blocks).

Step-by-step procedure:

1 If working in a group setting, assemble the participants in a circle, where they can comfortably sit and have plenty of personal space.

2 Carefully explain the purpose of the procedures that you are about to lead them through, so that they are familiar with what you wish to help them to achieve.

3   Answer any questions that the participants may have before you begin.

4   Administer a warm-up with shakers or other percussion instruments.

5   Provide a drum for each group member.

6   The leader of the group trains the group in a basic 4-beat rhythm, counting the beats "1-2-3-4."

7   The group members are then instructed to rest on one of the beats, starting with beat 4. After practicing this exercise, the group rests on beat 3 for the next round of drumming. The same procedure is followed for beat 2 and beat 1.

8   Next, the group is divided into two sections. One section rests on beat 4, while the other section rests on beat 2.

9   Finally, the group is divided into four groups by numbering off "1-2-3-4." All of the 1s drum only on the first beat, the 2s beat only the second beat, the 3s drum only on the third beat, and the 4s beat only on the fourth beat. The leader initially counts the beats of each measure, so that the group members can easily follow the instructions. As the rhythm progresses, the leader stops counting the beats, requiring the group members to keep track of when they need to play.

10 After the exercise has been completed, ask the group to discuss the experience and identify what situations in their everyday lives will benefit from the exercise.

Application to everyday life: In social settings, the participants will be able to inhibit their behaviors appropriately.

Possible methods for measuring changes:

1   Immediately after taking part in the exercise, participants can be asked to rate on a 10-point scale their confidence in their ability to successfully inhibit behaviors when necessary.

2   A few weeks after taking part in this exercise, participants can be asked to describe, orally or in writing, situations where they were able to effectively inhibit their behavior when necessary.

23.5.7 **Taking responsibility**

NMT technique used: Musical executive function training (MEFT): problem solving, decision making.

Cognitive areas targeted: Executive function, social.

Brain system and function targeted: The frontal system that is associated with initiative, planning, and goal setting.

Goal of the exercise: To provide social support that will improve self-confidence.

Clientele description: Anyone who wishes to improve their ability to respond positively to life's challenges.

Setting: Group.

Equipment needed: Hand drums.

Step-by-step procedure:

1 Assemble the participants in a circle, where they can comfortably sit and have plenty of personal space.

2 Carefully explain the purpose of the procedure that you are about to lead them through, so that they are at ease with what you wish to achieve.

3 Answer any questions that the participants may have before you begin.

4 Distribute a drum to each group member.

5 Invite each participant to choose an issue in their life with which they are having difficulty.

6 Ask them to decide what steps they can take to overcome that difficulty.

7 Then ask them to visualize themselves successfully taking those steps.

8 Finally, ask them to confidently declare to the other group members "I can_____", accompanying their statement on their drum.

9 The remaining group members, using their drums, respond with "Yes you can!", "Of course you can!", or any other encouraging remark that the group decides to use.

10 After everyone has had the opportunity to share their confidence in their ability to respond to challenges, the group discusses the impact that the exercise has had on each person, and how it will influence their confidence in their ability to solve problems.

Application to everyday life: Having received social support for expressing their self-confidence, the participants in this exercise will be able to apply this feeling to real-life challenges.

Possible methods for measuring changes:

1 Immediately after taking part in the exercise, participants can be asked to rate on a 10-point scale their confidence in their ability to overcome the difficulty they mentioned in the exercise.

2 A few weeks after taking part in this exercise. participants can be asked to describe, orally or in writing, situations where they overcame difficulties or acted with increased confidence.

23.5.8 Creative problem solving

NMT technique used: Musical executive function training (MEFT): decision making.

Cognitive areas targeted: Attention, verbal, executive function, psychosocial.

Brain systems and functions targeted: Frontal executive function system, limbic system.

Goal of the exercise: To increase creative behavior, and to allow the participants to have fun.

Clientele description: Anyone who wishes to improve their creativity and to have fun.

Setting: Group.

Equipment needed: Accompaniment instrument (e.g. guitar, piano, autoharp), chalkboard or easel with a pad of paper to present the songs, and chalk or a marker to write on the board or paper.

Step-by-step procedure:

1 Assemble the participants where they can comfortably sit, have plenty of personal space, and can easily see the chalkboard or easel.

2 Carefully explain the purpose of the procedure that you are about to lead them through, so that they understand and are at ease with what you wish to achieve.

3 Answer any questions that the participants may have before you begin.

4 Before the group begins, prepare several songs by removing key words so that the group can "fill in the blank" with a word that is related but different. A variety of songs can be used, and the leader can vary the number of words substituted (from 100% to two or three). When blank spaces are left for the words, give instructions about the type of word to be substituted (e.g. plural noun, verb ending in -ing).

5 Introduce the idea of creativity to the group, encouraging them to have fun and to let new ideas emerge.

6 On the chalkboard or easel tablet, draw a blank line for each word to be substituted.

7 Keep the name of the song a secret until the participants have supplied the substitute words. This will add to the surprise and fun of the exercise.

8 After each line, write the type of word needed (e.g. noun, proper name, action word, descriptive word).

9 Ask the group for words to fill in the blanks for the song.

10 Lead the group in singing the song, including the new words.

11 After singing the song, allow the group to change any of the words they wish, to make the song more meaningful, funny, etc.

12 After finishing the exercise, move on to a new song.

Examples of "music-libs" include the following:

1 *Home on the Range*: "Oh give me a (noun), where the (noun) (verb), and the (plural noun) and the (plural noun) (verb). Where (adverb) is (verb, past tense), a (adverb) (noun), and the skies are not (adjective) all (noun)."

2 *You Are My Sunshine*: "You are my (noun), my only (same noun). You make me (emotion), when skies are (color). You'll never know (same noun), how much I (verb) you. Please don't (verb) my (same noun) away."

3 *Michael Row Your Boat Ashore*: "Michael (verb) your (object) ashore, hallelujah, Michael (same verb) your (same object) ashore, hallelujah."

4 *Twinkle, Twinkle, Little Star*: "Twinkle, twinkle, (adjective) (noun), how I wonder what you are. Up above the (noun) so (adjective). Like a (noun) in the sky. Twinkle, twinkle, (adjective) (noun), how I wonder what you are."

5 *She'll Be Comin' Round The Mountain*: "She'll be (verb) round the (noun) when she comes. She'll be (same verb) round the (same noun) when she comes. She'll be (same verb) round the (same noun), she'll be (same verb) round the (same noun), she'll be (same verb) round the (same noun) when she comes."

6 *The Old Gray Mare*: "The (adjective, color, noun), she ain't what she used to be, ain't what she used to be, ain't what she used to be. The (adjective, color, noun), she ain't what she used to be, many long years ago. Many long years ago, many long years ago. The (adjective, color, noun), she ain't what she used to be, many long years ago."

Application to everyday life: Participants will experience greater creativity in their everyday lives.

Possible methods for measuring changes:

1 Immediately after taking part in the exercise, participants can be asked to rate on a 10-point scale their confidence in their ability to be creative.

2 A few weeks after taking part in this exercise, participants can be asked to describe, orally or in writing, situations where they were able to be creative.

23.5.9 Creative decision making and reasoning: therapeutic music exercise for executive function improvement

NMT technique used: Musical executive function training (MEFT): problem solving, decision making, creativity, and reasoning.

Cognitive area targeted: Executive function.

Brain system and function targeted: Frontal lobes/executive system of the brain.

Goal of the exercise: This therapeutic music exercise involves a composition game in which the therapist guides the client through a live composition and performance process that uses EF tasks.

Clientele description: Anyone who wishes to improve their ability to create, reason, make decisions, and solve problems.

Setting: This exercise is usually conducted in individual sessions because such a setting supports the client's ability to focus on the components of EF without other stimuli or people present. However, it can also be adapted to a group setting where the client leads the group in performing his or her composition.

Equipment needed: Synthesizers with different play functions and tone banks, drums, percussion instruments (e.g. maracas, bells, wood blocks), and keyboard.

Step-by-step procedure:

1 The therapist guides the client through a structured music composition with questions and suggestions that require the client to use EF processes. At every step of building the composition, the client or a group directed by the client perform the composition.

2 The questions and suggestions of the therapist have to require the client to respond at each step of the composition process by using EF strategies with regard to decision making, problem solving, reasoning, comprehending, organizing, evaluating, creative thinking, etc.

3 The instruments used can include pitched and non-pitched percussion instruments, keyboards, and synthesizers.

4 Once the basic content and goal of the therapeutic music exercise have been explained to the client, the therapist typically starts an EF dialogue with questions and suggestions. For example:

- How would you like to start composing? Would you like to use a musical idea or an image, picture, or mood?
- What sounds express your idea?
- Will your piece include changes or follow one idea all the way through?
- What instrument(s) do you want to use?
- How do you want to choose sound types (melodies, sound clusters, rhythms, tempi, etc.)?
- Do you want to involve a group of players?
- How will the players know what to do?
- Will you conduct?

Synthesizers with different play functions and tone banks will allow the client to compose and to be physically involved in performing on live instruments. Synthesizers also allow storage of compositions so that the piece can be built gradually by adding to it over time.

Percussion instruments allow both group and individual performances. Individual set-ups may consist of a drum set for the client and a keyboard for the therapist. Group performance specifically adds the training component of social competence and leadership.

Depending on the level of functioning, the EF questions asked by the therapist may be closed or open-ended. An example of a closed question would be "I will play you two sad melodies. Which one do you like better for expressing your composition?" An example of an open-ended question would be "Tell me or show me how you want your sad melody to sound."

Application to everyday life: Participants who learn this exercise will be able to recognize when they have an impulse to behave inappropriately, tell themselves not to behave in that way, and then behave in a way that is appropriate for them.

Possible methods for measuring changes:

1 Immediately after taking part in the exercise, participants can be administered a questionnaire asking them to rate their confidence in their ability to reason, solve problems, or create something new.

2 A few weeks after taking part in this exercise, participants can be asked to describe, orally or in writing, situations where they effectively reasoned, solved problems, or created something new.

3 A formal psychological assessment of reasoning (e.g. the similarities subtest of the Wechsler Intelligence Test) or problem solving (e.g. the 20-question subtest of the Delis–Kaplan Executive Function System) can be administered to test executive function ability.

References

Bugos J A et al. (2007). Individualized piano instruction enhances executive function and working memory in older adults. *Aging & Mental Health, 11,* 464–71.

Burgess P W and Robertson I H (2002). Principles of the rehabilitation of frontal lobe function. In: D. T. Stuss and R. T. Knight (eds) *Principles of Frontal Lobe Functioning.* New York: Oxford University Press. pp. 557–72.

Ceccato, E. Caneva, P., and Lamonaca, D. (2006). Music therapy and cognitive rehabilitation in schizophrenic patients: a controlled study. *Nordic Journal of Music Therapy, 15,* 111–20.

Cicerone, K. D. et al. (2000). Evidence-based cognitive rehabilitation: recommendations for clinical practice. *Archives of Physical Medicine and Rehabilitation, 81,* 1596–615.

Gardiner, J. C. and Horwitz, J. L (2012). *Evaluation of a cognitive rehabilitation group featuring neurologic music therapy and group psychotherapy.* Unpublished manuscript.

Goldberg, E. (2001). *The Executive Brain: frontal lobes and the civilized mind.* New York: Oxford.

Gordon, W. A., Cantor, J., Ashman, T., and Brown, M. (2006). Treatment of post-TBI executive dysfunction: application of theory to clinical practice. *Journal of Head Trauma Rehabilitation, 21,* 156–67.

Hashimoto, J. et al. (2006). Examination by near-infrared spectroscopy for evaluation of piano performance as a frontal lobe activation task. *European Neurology, 55,* 16–21.

Hitchen, H., Magee, W. L., and Soeterik, S. (2010). Music therapy in the treatment of patients with neuro-behavioural disorders stemming from acquired brain injury. *Nordic Journal of Music Therapy, 19,* 63–78.

Lane-Brown, A. T. and Tate, R. L. (2009). Apathy after acquired brain impairment: a systematic review of non-pharmacological interventions. *Neuropsychological Rehabilitation, 19,* 481–516.

Malia, K. et al. (2004). *Recommendations for Best Practice in Cognitive Rehabilitation Therapy: acquired brain injury.* Exton, PA: Society for Cognitive Rehabilitation. www.societyforcognitiverehab.org/membership-and-certification/documents/EditedRecsBestPrac.pdf

Miller, B. L. and Cummings, J. L. (eds) (2007). *The Human Frontal Lobes: functions and disorders,* 2nd edition. New York: Guilford.

Miller, E. B. (2007). *Getting from psy-phy (psychophysiology) to medical policy via music and neurofeedback for ADHD children.* Doctoral dissertation. Bryn Mawr, PA: Bryn Mawr College, Graduate School of Social Work.

Schweizer, S., Hampshire, A., and Dalgleish, T. (2011). Extending brain training to the affective domain: increasing cognitive and affective executive control through emotional working memory training. *PLoS One, 6,* 1–7.

Stuss, D. T. and Knight, R. T. (eds) (2002). *Principles of Frontal Lobe Function.* New York: Oxford University Press.

Thaut, M. H. (2005). *Rhythm, Music, and the Brain: scientific foundations and clinical applications.* New York: Routledge.

Thaut, M. H. et al. (2009). Neurologic music therapy improves executive function and emotional adjustment in traumatic brain injury rehabilitation. *Annals of the New York Academy of Sciences, 1169*, 406–16.

Chapter 24

Musical Mnemonics Training (MMT)

James C. Gardiner and Michael H. Thaut

24.1 Definition

Memory is the ability to re-create information or scenarios in your mind, based on your past experiences. It is the cognitive skill that allows you to go backward in time to re-live anything you are able to re-create. There are times, however, after a neurological injury or illness, when memory can be disrupted or even lost. Cognitive rehabilitation specialists are often called on to help rebuild and restore memory. Music can play a special role in memory rehabilitation.

Mnemonics, according to Wilson (2009, p. 74), "are systems that enable us to remember things more easily." Mnemonics refer to *anything* that increases recall. Mnemonics may be verbal (e.g. making a reminder word from the first letters of the words we want to remember), visual (e.g. associating a face with a name), movement (e.g. the movements for the song *Itsy Bitsy Spider*), or musical (e.g. inserting the ideas that we want to learn into a familiar tune).

Musical mnemonics training (MMT) uses music as a mnemonic device to sequence and organize information and add meaning, pleasure, emotion, and motivation in order to enhance the person's ability to learn and recall the information involved (Thaut, 2005). MMT uses rhythms, songs, rhymes, chants, etc., to enrich learning and to increase our chances of successful remembering.

24.1.1 Overview of different types of memory

The following is a basic overview of different types of memory. There are also additional ways to classify the various types of memory.

- *Working memory* keeps information in mind for a few seconds until it is no longer needed (e.g. recalling the name of a website from the time someone tells you about it until you type it into your browser).

- *Semantic memory* recalls information about the world (e.g. recalling the names of the world's continents).

- *Episodic memory* recalls personal experiences and events (e.g. remembering what you did on your 16th birthday).

♦ The *perceptual representation system (PRS)* analyzes and compares new information with information that you already know (e.g. you hear that Pluto is no longer a planet; your PRS still recalls Pluto as a planet, so you revise your memory of the planets in the solar system).

♦ *Procedural memory* learns and recalls motor and cognitive skills (e.g. when playing the guitar, your motor system remembers how to move your fingers, hands, arms, etc., in order to play music). This type of memory is often referred to as "muscle memory."

♦ *Prospective memory* reminds people to perform particular actions at the right moment (e.g. remembering to attend a concert on a particular date).

24.2 **Target populations**

MMT is useful for improving memory in a variety of populations, including patients who have experienced traumatic brain injury, stroke, brain tumor, multiple sclerosis, Parkinson's disease, anoxia, exposure to toxins, or other neurological diseases or injuries. Memory rehabilitation can help people with dementia to become more alert and recall autobiographical information that they have associated with music. In addition, episodic, recognition, and procedural memory training have been found to be effective in patients with Alzheimer's disease. MMT is also useful for strengthening memory skills in wellness training, when healthy individuals wish to improve their recall.

24.3 **Research summary**

Participation in a rehabilitation program with remediation and compensation has been shown to improve both visual and verbal memory. Ho and Bennett (1997) found that patients with mild-to-moderate traumatic brain injury who participated in a cognitive rehabilitation program for a median of 59 sessions showed significant improvement in verbal learning and complex visual memory. In a study by Thickpenny-Davis and Barker-Collo (2007), adults with traumatic brain injury or cerebrovascular accident who participated in memory rehabilitation showed significant improvement in delayed memory for words and figures, and maintained this improvement for at least 1 month.

Learning memory strategies is helpful (Gordon et al., 2006). Berg et al. (1991) studied memory treatment consisting of "well-known principles of memory functioning" with regard to everyday functioning compared with a control group that was given memory tasks and games. The results showed that those who learned a memory strategy improved in memory significantly more than the control group, and the results were maintained throughout a 4-month follow-up.

Visual imagery training effectively improves memory for stories and appointments. Kaschel et al. (2002) demonstrated that visual imagery memory training over a period of 10 weeks resulted in improved memory for stories and appointments, and the results were maintained over a 3-month period of time.

Glisky and Glisky (2002) reviewed the literature on memory rehabilitation and reported four successful approaches:

1 *Practice and rehearsal.* Although simply practicing memorization does not normally improve memory skills in people with neurological impairment, focusing on practicing recall of information that is meaningful and needed in everyday life can be useful. In addition, using "spaced retrieval" or increasing the amount of time between attempts to recall the information can be helpful.

2 *Mnemonic strategies.* Patients with severe neurological injuries or illnesses may have difficulty learning mnemonic strategies. However, when directed at a particular daily memory need (e.g. learning names), visual imagery has been found to be success-ful. Chaining, or linking pieces of information to be remembered into a meaningful order (e.g. remembering a schedule or a series of steps that are needed to accomplish a job), has been found to help to increase memory (Glisky and Schacter, 1989). A useful method for increasing memory for reading materials is the SQ3R (Robinson, 1970) or PQRST approach. This involves Previewing the materials to be read, asking Questions about the information, Reading the passage, Stating the answers to the questions, and Testing recall of the materials that were read. Wilson (2009) found that the PQRST method was effective with neurological rehabilitation.

3 *External aids and environmental supports.* Memory rehabilitation in this area includes labeling physical areas in the person's environment (e.g. cupboards, rooms), and using notebooks, alarms, timers, calendars, diaries, or electronic devices such as smart phones to keep necessary information at hand.

4 *Domain-specific learning*:

   a *Implicit memory* refers to the recalling of information that has been learned earlier in life, without recalling the setting in which it was learned. Schacter et al. (1993) concluded that priming (giving cues or hints to help someone to recall previously learned information) can help even individuals with severe memory loss to learn new information by pairing it with ideas or movements that they have thoroughly learned in the past. An example of implicit memory training is introducing a song that the injured person learned in the past, and then linking new information with that familiar song so that the new information will be remembered when the song is recalled.

   b *Errorless learning (EL)* is also a powerful domain-specific technique. It provides cues early in the learning process, so that the learner never fails to correctly recall the information. The cues are gradually withdrawn, so that memory strengthens over time and eventually the cues become unnecessary. Wilson (2009) studied patients with brain injuries and found that errorless learning was superior to learning by errors and mistakes. In a single-subject study, Dewar and Wilson (2006) improved the patient's ability to recognize faces through errorless learning and vanishing cues. There was evidence of continued success with new faces, and the new learning was maintained over time.

After completing an exhaustive review of the literature on cognitive rehabilitation after brain injury, Cicerone et al. (2011) recommended cognitive rehabilitation training of memory, as well as comprehensive rehabilitation after traumatic brain injury. Gordon et al. (2006) also endorsed compensatory training as an effective memory remediation strategy. Recommendations for best practice in cognitive habilitation therapy (Malia et al., 2004) include compensatory memory training and the need for training to be functionally oriented so that it can be applied to real-life situations.

Music enhances the functioning of the brain areas that are used for learning. Peterson and Thaut (2007) measured brain waves with electroencephalography (EEG) and found that music enhanced the networks used for verbal learning in the frontal lobes of the brain.

Chan et al. (1998) and Ho et al. (2003) discovered that students with musical training through experience in a band or orchestra, and through individual music lessons, had significantly better verbal memory, but not better visual memory, than their non-musical schoolmates.

Access to verbal knowledge was improved by music in a patient suffering from severe memory deficits (Baur et al., 2000). Melody and rhythm have also been shown to improve recall of ideas. Wallace and Rubin (Rubin and Wallace, 1990; Wallace, 1994; Wallace and Rubin, 1988, 1991), having studied the effects of melody and rhythm on ability to recall verbal information, established that melodies can provide cues to help to recall the words of a song. They found that melody and rhythm were superior to spoken presentations in helping to recall ideas presented.

Music has been shown to successfully improve memory in patients with dementia. Listening to classical music enhanced recall of episodic memory (Irish et al., 2006), and listening to song lyrics enhanced recognition of the lyrics later (Simmons-Stern et al., 2010) among patients with Alzheimer's disease. Songwriting improved memory skills among elderly people with dementia (Hong and Choi, 2011). Virtual-reality training plus music listening were shown to improve memory in a patient with Alzheimer's disease (Optale et al., 2001).

Singing has also been found to improve memory for names and for other verbal information. Carruth (1997) demonstrated that using singing helped nursing home patients with memory problems to enhance their memory for names of people. Thaut et al. (2005) investigated the relative effectiveness of spoken and musical (singing) presentations on the recall of verbal information, and they measured both EEG and memory recall. Their results showed superior learning and memory for the musical condition. In another study by Thaut et al. (2008), patients with multiple sclerosis performed better on word order memory when the words were presented through singing than they did when the words were spoken. Thaut (2010) reported that the stimulation by music of shared and parallel systems in the brain allows music to improve cognitive functions, including memory. Iwata (2005) discovered that when learning a foreign language, active participation with both singing and signing enhanced learning compared with a more passive approach. Musical mnemonics training also helped to facilitate verbal learning (Moore et al., 2008).

Rhythm has been shown to improve working memory for numbers. Silverman (2012) found that when information to be recalled was paired with rhythm, the recall was greater than when rhythm was not involved. Morton et al. (1990) also established that exposure to music improved ability to recall digits.

Listening to music also enhances memory. Sarkamo et al. (2008) found that stroke patients who listened to music showed significantly greater improvement in memory than stroke patients who listened to audio books or engaged in standard stroke rehabilitation.

A cognitive rehabilitation program featuring NMT showed improvement in both visual and verbal memory. Gardiner and Horwitz (2012) studied the outcomes of 22 patients with traumatic brain injuries who participated in an average of 53 sessions using NMT and psycho-educational group psychotherapy. The participants showed significant improvements in verbal learning, verbal recall, and visual recall.

In his summary of the musical mechanisms that promote memory, Thaut stated that "music can function as an excellent memory template to organize verbal materials during non-musical declarative or procedural learning" (Thaut, 2005, p. 75). His theoretical framework explains how musical stimuli improve brain functioning:

1 Music provides immediate stimulation and structure to the brain.

2 It introduces timing, grouping, and synchronization for better organization.

3 It recruits shared or parallel brain systems to assist in finishing the work at hand.

4 Finally, music adds emotion and motivation to the process.

24.4 **Therapeutic mechanisms**

Figure 24.1 provides a summary of the principles and techniques for memory improvement, presented in acronym form to help the reader to recall the principles.

24.5 **Clinical protocols**

24.5.1 **Memory for names: rhythm and chanting**

NMT technique used: Musical mnemonics training (MMT).

Brain system and function targeted: Memory system, including the prefrontal lobes, hippocampus, limbic system, and cerebellum.

Goal of the exercise: Participants will be able to recall the names of the other group members after the session. Their ability to recall the names of new people they meet after the session will also be increased.

Clientele description: Anyone who wishes to improve their memory skills.

Setting: Group.

Equipment needed: Drums, percussion instruments (e.g. maracas, bells, wood blocks).

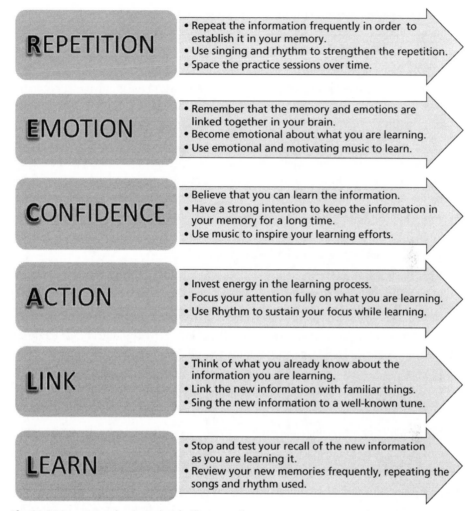

Fig. 24.1 Memory mechanisms that facilitate recall.

Step-by-step procedure:

1 Assemble the participants in a circle, where they can comfortably sit and have plenty of personal space.

2 Carefully explain the goal of the procedure you are about to lead them through, so that they are at ease with what you wish to achieve.

3 Answer any questions that the participants may have before you begin.

4 Distribute the rhythm instruments to the participants.

5 Warm up the group with rhythm practice.

6 Demonstrate how rhythms can be applied to names (e.g. George Washington, John F. Kennedy, or names of admired individuals suggested by group members).

7 The leader demonstrates how their own name can be learned by clearly stating their name, starting a rhythm that matches their name, saying their name repeatedly to the rhythm, inviting the group to join in by drumming the rhythm and chanting the leader's name, and bringing the process to a close.

8 Each group member is then invited to teach their name to the group by clearly stating their name, making up a rhythm for their name, leading the group in chanting their name to the rhythm, and stopping the group with a signal when they have finished.

9 When learning the names of other group members, each participant is asked to look at the person whose name is being learned, carefully study the features of the person's face, follow the rhythm on his or her own musical instrument, and chant the person's name.

10 After three or four group members have presented their names, the leader guides the group in a review of the names that have been learned so far. The review is initiated periodically until the exercise has been completed.

11 After the learning has been completed, the participants can be given the opportunity to recite the names of all the group members, in order to test their new memory skills.

Variations: Ask each person to form an association device for their name and present it to the group musically, with action included. For example, Tony could drum his name and after the first beat point to his toe and after the second beat point to his knee.

Application to everyday life: The memory principles of action, repetition, rhythm, and spaced rehearsals can be applied to other learning and memory tasks, such as recalling a schedule or learning the name of a new acquaintance.

Possible methods for measuring changes:

1 Immediately after taking part in the exercise, participants can be asked to rate on a 10-point scale their confidence in their ability to remember information.

2 A few weeks after taking part in this exercise, participants can be asked to describe, orally or in writing, situations where they were able to more effectively remember information.

3 Participants can be administered a standardized memory test to measure their skills before and after taking part in the musical exercise.

24.5.2 Remembering a list

NMT technique used: Musical mnemonics training (MMT): declarative mnemonics, semantic and episodic memory.

Brain system and function targeted: Memory consolidation and recall system involving the bilateral temporal lobes, limbic system, and cerebellum.

Goal of the exercise: Participants will be able to recall a list of words, such as a shopping list.

Clientele description: Anyone who wishes or needs to improve their semantic memory skills.

Setting: Individual or group.

Equipment needed: A chalkboard or sketch pad on which to write words, a variety of percussion instruments, and a musical instrument such as a guitar, piano, or autoharp to accompany group singing.

Step-by-step procedure:

1 If working in a group setting, assemble the participants where they can comfortably sit, have plenty of personal space, and are able to see the words presented.

2 Carefully explain the goal of the procedure you are about to lead them through, so that they understand and are at ease with what you wish to achieve.

3 Answer any questions that the participants may have before you begin.

4 Distribute the rhythm instruments to the participants.

5 Warm up the group with rhythm practice.

6 Introduce the group to the following list of 15 words to be learned in the session: dog, sky, lake, tree, flag, car, dress, train, quilt, apple, cup, penny, sunshine, road, boot.

7 If the group wishes, they can make up the list of words (such as a shopping list), so that it will be meaningful to them.

8 Make up a lively rhythm which will be fun to play and that includes all 15 words.

9 Lead the group in repeatedly chanting the words to the rhythm and accompanying the rhythm with their instruments.

10 Ask the group to recite the list of words.

11 Allow the group to rest by singing a song that is unrelated to the words.

12 Ask them to recite the list of words again.

13 Reintroduce the list of words in a song that is lively and fun to perform.

14 Teach the song to the group members and repeat it several times, as they use their instruments.

15 Ask them to recite the list of words.

16 Reorganize the words into a meaningful order (e.g. place the dog in a dress in a car by a lake near an apple tree with a train going by with a flag quilt waving from the back).

17 Make up a new song about the newly ordered words.

18 Teach the song to the group members and repeat it several times, as they use their instruments.

19 Ask them to recite the list of words.

Application to everyday life: Ask the participants to discuss how they will be able to learn, retain and use new information, such as a shopping list, that they encounter in everyday life.

Possible methods for measuring changes:

1 Immediately after taking part in the exercise, participants can be asked to rate on a 10-point scale their confidence in their ability to learn, retain, and use new information.

2 A few weeks after taking part in this exercise, participants can be asked to describe, orally or in writing, situations where they needed to recall information, and whether or not they were able to do so.

3 Participants can be administered a standardized memory test to measure their memory skills before and after taking part in the musical memory exercise.

24.5.3 Peg list memory

NMT technique used: Musical mnemonics training (MMT): declarative mnemonics, semantic memory.

Brain system and function targeted: Memory systems in the brain, including the bilateral temporal lobes, hippocampus, limbic system, and cerebellum.

Goal of the exercise: Participants will be able to recall a list of recently learned verbal information, such as a shopping list.

Clientele description: Anyone who wishes to improve their memory skills.

Setting: Individual or group.

Equipment needed: Accompaniment instrument (guitar, piano, or autoharp), drums, percussion instruments (e.g. maracas, bells, wood blocks).

Step-by-step procedure:

1 If working in a group, assemble the participants in a circle, where they can comfortably sit and have plenty of personal space.

2 Carefully explain the goal of the procedure you are about to lead them through, so that they are at ease with what you wish to achieve.

3 Answer any questions that the participants may have before you begin.

4 Teach the group how to use the body peg list, by associating and chaining information with something familiar. For example, suppose that you wish to buy eggs, and want to remember them by associating them with your hair. Imagine that you break several eggs on top of your head and let their contents soak into your hair. The senses and emotional reactions to the image will make the memory very strong.

5 The pegs on the body peg list are the hair, eyes, nose, mouth, chin, shoulders, waist, thighs, knees, and feet.

6 Ask the group to construct a shopping list of 10 items.

7 Once the 10 items have been chosen by the group, improvise a song and teach it to them, placing the items in the blanks below:

8 "I have _____ in my hair and _____ in my eyes, and I have some _____ in my nose. I have _____ in my mouth and ___ on my chin, and my shoulders carry some _____. _____ are hanging from my waist, _____ are on my thighs, with _____ on my knees, and _____ between my toes."

9 Practice the song several times, with the group singing together and using percussion instruments to provide the rhythm.

10 Ask the group to recall the 10 items, first using the song, and then without the song.

Application to everyday life: Participants will be able to use the body peg song in everyday life to learn a list of procedures, shopping items, etc.

Possible methods for measuring changes:

1 Immediately after taking part in the exercise, participants can be asked to rate on a 10-point scale their confidence in their ability to remember important information.

2 A few weeks after taking part in this exercise, participants can be asked to describe, orally or in writing, situations where they were able to learn and retain new information.

3 Participants can be administered a standardized memory test to measure their skills before and after taking part in the musical exercise.

24.5.4 Episodic memory

NMT technique used: Musical mnemonics training (MMT): episodic memory.

Brain system and function targeted: Memory systems in the brain, including the bilateral temporal lobes, hippocampus, limbic system, and cerebellum.

Goal of the exercise: Participants will be able to recall additional important and meaningful information from their past life.

Clientele description: Anyone who wishes to revive memories of past experiences.

Setting: Group.

Equipment needed: Drums, percussion instruments (e.g. maracas, bells, wood blocks).

Step-by-step procedure:

1 Assemble the participants in a circle, where they can comfortably sit and have plenty of personal space.

2 Carefully explain the purpose of the procedure that you are about to lead them through, so that they are at ease with what you wish to achieve.

3 Answer any questions that the participants may have before you begin.

4 Ask each participant or a family member to make a list of important events in their past life.

5 Hand out the rhythm instruments to the group members.

6 Ask each group member to choose an important event from their past. Using rhythm instruments, the group develops a chant to commemorate that event (e.g. "In 1963, I went to Vietnam").

7 If group members have a difficult time recalling events, the leader can play music that was popular between 15 and 25 years after the year of their birth. The music will be used to bring back memories of their late teens and early adulthood.

8 Continue until each group member has had the opportunity to participate.

9 Discuss the outcome with the group. What memories were brought back by listening to the important events of the other group members?

Application to everyday life: This exercise can help participants to recall memories that they need to deal with in counseling or when exploring the meaning of their life.

Possible methods for measuring changes:

1 A few weeks after taking part in this exercise, participants can be asked to describe, orally or in writing, situations where they felt, thought, or acted differently as a result of recalling memories from their past.

2 Participants can be administered a brief emotional adjustment questionnaire such as the Brief Symptom Inventory 18 to measure their emotions before and after taking part in the musical exercise.

24.5.5 Memory for rhythms

NMT technique used: Musical mnemonics training (MMT).

Brain system and function targeted: Memory system, including the prefrontal lobes, hippocampus, and cerebellum.

Goal of the exercise: Participants will improve their ability to recall and name a behavioral process.

Clientele description: Anyone who wishes to improve their memory skills.

Setting: Individual or group.

Equipment needed: Drums, percussion instruments (e.g. maracas, bells, wood blocks).

Step-by-step procedure:

1 If a group is involved, assemble the participants in a circle, where they can comfortably sit and have plenty of personal space.

2 Carefully explain the purpose of the procedure that you are about to lead them through, so that they are at ease with what you wish to help them to achieve.

3 Answer any questions that the participants may have before you begin.

4 Conduct a warm-up with shakers, so that the participants feel comfortable with rhythms.

5 The leader introduces a rhythm to the group and gives a name to the rhythm. It is helpful if the rhythm and the name are closely related, and if the name is meaningful to the group (e.g. the name of a local attraction) or is related to the purpose of the group (e.g. one of my former groups named themselves the "Rhythm Builders" and built a signature rhythm associated with that name).

6 After practicing the leader's rhythm, the group members are encouraged to choose a meaningful name and to construct a rhythm around that name.

7 The group practices the rhythm while reciting the name or phrase associated with it.

8 After trying several rhythms, the group chooses one of these and practices it at length. They are asked to remember both the rhythm and its name.

9 The group engages in other activities, unrelated to the rhythm.

10 The leader periodically returns to the rhythm by asking the group to recall the name of the rhythm and to demonstrate their memory of the rhythm.

11 If the group meets again at subsequent meetings, the rhythm can be brought up so that the memory can be renewed.

12 Other rhythms can be created by the group, named, and made part of the developing culture of the group.

Application to everyday life: The memory principles of action, repetition, rhythm, and spaced rehearsals can be applied to other learning and memory tasks, such as recalling a schedule or learning the name of a new acquaintance.

Possible methods for measuring changes:

1 Immediately after taking part in the exercise, participants can be asked to rate their confidence in their ability to remember information.

2 A few weeks after taking part in the exercise, participants can be asked to describe, orally or in writing, situations where they were able to more effectively remember information.

3 Participants can be administered a standardized memory test to measure their skills before and after taking part in the musical exercise.

24.5.6 Name that tune: individual and "free for all"

NMT techniques used: Musical mnemonics training (MMT): declarative mnemonics, semantic and episodic memory.

Cognitive areas targeted: Declarative memory.

Brain system and function targeted: Temporal lobe memory retrieval systems, frontal lobe attention systems, limbic system, and prefrontal executive function systems for problem solving and initiation.

Goal of the exercise: Participants will be able to listen attentively to important information, make appropriate decisions about the information, and initiate communications about those decisions.

Clientele description: Anyone who wishes to improve their memory and communication skills.

Setting: Group.

Equipment needed: Recorded music player (e.g. CD player, MP3 player) and a wide variety of recorded songs.

Step-by-step procedure: individual

1 Assemble the participants where they can comfortably sit, hear the recorded music, and have adequate personal space.

2 Carefully explain the purpose of the procedure that you are about to lead them through, so that they are at ease with what you wish to achieve.

3 Answer any questions that the participants may have before you begin.

4 Group members take turns at sitting in the "Hot Seat" (which can be designated as the chair they are already sitting in), where they listen to one song and are asked to recall the title, artist, and (if appropriate) composer of the song.

5 One point is awarded for each correct answer (i.e. title, artist, and composer), so a maximum total of three points is possible for each song presented.

6 If the participant does not know any of the answers, they can ask the audience (i.e. the other group members), and choose what they think is the best answer from the audience. If it is correct, they are awarded a point for each correct answer.

7 If the audience members give an incorrect answer, the contestant is then given two or three possible answers, and if they guess the right one, they can still be awarded a point.

8 After all of the group members have been given an equal number of opportunities in the "Hot Seat", the points are tallied. The person with the highest number of points is the winner.

Step-by-step procedure: free for all

1 The group members listen to a song and are asked to recall the title, artist, and (if appropriate) composer of the song.

2 The first person to raise their hand is called on to give an answer to these questions.

3 One point is awarded for each correct answer (title, artist, and composer).

4 If the person gives any incorrect information, other group members are given the opportunity to raise their hands to provide the correct answer.

5 An alarm will be set to go off when the allotted time for the session is up. The person with the most points when the alarm sounds is the winner.

Variations:

1 Present the group with different categories of music (e.g. big band, country and western, rock 'n' roll, classical, blues, gospel, jazz, Latin). When each person takes the "Hot Seat", they have to try to identify a song played from the category that they choose.

2 Extra points can be given for trivia about the song, such as the year in which it was written, the name of a movie in which it featured, or the name of another artist who has recorded it.

3 If the song title is included in the lyrics of the song, the group leader (with forewarning to the group) points to the music speakers (or signals in some other way) at the time when the title is being sung, to give the participants a cue to concentrate on the music lyrics and thus identify the title.

4 Provide paper and pencils for the participants, so that all of the responses can be written down.

5 If there is no recall of a song by the group or individual, use priming to help them to recall the answers. For example, if the song is *My Way* by Frank Sinatra, the leader may use hints such as "The song title starts with M" or "The song title has two words, starting with M and W" or "The artist is nicknamed 'Blue Eyes.'"

Application to everyday life: This exercise is designed to increase the participants' alertness and their memory-searching, initiation, decision-making, and communication skills. These skills should benefit them in a variety of everyday settings, such as recalling their family history and communicating it to close family members, or recalling information learned from reading in order to help complete a group project.

Possible methods for measuring changes:

1 Immediately after taking part in the exercise, participants can be asked to rate on a 10-point scale their confidence in their ability to remember important information, make decisions, and communicate the results of those decisions.

2 Participants can be administered a standardized memory test to measure their skills before and after taking part in the musical exercise.

24.5.7 **Prospective memory**

NMT technique used: Musical mnemonics training (MMT): declarative mnemonics, semantic and prospective memory.

Brain system and function targeted: A combination of the memory system in the bilateral temporal lobes and the initiation center in the prefrontal cortex.

Goal of the exercise: Participants will be able to perform an action in the future, at the time when the action is intended.

Clientele description: Anyone who wishes to improve their prospective memory skills.

Setting: Individual or group.

Equipment needed: Drums, percussion instruments (e.g. maracas, bells, wood blocks).

Step-by-step procedure:

1 If you are working in a group setting, assemble the participants in a circle, where they can comfortably sit and have plenty of personal space.

2 Carefully explain the purpose of the procedure that you are about to lead them through, so that they are at ease with what you wish to help them to achieve.

3 Answer any questions that the participants may have before you begin.

4 Distribute the rhythm instruments to the participants.

5 Choose a future event (e.g. next week's group, or an appointment or task).

6 Establish a rhythm based on a phrase such as "I come to group next Wednesday at three!" or "I winterize my home by October 1."

7 Teach the group how to use this technique to recall an appointment that they need to attend or a task that they need to remember to do.

8 Each person in turn states an important event in their near future.

9 Together the group perform a rhythm, but only the person who needs to recall the event will chant the date and time of the event.

10 The process continues until each person has had the opportunity to memorize an event with rhythm.

11 Finally, the group discusses how the technique can be used in everyday life.

Application to everyday life: Participants will be able to use their prospective memory skills to remember to attend appointments, perform maintenance on machines, schedule medical care appointments, etc.

Possible methods for measuring changes:

1 Immediately after taking part in the exercise, participants can be asked to rate on a 10-point scale their confidence in their ability to remember important appointments or tasks that they need to complete in the future.

2 A few weeks after taking part in this exercise, participants can be asked to describe, orally or in writing, situations where they were able to recall needed information in order to act appropriately.

3 Participants can be administered a standardized memory test to measure their skills before and after taking part in the musical exercise.

References

Baur, B. et al. (2000). Music memory provides access to verbal knowledge in a patient with global amnesia. *Neurocase*, 6, 415–21.

Berg, I. J., Koning-Haanstra, M., and Deelman, B. G. (1991). Long-term effects of memory rehabilitation: a controlled study. *Neuropsychological Rehabilitation*, 1, 97–111.

Carruth, E. K. (1997). The effects of singing and the spaced retrieval technique on improving face-name recognition in nursing home residents with memory loss. *Journal of Music Therapy*, 34, 165–86.

Chan, A. S., Ho, Y. C., and Cheung, M. C. (1998). Music training improves verbal memory. *Nature*, 396, 128.

Cicerone, K. D. et al. (2011). Evidence-based cognitive rehabilitation: updated review of the literature from 2003 through 2008. *Archives of Physical Medicine and Rehabilitation*, 92, 519–30.

Dewar, B. and Wilson, B. A. (2006). Training face identification in prosopagnosia. *Brain Impairment*, 7, 160.

Gardiner, J. C. and Horwitz, J. L. (2012). *Evaluation of a cognitive rehabilitation group featuring neurologic music therapy and group psychotherapy*. Unpublished manuscript.

Glisky, E. L. and Schacter, D. L. (1989). Extending the limits of complex learning in organic amnesia: computer training in a vocational domain. *Neuropsychologia*, 25, 107–20.

Glisky, E. L. and Glisky, M. L. (2002). Learning and memory impairments. In: P. J. Eslinger (ed.) *Neuropsychological Interventions: clinical research and practice*. New York: Guilford. pp. 137–62.

Gordon, W. A. et al. (2006). Traumatic brain injury rehabilitation: state of the science. *American Journal of Physical Medicine and Rehabilitation*, 85, 343–82.

Ho, M. R. and Bennett, T. L. (1997). Efficacy of neuropsychological rehabilitation for mild-moderate traumatic brain injury. *Archives of Clinical Neuropsychology, 12,* 1–11.

Ho, Y. C., Cheung, M. C., and Chan, A. S. (2003). Music training improves verbal but not visual memory: cross-sectional and longitudinal explorations in children. *Neuropsychology, 17,* 439–50.

Hong, I. S. and Choi, M. J. (2011). Songwriting oriented activities improve the cognitive functions of the aged with dementia. *Arts in Psychotherapy, 38,* 221–8.

Irish, M. et al. (2006). Investigating the enhancing effect of music on autobiographical memory in mild Alzheimer's disease. *Dementia and Geriatric Cognitive Disorders, 22,* 108–20.

Iwata, K. (2005). *The effect of active and passive participation with music on the foreign language acquisition and emotional state of university students.* Master's Thesis. Tallahassee, FL: Florida State University.

Kaschel, R. et al. (2002). Imagery mnemonics for the rehabilitation of memory: a randomised group controlled trial. *Neuropsychological Rehabilitation, 12,* 127–53.

Malia, K. et al. (2004). *Recommendations for Best Practice in Cognitive Rehabilitation Therapy: acquired brain injury.* Exton, PA: Society for Cognitive Rehabilitation. http://www.societyforcognitiverehab. org/membership-and-certification/documents/EditedRecsBestPrac.pdf

Moore, K. S. et al. (2008). The effectiveness of music as a mnemonic device on recognition memory for people with multiple sclerosis. *Journal of Music Therapy, 45,* 307–29.

Morton, L. L., Kershner, J. R., and Siegel, L. S. (1990). The potential for therapeutic applications of music on problems related to memory and attention. *Journal of Music Therapy, 26,* 58–70.

Optale, G. et al. (2001). Music-enhanced immersive virtual reality in the rehabilitation of memory-related cognitive processes and functional abilities: a case report. *Presence: Teleoperators and Virtual Environments, 10,* 450–62.

Peterson, D. A. and Thaut, M. H. (2007). Music increases frontal EEG coherence during verbal learning. *Neuroscience Letters, 412,* 217–21.

Robinson, F. B. (1970). *Effective Study.* New York: Harper & Row.

Rubin, D. C. and Wallace, W. T. (1990). Rhyme and reason: analyses of dual-retrieval cues. *Journal of Experimental Psychology: Learning, Memory, and Cognition, 15,* 698–709.

Sarkamo, T. et al. (2008). Music listening enhances cognitive recovery and mood after middle cerebral artery stroke. *Brain, 131,* 866–76.

Schacter, D. L., Chiu, C. Y. P., and Oshsner, K. N. (1993). Implicit memory: a selective review. *Annual Review of Neuroscience. 16,* 159–82.

Schacter, D. L., Wagner, A. D., and Buckner, R. L. (2000). Memory systems of 1999. In: E. Tulving and F. I. M. Craik (eds) *The Oxford Handbook of Memory.* Oxford: Oxford University Press. pp. 627–43.

Silverman, M. J. (2012). Effects of melodic complexity and rhythm on working memory as measured by digit recall performance. *Music and Medicine, 4,* 22–7.

Simmons-Stern, N. R., Budson, A. E., and Ally, B. A. (2010). Music as a memory enhancer in patients with Alzheimer's disease. *Neuropsychologia, 40,* 3164–7.

Thaut, M. H. (2005). *Rhythm, Music, and the Brain: scientific foundations and clinical applications.* New York: Routledge.

Thaut, M. H. (2010). Neurologic music therapy in cognitive rehabilitation. *Music Perception, 27,* 281–5.

Thaut, M. H., Peterson, D. A., and McIntosh, G. C. (2005). Temporal entrainment of cognitive functions: musical mnemonics induce brain plasticity and oscillatory synchrony in neural networks underlying memory. *Annals of the New York Academy of Sciences, 1060,* 243–54.

Thaut, M. H., Peterson, D. A., Sena, K. M, and Mcintosh, G. (2008). Musical structure facilitates verbal learning in multiple sclerosis. *Music Perception, 25,* 325–30.

Thickpenny-Davis, K. L. and Barker-Collo, S. L. (2007). Evaluation of a structured group format memory rehabilitation program for adults following brain injury. *Journal of Head Trauma Rehabilitation, 22,* 303–13.

Wallace, W. T. (1994). Memory for music: effect of melody on recall of text. *Journal of Experimental Psychology, 20,* 1471–85.

Wallace, W. T. and Rubin, D. C. (1988). "The Wreck of the Old 97": a real event remembered in song. In: U. Neisser and E. Winograd (eds) *Remembering Reconsidered: ecological and traditional approaches to the study of memory.* Cambridge, UK: Cambridge University Press. pp. 283–310.

Wallace, W. T. and Rubin, D. C. (1991). Characteristics and constraints in ballads and their effect on memory. *Discourse Processes, 14,* 181–202.

Wilson, B. A. (2009). *Rehabilitation of Memory,* 2nd edition. New York: Guilford.

Chapter 25

Musical Echoic Memory Training (MEM)

Michael H. Thaut

25.1 Definition

Echoic memory is the earliest stage of auditory memory formation, and it operates like a sensory memory register, its function being to retain immediate auditory information that a person has just perceived until it can be processed more elaborately in working memory. Another function of echoic memory is to hold auditory information in the sensory register until a subsequent sound is heard which then assigns meaning to the first sound, as in rapid processing of speech sound sequences. Echoic memory is very short, and is defined as anywhere within the range of 2–4 seconds. However, it is considerably longer than iconic memory for visual information, which lasts less than 1000 milliseconds, or haptic memory for touch, which lasts for a maximum of 2 seconds. Echoic memory is longer than iconic memory because most salient visual information continues to be present for repeated scanning, whereas auditory information —due to its temporal waveform nature— can never be re-scanned unless it is actually repeated (Cowan, 1988).

Musical echoic memory training uses the immediate recall of musical sounds presented by singing, instrumental playing, or recorded music to retrain echoic memory.

25.2 Target populations

The main target populations for echoic memory training are patients with auditory memory dysfunction due to stroke in the dorsolateral prefrontal or temporal-parietal cortex, patients with traumatic brain injury, cochlear implant users, children with developmental language disorders and autism, and patients with dementia (Pekkonen et al., 1994) or schizophrenia (Javitt et al., 1997).

25.3 Research summary

In the 1960s, following the research on visual sensory memory storage, echoic memory as its counterpart for auditory sensory memory was investigated, and the actual term *echoic memory* was coined (Neisser, 1967; Sperling, 1963). Based on Baddeley's model of working memory, there is a phonological loop that processes auditory information in two steps. The first step is a phonological store with the capacity to hold auditory information in sensory register for up to 4 seconds before the information decays. This "store" or "auditory holding tank" constitutes the echoic memory process. The second proposed step would be a sub-vocal rehearsal process which would refresh the information and keep a memory trace in existence that could eventually be integrated into the working memory, which retains information for about 20–30 seconds (Baddeley et al., 2009). However, since music creates essentially non-verbal forms of auditory memory, it may constitute an independent part of the phonological loop.

The storage for auditory sensory memory has been found in the primary auditory cortex contralateral to the ear of presentation. If the echoic memory system is stimulated by free-field stimuli to both ears, the primary auditory cortex in both hemispheres is stimulated. Attentional control and the subsequent steps in the phonological loop to transfer information into working memory link the auditory cortex to the ventrolateral prefrontal cortex (Broca's area on the left hemisphere and Broca's analog in the right hemisphere) for sub-vocal rehearsal, the premotor cortex for rhythmic organization, and the posterior parietal cortex for spatial localization and temporal pattern discrimination (Alain et al., 1998).

Musical research on echoic memory has been sparse so far. However, some basic auditory research has yielded important findings (Naatanen et al., 1989). Inui et al. (2010) have shown that the single presentation of a sound is enough to create a memory trace shown as a distinct cortical response in the superior temporal gyrus (auditory cortex). Several studies have shown the engagement of echoic memory processes to musical stimulation (Koelsch, 2011; Koelsch et al., 1999; Kubovy and Howard, 1976).

Auditory (echoic) memory training that discriminated between two different pitch patterns showed neurophysiological changes in brain-wave patterns associated with early auditory sensory memory (Atienza et al., 2002).

A clinical research study on post-stroke patients showed that daily listening to music or audio books improved their echoic memory (Saerkaemoe et al., 2010).

25.4 **Therapeutic mechanisms**

During the initial stages of auditory memory processing, the inner ear converts sound waves into trains of nerve impulses that represent the basic features of acoustical vibrations such as frequency (pitch), amplitude (loudness), and waveform (presence or absence of vibrations in the harmonic spectrum creating the perception of timbre). These sensory data are then perceptually organized into single coherent acoustical events forming an echoic memory. Music is a harmonically complex sound language, with a rich acoustical wave spectrum. Echoic memories in music consist of multiple simultaneously sounding vibration patterns with distinct frequencies and amplitudes that are perceptually fused or bound together. Thus music creates an enriched auditory environment to stimulate the auditory sensory register and create perceptual organization for echoic memory formation.

25.5 **Clinical protocols**

25.5.1 **Therapeutic Music Exercise 1**

Sing a song or play a recorded song, stop the song at random places, and ask the patient which was the last word or phoneme they heard in the song.

25.5.2 **Therapeutic Music Exercise 2**

Repeat Exercise 1 but create ambient background sounds as a distractor during the song presentation.

25.5.3 **Therapeutic Music Exercise 3**

Repeat Exercise 1, but ask the patient to repeat the last two, three, or four words that they heard in the song before it stopped.

25.5.4 **Therapeutic Music Exercise 4**

Play two close pitches immediately behind each other on a keyboard or pitched percussion instrument, and ask the patient whether the two sounds were the same or different.

25.5.5 **Therapeutic Music Exercise 5**

Play a sequence of random pitches or a familiar melody, stop at a random place and ask the patient to hum, sing, or play back the last note (or the last two, three, or four notes).

References

Alain C, Woods D L, and Knight R T (1998). A distributed cortical network for auditory sensory memory in humans. *Brain Research, 812,* 23–37.

Atienza M, Cantero JL, and Dominguez-Marin E (2002). The time course of neural changes underlying auditory perceptual learning. *Learning & Memory, 9,* 138–50.

Baddeley A D, Eysenck M W, and Anderson M (2009). *Memory.* New York: Psychology Press.

Cowan N (1988). Evolving conceptions of memory storage, selective attention and their mutual constraints within the human information-processing system. *Psychological Bulletin, 104,* 163–91.

Inui K et al. (2010). Echoic memory of a single pure tone indexed by change-related brain activity. *BMC Neuroscience, 11,* 135.

Javitt D C et al. (1997). Impaired precision but normal retention of auditory sensory (echoic) memory information in schizophrenia. *Journal of Abnormal Psychology, 106,* 315–24.

Koelsch S (2011). Toward a neural basis of music perception – a review and updated model. *Frontiers in Psychology, 2,* 110.

Koelsch S, Schroeger E, and Tervaniemi M (1999). Superior pre-attentive auditory processing in musicians. *Neuroreport, 10,* 1309–13.

Kubovy M and Howard F P (1976). Persistence of a pitch-segregating echoic memory. *Journal of Experimental Psychology: Human Perception and Performance, 2,* 531–7.

Naatanen R et al. (1989). Do event-related potentials reveal mechanisms of the auditory sensory memory in the human brain? *Neuroscience Letters, 98,* 217–21.

Neisser U (1967). *Cognitive Psychology.* New York: Appleton-Century-Crofts.

Pekkonen E et al. (1994). Auditory sensory memory impairment in Alzheimer's disease: an event-related potential study. *Neuroreport, 5,* 2537–40.

Saerkaemoe T et al. (2010). Music and speech listening enhance the recovery of early sensory processing after stroke. *Journal of Cognitive Neuroscience, 22,* 2716–27.

Sperling G (1963). A model for visual memory tasks. *Human Factors, 5,* 19–31.

Chapter 26

Associative Mood and Memory Training (AMMT)

Shannon K. de l'Etoile

26.1 Definition

Associative mood and memory training (AMMT) is a cognitive rehabilitation technique that uses music to enhance memory processes in three ways—by producing a mood-congruent state to facilitate memory recall, by activating associative mood and memory networks to access long-term memories, and by instilling a positive mood at both encoding and recall to enhance learning and memory function (Gardiner, 2005; Hurt-Thaut, 2009; Thaut et al., 2008).

With regard to memory processes that are relevant to AMMT, encoding involves the way in which details and information are initially experienced, whereas representation pertains to how information is stored in memory (Schwartz, 2011a). Retrieval involves recovering information from long-term memory and bringing it into consciousness for examination in working memory. Various types of memories can exist within long-term storage. Implicit memories include information and skills that are utilized automatically or without conscious effort, such as remembering how to drive a car (Lim and Alexander, 2007). Explicit memories require conscious recall of information and events, and may be either semantic or episodic.

Semantic memories pertain to general knowledge of the world, such as facts, figures, principles, and rules. Episodic memories consist of long-term memory for personal experiences, including significant life events that happened years ago (e.g. one's wedding), or less important events that may have occurred within the last few hours (e.g. walking the dog this morning) (Lim and Alexander, 2007; Schwartz, 2011a). Knowing the specific street address of one's first home is a self-referential semantic memory, whereas remembering significant events which occurred at that location, such as family holidays, constitutes episodic memories. Combined, self-referential semantic memories and episodic memories constitute autobiographical memories (Birren and Schroots, 2006; Conway and Pleydell-Pearce, 2000; Schwartz, 2011a).

By promoting an awareness of self in place and time, autobiographical memories contribute to a sense of reason and meaning in life as needed to structure daily activities and anticipate future events (Foster and Valentine, 2001; O'Rourke et al., 2011). Consequently, the ability to encode, retain, and recall autobiographical memories is critical to other cognitive functions, such as planning and problem solving (Berry et al., 2010; Buijssen, 2005). The goal of AMMT is for patients to improve their cognitive functioning by recalling previous autobiographical memories and, if possible, establishing new ones.

26.2 Target populations

The clinical populations most in need of AMMT include individuals with neurologically based memory disorders, as well as individuals who need to recall long-term memories as part of life review. Memory disorders represent a prevalent, persistent, and debilitating consequence of neurologic injury (Glisky, 2004). Such deficits typically result from damage to brain structures implicated in memory function, including the medial temporal lobes, diencephalon, frontal lobes, and basal forebrain. Damage to these areas can produce amnesia, which primarily affects encoding of new information into episodic memory, and may also interfere with retrieval of both episodic and semantic memories (Schwartz, 2011b).

Anterograde amnesia limits the ability to form new memories following brain damage, and can vary from mild to severe. When brain damage is permanent, so is the memory loss (Glisky, 2004; Schwartz, 2011b). Conversely, retrograde amnesia impairs the recall of events and information encountered prior to an injury. The time period that is affected varies greatly from one patient to another, and may range from minutes to years. Patients may still be able to learn new information and, provided the brain damage is not permanent, the period of retrograde loss will gradually diminish (Schwartz, 2011b). Older memories are likely to be recovered first, and more recent memories (i.e. those occurring closer in time to the injury) emerge next. Some patients may also experience global amnesia, consisting of both anterograde and retrograde memory deficits.

Amnestic disorders and other episodic memory impairments can result from traumatic brain injury, tumors, stroke, multiple sclerosis, or dementia (Fischer, 2001; Glisky, 2004; Lim and Alexander, 2007). Perhaps the most devastating of all memory disorders, dementia is characterized by multiple cognitive deficits, including a degeneration of attention, language, perception, and memory (American Psychiatric Association, 2000; Sweatt, 2003). Dementia most commonly results from Alzheimer's disease, but can be associated with a general medical condition (e.g. HIV disease) or other neurologic disorder (e.g. stroke, Parkinson's disease) (American Psychiatric Association, 2000; Robottom et al., 2010).

Patients with dementia have difficulty encoding information as needed for transfer from short-term to long-term memory. Therefore they struggle to learn new material, and may forget and have difficulty recalling previously learned information (American Psychiatric Association, 2000; Buijssen, 2005). In the early stages of dementia, patients may have problems recalling daily experiences, such as memory for a spatial location and names of new people (Sweatt, 2003). Consequently, they may lose valuable items (e.g. purse, keys), or become lost in a familiar neighborhood. In dementia's final stages, patients may demonstrate profound memory loss and will not be able to read or write, or comprehend a movie or television show. Ultimately, patients become verbally incoherent, struggle to recognize familiar individuals, and may forget their own occupation, birthday, or name (American Psychiatric Association, 2000; Sweatt, 2003).

Typically aging older adults may also benefit from AMMT, due to gradual deterioration in the brain areas that are needed for memory functions (e.g. hippocampus, prefrontal lobe), which contributes to functional memory impairments, including weak encoding, decreased ability to ignore irrelevant information, difficulty in sustaining attention, and diminished processing speed (Hoyer and Verhaeghen, 2006; Schenkenberg and Miller, 2000; Schwartz, 2011c). Starting at around the age of 60 years, older adults may have difficulty recalling episodic memories and remembering the context of past events, such as time and place (Berry et al., 2010; Hill and Bäckman, 2000; Hoyer and Verhaeghen, 2006; Sweatt, 2003). They may also show deficits in learning and remembering new information, including names, events, and spatial details (Hill and Bäckman, 2000; Sweatt, 2003).

One other population appropriate for AMMT is that of patients with terminal illness who may not experience memory deficits per se, but who need to put their life experiences into perspective and grieve their impending losses (Connor, 2009; Salmon, 1993; Soltys, 2007). For these patients, memory recall is part of a life-review process through which they identify patterns of meaning and discover ways of coping with their illness.

26.3 **Research summary**

Previous research on mood and memory has identified two important concepts that support AMMT. The first concept is mood-congruent memory, which pertains to encoding or recalling information that matches one's current mood (Eich and Schooler, 2000; Schwartz, 2011a). For instance, when in a positive mood, one is more likely to recall memories of happy events from the past. One may also be more attentive to information that has a positive affective valence, and therefore these details are more likely to be stored to memory.

The second concept is state-dependent memory, which occurs when material encoded in a particular state is remembered better if the same state is experienced at recall (Eich and Schooler, 2000; Schwartz, 2011a). Episodic memories in particular are typically encoded within a particular spatial and temporal context (i.e. a specific time and place), as well as within the context of one's current mood (Schacter and Tulving, 1994; Schwartz, 2011a). Thus "state" may pertain to a physical location, time of day or year, or one's current mood. When mood constitutes the state that influences encoding and recall, the term "mood state-dependent memory" is most appropriate. Accordingly, memory retrieval is enhanced when mood at recall matches mood at encoding.

Bower (1981) further explains these concepts through his *associative network theory of memory and emotion*. Human memory consists of an associative network in which events are recorded in connection with concepts that describe the event. For instance, memory for a certain event (e.g. one's college graduation ceremony) may be stored in association with other aspects of that event, such as the weather (e.g. a sunny day), the location (e.g. a large auditorium on a college campus), and other people who attended the event (e.g. family, friends, classmates). These details are established in connection with one another as semantic nodes within the associative network.

Recalling the event involves activating the network—a process that is analogous to an electrical system. Activation of a particular node may spread to associated concepts or nodes, eventually leading to recall of the event. For example, on a sunny day, one may experience activation of the "sunny-day" node. This activity could spread to nearby nodes, such as the memory for a large auditorium, or class peers last seen in that auditorium. With sufficient activation of associated nodes, the full memory of college graduation is successfully recalled.

A significant life event such as college graduation is likely to be associated with certain emotions, such as excitement and apprehension about the future, or relief and pride that a major accomplishment has been realized. The event "college graduation" is thus stored in memory in association with these emotional states. Emotions are also represented as specific memory nodes that are connected with other concept nodes in the network. When activation of an emotion node exceeds a particular threshold, even years after the event, the excitation travels to associated nodes, thus further enhancing recall of the event. Combining the activation of an emotion node with other cues is likely to elevate the total activation of the network, thus bringing memory for the event into one's consciousness.

Bower's theory clarifies the importance of emotions in memory recall, thus explaining mood state-dependent memory effects. Researchers further state that mood state-dependent recall is more likely to occur when the event stored in memory is believed to have caused the associated emotion, and when mood is intense enough to influence learning, memory, and attention—a process known as affective infusion (Bower and Forgas, 2000; Eich and Schooler, 2000; Forgas, 1995). Essentially, current mood may provide an affective bias for what information is encoded and retrieved. Mood state-dependent effects are therefore likely to occur during a strong, stable, and sincere mood, and when affect infusion is high during both encoding and recall (Bower and Forgas, 2000; Eich and Schooler, 2000; Forgas, 1995).

26.3.1 **Musical mood induction**

Various mood induction techniques exist, such as hypnosis, success/failure paradigms (e.g. winning or losing at computer games), and mood posturing (e.g. making facial expressions or assuming body postures consistent with certain moods). Other techniques include listening to a sad story, reading self-referent statements pertaining to happy or sad experiences (e.g. the Velten Mood Induction Procedure, or VMIP), or listening to music (e.g. musical mood induction procedures, or MMIP) (Albersnagel, 1988; Bower, 1981; Davies, 1986; Eifert et al., 1988; Gerrards-Hesse et al., 1994; Martin, 1990). In comparison with the VMIP, MMIP have demonstrated reliable and superior effects.

MMIP tend to produce a more intense and longer-lasting mood change than the VMIP (Albersnagel, 1988), while avoiding demand characteristics or gender differences (Clark and Teasdale, 1985; de l'Etoile, 2002; Pignatiello et al., 1986). They also achieve a higher success rate than the VMIP, which may only be effective with around 60% of participants (Clark, 1983; de l'Etoile, 2002; Gerrards-Hesse et al., 1994; Rachman, 1981). Overall, MMIP can produce a mood sufficient for mood state-dependent effects, and can elicit meaningful shifts in mood for the same individuals repeatedly over time (Eich and Schooler, 2000; Hernandez et al., 2003).

Effective MMIP involves active music listening and making a concerted effort to use the music to change mood. Passive music listening will typically not change or intensify mood state to the degree required for mood-based memory effects. In MMIP, researchers often provide specific instructions for participants, such as "Try to determine the mood of this piece, and move yourself into that mood" or "Get into the feeling of the music" (Clark and Teasdale, 1985; de l'Etoile, 2002; Hernandez et al., 2003). Other examples include "Listen carefully to the music, saturate yourself with the mood of the music, and try to stay in that mood" (Martin and Metha, 1997). When applied correctly, MMIP produce a mood of sufficient intensity to activate associative memory networks, thereby providing access to mood-congruent information and promoting recall of mood state-dependent memories (Thaut, 2002).

26.3.2 **Musical mood induction and mood state-dependent memory**

Musical mood induction procedures have generated mood state-dependent effects in both typical and clinical populations. In healthy adults, MMIP improved word retrieval (de l'Etoile, 2002; Thaut and de l'Etoile, 1993) and recall of autobiographical memories (Cady et al., 2008; Janata et al., 2007; Martin and Metha, 1997). Both younger and older adults experienced strong emotional reactions to music that correlated with retrieval of long-term memories (Alfredson et al., 2004; Knight et al., 2002; Schulkind et al., 1999). Older adults also maintained strong emotional reactions to music over long intervals of time (i.e. from their youth), and retrieved information from longer retention intervals than young adults, which suggests that the effect of emotion on memory may strengthen over time (Schulkind et al., 1999).

For dementia patients, memory for music appears to remain intact even in the later stages of the disease (Cuddy and Duffin, 2005; Prickett and Moore, 1991). Dementia patients displayed significantly better recall of autobiographical memories after a music listening condition than after other auditory conditions, such as ambient noise or silence (Foster and Valentine, 2001; Irish et al., 2006). Researchers explain that the music may have modulated patient arousal and attention, thus enhancing recall effects. Dementia patients have also shown an ability to learn new songs better than they could learn new verbal material (e.g. poems), and demonstrated long-term retention of new music (Prickett and Moore, 1991; Samson et al., 2009). Researchers explain that music perception utilizes a widely distributed cortical network as well as certain subcortical structures. For patients with Alzheimer's disease, stronger cortical areas may support and reinforce weaker ones during music processing (Cuddy and Duffin, 2005). In addition, subcortical structures needed for music perception are typically spared from the deterioration of Alzheimer's disease.

26.4 **Therapeutic mechanisms**

Brain imaging technology provides further evidence for affective and cognitive interactions relative to music. Findings indicate that experiencing positive affect involves a left lateralized circuit which links subcortical limbic structures, such as the amygdala and nucleus accumbens, with dorsal prefrontal structures, including the left side dorsolateral prefrontal cortex and dorsal anterior cingulate cortex (Ashby et al., 1999; Breiter et al., 2001; Dolan, 2002; Whittle et al., 2006). These areas receive rich dopaminergic projections, thus establishing their role as reward-related structures. Meanwhile, negative affective responses result from activation of subcortical limbic structures, including the amygdala and ventral anterior cingulate cortex, and their connections with right hemisphere structures, including the hippocampus, dorsal anterior cingulate cortex, and dorsolateral prefrontal cortex. The amygdala in particular helps to create and store long-term memories, especially those with high affective salience (Cahill et al., 1996; Dolan, 2002).

Research findings reveal that these same structures are involved during music listening, most notably when making an emotional judgment or response. Studies involving healthy young adults have demonstrated that listening to music as an affective task activates an interconnected network of both subcortical and cortical brain structures, including the ventral striatum, nucleus accumbens, amygdala, insula, hippocampus, hypothalamus, ventral tegmental area, anterior cingulate, orbitofrontal cortex, and ventral medial prefrontal cortex (Blood et al., 1999; Blood and Zatorre, 2001; Brown et al., 2004; Menon and Levitin, 2005). Patterns of neural activity observed during emotional response to music have also been noted in response to other euphoria-producing stimuli, including food, sexual activity, and drugs of abuse (Bardo, 1998; Berridge and Robinson, 1998; Gardner and Vorel, 1998). Thus music processing recruits brain regions that are typically involved in affective experiences, including pleasure and reward, and may induce specific mood states (Menon and Levitin, 2005).

The dopaminergic mesocorticolimbic system that is activated during affective music listening tasks may also play a role in memory functions (Ashby et al., 1999). Specifically, increased levels of dopamine enhance a number of cognitive functions, including alertness, information-processing speed, attention, and memory (Schück et al., 2002). Thus, affective musical tasks can recruit areas that link affective and cognitive processes, including memory (Blood et al., 1999; Brown et al., 2004; Menon and Levitin, 2005).

In one study, a musical task involving affective judgment produced activation of the rostral medial prefrontal cortex (RMPFC) (Janata, 2005), a structure that is also implicated in tasks pertaining to music and retrieval of autobiographical memories (Platel et al., 2003). In patients with Alzheimer's disease, rostral and ventral portions of the medial prefrontal cortex are among the last to atrophy (Thompson et al., 2003). Consequently, patients with Alzheimer's disease may still respond positively to familiar music (Janata, 2005). Ultimately, the RMPFC may represent a critical area for the integration of music and autobiographical memories.

Researchers have explored emotions, music, and memories in older adults and clinical populations. While listening to self-selected emotionally significant music that elicited recall of associated memories, older adults showed increased right temporal lobe activation, thus revealing neural mechanisms that link music perception, emotional responses, and memories (Alfredson et al., 2004). In addition, patients with epilepsy and auditory agnosia displayed comparable brain activation to healthy young adults during music listening, and could appreciate and respond emotionally to music (Dellacherie et al., 2009; Matthews et al., 2009). Furthermore, stroke patients who listened to preferred music demonstrated significantly greater cognitive recovery in verbal memory and focused attention in comparison with patients who listened to audio books or who had no listening material (Sarkamo et al., 2008). The music listening group also showed a less depressed and confused mood than the other two patient groups. Researchers conclude that the cognitive improvements appeared to be mediated by the positive mood induced by daily music listening.

To summarize, the brain structures that are activated during emotional responses to music are also involved in reward and pleasure circuitry, and thus music is an appropriate stimulus for mood induction. In addition, the brain areas that are used for focused music listening are also implicated in tasks involving the synthesis of affective and cognitive activity, such as the recall of memories with high levels of emotional arousal. As a highly salient emotional stimulus, music appears to activate an amygdala-based neural network that plays a major role in the processing of emotional stimuli (Thaut, 2010). Using music to activate this network provides an emotional context for cognitive activity, and reinforces the emotional salience of memory content. These scientific mechanisms support the use of music to induce mood, thereby promoting mood-congruent memory recall as well as retrieval of mood state-dependent memories.

26.5 **Clinical protocols**

AMMT involves using music to induce a specific mood state that is associated with material stored in long-term memory, specifically autobiographical memories that pertain to the self and one's past experiences. Through focused music listening, the patient experiences a shift in mood, or intensification of their current mood, which then activates an associative memory network, creating access to memories of information or events from the past. Thus AMMT constitutes a method for engaging in reminiscence or life review.

By definition, reminiscence involves creating an account of the past that may include events, thoughts, and feelings (Bulechek et al., 2008; Soltys, 2007). When applied systematically, reminiscence evolves into life review, in which recall of autobiographical memories is used to maintain or acquire coping strategies and make critical decisions about the future (Garland and Garland, 2001a; Soltys, 2007).

Life review may benefit patients with amnestic disorders or other episodic memory deficits, and is also recommended for people of any age who are approaching the end of life and need to put their life experiences into perspective (Butler, 1963; Haight and Burnside, 1993; Koffman, 2000; Kunz, 2002; Stinson, 2009; Walker and Adamek, 2008).

Life review may be best considered within the context of life-span developmental theory (Garland and Garland, 2001a; Giblin, 2011). According to Erikson (1959), personality and sense of self evolve in stages during which specific conflicts must be addressed and mastered. The conflict experienced in older adulthood or at the end of life is that of despair versus integrity, and involves struggling between feelings of regret and bitterness, and feelings of acceptance of the decisions one has made and the life one has lived (Erikson, 1997). Life review can help to resolve this conflict, leading to effective adaptation to aging or terminal illness (Birren and Schroots, 2006; Garland and Garland, 2001b; Koffman, 2000; Middleton and Edwards, 1990; O'Rourke et al., 2011; Soltys, 2007).

Life review may not be appropriate for individuals with severe intellectual disability, or who have obsessive thought patterns and are likely to fixate on negative events in a non-productive manner (Garland and Garland, 2001b). In addition, some patients with dementia may be capable of reminiscing, but due to difficulties with time orientation they may struggle to connect past events with the present. For these patients, recall of past events may be a sufficient therapeutic goal, whereas achieving insight about present and future events may not be possible.

26.5.1 Guidelines for selection of music

When selecting music for AMMT, clinicians should consider patient demographics. Older adults prefer music that was popular during their young adult years, and are more likely to show stronger emotional responses to this music (Bartlett and Snelus, 1980; Gibbons, 1977; Hanser et al., 2011; Jonas, 1991; Lathom et al., 1982; Schulkind et al., 1999). Memories from this time period pertain to events relating to identity, including novel events with high emotional salience, and are often recalled with greater frequency and vividness (Birren and Schroots, 2006; Rubin et al., 1998). Furthermore, most older adults tend to remember positive events more than negative ones, and older women are likely to recall memories related to family and health, whereas older men recall more work-related memories. Patients with dementia demonstrate better recall for life events experienced prior to disease onset as well as significant life events with high emotional arousal (Buijssen, 2005).

Another factor to consider is the patient's familiarity with the music. In certain situations, a piece of music may be stored within an associative network along with other semantic concepts and emotions (Krumhansl, 2002). For example, "Ode to Joy" may have been played at a patient's wedding—a significant life event that is likely to be associated with strong emotions. Hearing this piece at a later time would activate the patient's associative network containing wedding-day memories. Simultaneously, emotions from the wedding existing as nodes within the same network would also be activated. These two powerful cues in combination would then activate additional nodes, enabling the patient to recall specific details of wedding-day activities. Familiar musical pieces associated with more general time periods, as opposed to specific events, can also lead to effective recall in much the same manner (Krumhansl, 2002).

By contrast, patients do not necessarily need to know a particular piece of music in order to have an emotional response that leads to memory retrieval (Janata et al., 2007). If patients can recognize the artist, style, or genre of music, or can place the music as belonging within a certain cultural or historic context, these cues will often be sufficient for inducing mood associated with memories of past events (J. Goelz, personal communication, 31 January 2012; Janata et al., 2007). For example, a patient may have a strong preference for songs made famous by Frank Sinatra in the 1950s. When hearing a Sinatra recording that was less popular during that same time period, and that is therefore less familiar, the patient may still recognize the piece as being "Sinatra-ish", and therefore experience a mood response sufficient for memory recall. Even without such stylistic cues, the intrinsically emotional nature of any given musical piece can lead to successful mood induction (Krumhansl, 2002).

26.5.2 Guidelines for AMMT session planning and implementation

Clinicians should carefully consider session format and frequency. For some patients, participating in a group format promotes therapeutic mood change and memory recall (Suzuki, 1998). In addition, discovering common experiences with other group members can promote a shared identity or sense of belonging that further contributes to sense of self as needed for effective coping and decision making (Birren and Schroots, 2006; Cheston and Bender, 1999; Middleton and Edwards, 1990). However, in the advanced stages of dementia, optimal results may be better achieved via individualized treatment in which the therapist interacts with the patient on a one-to-one basis with close physical proximity (Prickett and Moore, 1991). Greater therapeutic gains are also more likely when sessions take place frequently, perhaps on a daily basis or at least two to three times per week.

With regard to music presentation, clinicians should first identify life events and time periods that are significant to each patient (i.e. college years, marriage, family, career, etc.) (Grocke and Wigram, 2007), and then select music associated with such events, or their respective moods. Music should be sequenced within or across sessions to match the temporal order of life events. Since autobiographical memories tend to be organized in the same sequence as they originally occurred, recall is more efficient when retrieval cues correspond to this temporal order (Anderson and Conway, 1997). Music may be played from recordings or presented live, and patients can then listen or sing along to it (Grocke and Wigram 2007). The most important variable to consider with regard to recorded music versus a live performance is the music's ability to effectively induce mood.

Prior to music presentation, the clinician should encourage active, focused listening in order for musical mood induction to occur. Helpful suggestions include "Let yourself move into the mood of the music", or "Figure out the mood of this piece, and put yourself in that mood", or "Stay with that mood." In addition, patients may think about events that match the mood of the music (Eich and Schooler, 2000). Patients do not need an emotional label for the music, as leaving the emotional interpretation of the music open-ended allows for subjective responses that may be more meaningful than what the therapist could have anticipated.

Clinicians should discretely monitor patient behavior for affective response during music listening, and then provide a moment of reflective silence after the music has ended (Grocke and Wigram, 2007). The therapist should then help the patients to verbally process their responses to the music by utilizing the following format (adapted from a lecture given on 1 March 2011 by S. de l'Etoile; J. Goelz, personal communication, 31 January 2012; Grocke and Wigram, 2007; Thaut, 1999).

26.5.2.1 Level 1: Orienting

Questions or suggestions are designed to orient patients to the music they have just heard or sung, thus verifying reality orientation and attention to the music. Examples include:

> *What was that song about?*
> *What were some of the words?*
> *What do you like about this song?*
> *What do you think about this musical artist/composer?*

26.5.2.2 Level 2: Recall

Questions and comments prompt patients to share their affective responses to the song, as well as their associated personal experiences (i.e. memories). Examples include:

> *What were you feeling as you listened to/sang this song?*
> *What thoughts or images came to mind as you were listening?*
> *What does the song remind you of?*
> *What are you thinking now, after listening to that song?*

26.5.2.3 Level 3: Application

The therapist helps patients to determine the meaning of their memories and apply that knowledge to their current life situation. Patients may retrieve a valuable insight, remember how they managed a particular crisis, or experience satisfaction from previous accomplishments. Recalling this information not only helps patients to improve memory function, but also enables them to cope with current difficulties and meet the developmental tasks of aging, as needed. Examples include:

> *What is most meaningful to you about that time in your life?*
> *What did you find most difficult (or most pleasing) about that event?*
> *What did you learn from that experience?*
> *What advice would you give to someone today, going through that same circumstance?*

Questions should be tailored to meet each patient's specific needs, and also reflect emotions and thoughts triggered by the music.

Verbal processing must accommodate each patient's capacity for insight and reality orientation. If patients are limited in this regard, then questions at Levels 1 and 2 may be sufficient, whereas proceeding to Level 3 may be difficult and confusing. In addition, if a patient cannot verbalize memories that are being elicited, family members can share their own memories and emotions that specifically involve the patient.

26.5.3 Clinical example of associative mood and memory training (AMMT)

The following example demonstrates how AMMT can be used with a patient who has memory recall deficits.

Case study

Helen is an older woman who is widowed and has vascular dementia due to having experienced multiple strokes. Her adult children report that she now needs more supervision, as she has wandered into the neighborhood and become lost on several occasions, and has many times left the stove turned on after preparing a meal. Helen now attends an adult day-care program that provides meals and structured activities on weekdays. In the evenings and at weekends she stays with her daughter and her daughter's husband, who both care for her. Before Helen's dementia progresses to an advanced stage, she needs opportunities to engage in meaningful life review.

The music therapist determines that Helen was born in 1947 and was thus a young adult during the mid to late 1960s. Consequently, the therapist selects love songs that were popular at that time to help Helen recall memories related to romantic relationships from her young adulthood. Such relationships represent significant life events and are likely to have high emotional salience. Thus mood induction through music is likely to activate associative memory networks containing information about these experiences.

The therapist begins by playing the guitar and singing "Build Me Up Buttercup", which was made popular by The Foundations in 1968. Helen is encouraged to sing along, and to determine the mood of the song. Although this song has many upbeat qualities (e.g. major key, fast tempo, engaging pop style), the lyrics depict feelings of frustration with a significant other who repeatedly breaks promises. After singing the song, the therapist engages Helen in verbal processing as follows:

Level 1: Orienting

* *What was the nickname used in the song?*
* *What is the singer trying to say to "Buttercup"?*
* *What was the mood of this song?*

Level 2: Recall

* *When have you felt the same way?*
* *Tell me about [this time, this person].*

Level 3: Application

* *What did you learn from dating [that person]?*
* *What advice would you give to someone today, who might be in a similar dating situation?*

In the same or a subsequent session, the therapist plays a recording of "Sweet Caroline;" a song made famous by Neil Diamond in 1969. The therapist encourages Helen to focus on the mood of the piece, and to think of events that match the mood. This particular song also projects a positive mood and has a rousing chorus in which the melodic line is punctuated with a strong brass presence, making it especially memorable. After playing the recording, the therapist presents the following comments and questions to Helen:

Level 1: Orienting

+ *I heard another nickname in this song. What was it?*
+ *I wonder if you can also tell me the name of the man who is singing this song.*
+ *What is Neil Diamond saying to "Caroline"?*
+ *What do you think Neil Diamond is feeling, as he says this?*

Level 2: Recall

+ *What are you feeling now, after listening to the song?*
+ *What images or thoughts come to mind, with this feeling?*

Level 3: Application

+ *What was important to you about that time in your life?*

Subsequently, the therapist plays the keyboard and sings "I Got You Babe", which was the signature song of the pop duo Sonny and Cher, topping the charts in 1965. This song projects a cheerful, optimistic mood through its instrumental arrangement, highly repetitive refrain, and lyrics that depict a supportive and loving relationship.

Level 1: Orienting

+ *I think I heard another nickname in this song. What was it?*
+ *What do you think of the lyrics "I got you, babe"? What do these lyrics mean?*

Level 2: Recall

+ *What is it like to be called "babe", or another nickname? For example, what feeling did you have when [your boyfriend/husband] called you by this special name?*
+ *Tell me about a nickname you had for [a boyfriend/husband].*
+ *What made that person special to you?*

Level 3: Application

+ *What was the best part about having a [boyfriend/husband]?*
+ *What was the worst part?*
+ *What do you value most about that relationship?*

References

Albersnagel, F. A. (1988). Velten and musical mood induction procedures: a comparison with accessibility of thought associations. *Behavior Research and Therapy, 26*, 79–96.

Alfredson, B. B., Risberg, J., Hagberg, B., and Gustafson, L. (2004). Right temporal lobe activation when listening to emotionally significant music. *Applied Neuropsychology, 11*, 161–6.

American Psychiatric Association (2000). Delirium, dementia, and amnestic and other cognitive disorders. In: *Diagnostic and Statistical Manual of Mental Disorders*, 4th edition, text revision. Washington, DC: American Psychiatric Association. pp. 135–80.

Anderson, S. J. and Conway, M. A. (1997). Representation of autobiographical memories. In: M. A. Conway (ed.) *Cognitive Models of Memory*. Cambridge, MA: MIT Press. pp. 217–46.

Ashby, F. G., Isen, A. M., and Turken, A. U. (1999). A neuropsychological theory of positive affect and its influence on cognition. *Psychological Review, 106*, 529–50.

Bardo, M. T. (1998). Neuropharmacological mechanisms of drug reward: beyond dopamine in the nucleus accumbens. *Critical Reviews in Neurobiology, 12*, 37–67.

Bartlett, J. C. and Snelus, P. (1980). Lifespan memory for popular songs. *American Journal of Psychology, 93*, 551–60.

Berridge, K. C. and Robinson, T. E. (1998). What is the role of dopamine in reward: hedonic impact, reward learning, or incentive salience? *Brain Research Review, 28*, 309–69.

Berry, J. et al. (2010). Memory aging: deficits, beliefs, and interventions. In: J. Cavanaugh and C. K. Cavanaugh (eds). *Aging in America. Volume I. Psychological aspects*. Oxford, UK: Praeger Perspectives. pp. 255–99.

Birren, J. E. and Schroots, J. J. F. (2006). Autobiographical memory and the narrative self over the life span. In: J. E. Birren and K. W. Schaie (eds) *Handbook of the Psychology of Aging*, 6th edition. New York: Academic Press. pp. 477–98.

Blood, A. J. and Zatorre, R. J. (2001). Intensely pleasurable responses to music correlate with activity in brain regions implicated in reward and emotion. *Proceedings of the National Academy of Sciences of the USA, 98*, 11818–23.

Blood, A. J., Zatorre, R. J., Bermudez, P., and Evans, A. C. (1999). Emotional responses to pleasant and unpleasant music correlate with activity in paralimbic brain regions. *Nature Neuroscience, 2*, 382–7.

Bower, G. H. (1981). Mood and memory. *American Psychologist, 36*, 129–48.

Bower, G. H. and Forgas, J. P. (2000). Affect, memory, and social cognition. In: E. Eich et al. (eds) *Cognition and Emotion*. New York: Oxford University Press. pp. 87–168.

Breiter, H. C. et al. (2001). Functional imaging of neural responses to expectancy and experience of monetary gains and losses. *Neuron, 30*, 619–39.

Brown, S., Martinez, M. J., and Parsons, L. M. (2004). Passive music listening spontaneously engages limbic and paralimbic systems. *Neuroreport, 15*, 2033–7.

Buijssen, H. (2005). The simple logic behind dementia. In: *The Simplicity of Dementia: a guide for family and carers*. London: Jessica Kingsley Publishers. pp. 21–50.

Bulechek, G., Butcher, H., and Dochterman, J. (2008). Reminiscence therapy. In: G. Bulechek, H. Butcher, and J. Dochterman (eds). *Nursing Intervention Classification (NIC)*, 5th edition. St Louis, MO: Mosby-Elsevier. pp. 608–9.

Butler, R. N. (1963). The life review: an interpretation of reminiscence in old age. *Psychiatry Journal for the Study of Interpersonal Processes, 26*, 65–76.

Cady, E. T., Harris, R. J., and Knappenberger, J. B. (2008). Using music to cue autobiographical memories of different lifetime periods. *Psychology of Music, 36*, 157–78.

Cahill, L., Haier, R. J., and Fallon, J. (1996). Amygdala activity at encoding correlated with long-term, free recall of emotional information. *Proceedings of the National Academy of Sciences of the USA, 93*, 8016–21.

Cheston, R. and Bender, M. (1999). Managing the process of loss. In: *Understanding Dementia: the man with the worried eyes*. London: Jessica Kingsley Publishers. pp. 168–87.

Clark, D. M. (1983). On the induction of depressed mood in the laboratory: evaluation and comparison of the Velten and musical procedures. *Advances in Behavior Research and Therapy, 5*, 27–49.

Clark, D. M. and Teasdale, J. D. (1985). Constraints on the effects of mood on memory. *Journal of Personality and Social Psychology, 48*, 1595–608.

Connor, S. R. (2009). Psychological and spiritual care. In: *Hospice and Palliative Care: the essential guide*, 2nd edition. New York: Routledge. pp. 55–73.

Conway, M. A. and Pleydell-Pearce, C. W. (2000). The construction of autobiographical memories in the self-memory system. *Psychological Review, 107,* 261–88.

Cuddy, L. L. and Duffin, J. (2005). Music, memory, and Alzheimer's disease: is music recognition spared in dementia, and how can it be assessed? *Medical Hypotheses, 64,* 229–35.

Davies, G. (1986). Context effects on episodic memory: a review. *Cahiers de Psychologie Cognitive, 6,* 157–74.

de l'Etoile, S. K. (2002). The effect of a musical mood induction procedure on mood state-dependent word retrieval. *Journal of Music Therapy, 39,* 145–60.

Dellacherie, D. et al. (2009). The birth of musical emotion: a depth electrode case study in a human subject with epilepsy. *Annals of the New York Academy of Sciences, 1169,* 336–41.

Dolan, R. J. (2002). Emotion, cognition, and behavior. *Science, 298,* 1191–4.

Eich, E. and Schooler, J. W. (2000). Cognition/emotion interactions. In: E. Eich et al. (eds) *Cognition and Emotion.* New York: Oxford University Press. pp. 3–29.

Eifert, G. H., Craill, L., Carey, E., and O'Connor, C. (1988). Affect modification through evaluative conditioning with music. *Behavior Research and Therapy, 26,* 321–30.

Erikson, E. H. (1959). Growth and crises of the healthy personality. In: *Psychological Issues: identity and the life cycle. Volume 1.* New York: International Universities Press, Inc. pp. 50–100.

Erikson, E. H. (1997). Major stages in psychosocial development. In: *The Life Cycle Completed: extended version.* New York: W. W. Norton & Company. pp. 55–82.

Fischer, J. S. (2001). Cognitive impairment in multiple sclerosis. In: S. D. Cook (ed.) *Handbook of Multiple Sclerosis,* 3rd edition. New York: Marcel Dekker, Inc. pp. 233–55.

Forgas, J. P. (1995). Mood and judgment: the affect infusion model (AIM). *Psychological Bulletin, 117,* 39–66.

Foster, N. A. and Valentine, E. R. (2001). The effect of auditory stimulation on autobiographical recall in dementia. *Experimental Aging Research, 27,* 215–28.

Gardiner, J. C. (2005). Neurologic music therapy in cognitive rehabilitation. In: M. H. Thaut (ed.) *Rhythm, Music, and the Brain: scientific foundations and clinical applications.* New York: Routledge. pp. 179–202.

Gardner, E. L. and Vorel, S. R. (1998). Cannabinoid transmission and reward-related events. *Neurobiology of Disease, 5,* 502–33.

Garland, J. and Garland, C. (2001a). Review in context. In: *Life Review in Health and Social Care: a practitioner's guide.* Philadelphia, PA: Brunner-Routledge. pp. 3–26.

Garland, J. and Garland, C. (2001b). Why review? In: *Life Review in Health and Social Care: a practitioner's guide.* Philadelphia, PA: Brunner-Routledge. pp. 27–45.

Gerrards-Hesse, A., Spies, K., and Hesse, F. W. (1994). Experimental inductions of emotional states and their effectiveness: a review. *British Journal of Psychology, 85,* 55–78.

Gibbons, A. C. (1977). Popular music preferences of elderly people. *Journal of Music Therapy, 14,* 180–89.

Giblin, J. C. (2011). Successful aging: choosing wisdom over despair. *Journal of Psychosocial Nursing, 49,* 23–6.

Glisky, E. L. (2004). Disorders of memory. In: J. Ponsford (ed.) *Cognitive and Behavioral Rehabilitation: from neurobiology to clinical practice.* New York: Guilford Press. pp. 100–28.

Grocke, D. and Wigram, T. (2007). Song lyric discussion, reminiscence, and life review. In: *Receptive Methods in Music Therapy: techniques and clinical applications for music therapy clinicians, educators, and students.* London: Jessica Kingsley Publishers. pp. 157–78.

Haight, B. and Burnside, I. (1993). Reminiscence and life review: explaining the difference. *Archives of Psychiatric Nursing, 7,* 91–8.

Hanser, S. B., Butterfield-Whitcomb, J., Kawata, M., and Collins, B. (2011). Home-based music strategies with individuals who have dementia and their family caregivers. *Journal of Music Therapy, 48*, 2–27.

Hernandez, S., Vander Wal, J. S., and Spring, B. (2003). A negative mood induction procedure with efficacy across repeated administrations in women. *Journal of Psychopathology and Behavioral Assessment, 25*, 49–55.

Hill, R. and Bäckman, L. (2000). Theoretical and methodological issues in memory training. In: R. D. Hill, L. Bäckman, and A. S. Neely (eds) *Cognitive Rehabilitation in Old Age.* New York: Oxford University Press. pp. 23–41.

Hoyer, W. J. and Verhaeghen, P. (2006). Memory aging. In: J. E. Birren and K. W. Schaie (eds) *Handbook of the Psychology of Aging,* 6th edition. New York: Academic Press. pp. 209–32.

Hurt-Thaut, C. (2009). Clinical practice in music therapy. In: S. Hallam, I. Cross, and M. Thaut (eds) *The Oxford Handbook of Music Psychology.* Oxford: Oxford University Press. pp. 503–14.

Irish, M. et al. (2006). Investigating the enhancing effect of music on autobiographical memory in mild Alzheimer's disease. *Dementia and Geriatric Cognitive Disorders, 22*, 108–20.

Janata, P. (2005). Brain networks that track musical structure. *Annals of the New York Academy of Sciences, 1060*, 111–24.

Janata, P., Tomic, S. T., and Rakowski, S. K. (2007). Characterization of music-evoked autobiographical memories. *Memory, 15*, 845–60.

Jonas, J. L. (1991). Preferences of elderly music listeners residing in nursing homes for art music, traditional jazz, popular music of today, and country music. *Journal of Music Therapy, 28*, 149–60.

Knight, B. G., Maines, M. L., and Robinson, G. S. (2002). The effects of sad mood on memory in older adults: a test of the mood congruence effect. *Psychology and Aging, 17*, 653–61.

Koffman, S. D. (2000). Introduction. In: *Structured Reminiscence and Gestalt Life Review.* New York: Garland Publishing, Inc. pp. 3–14.

Krumhansl, C. L. (2002). Music: a link between cognition and emotion. *Current Directions in Psychological Science, 11*, 45–50.

Kunz, J. A. (2002). Integrating reminiscence and life review techniques with brief, cognitive behavioral therapy. In: J. D. Webster and B. K. Haight (eds) *Critical Advances in Reminiscence Work: from theory to application.* New York: Springer Publishing Company. pp. 275–88.

Lathom, W. B., Petersen, M., and Havlicek, L. (1982). Musical preferences of older people attending nutritional sites. *Educational Gerontology, 8*, 155–65.

Lim, C. and Alexander, M. P. (2007). Disorders of episodic memory. In: O. Godefroy and J. Bogousslavsky (eds) *The Behavioral and Cognitive Neurology of Stroke.* New York: Cambridge University Press. pp. 407–30.

Martin, M. (1990). On the induction of mood. *Clinical Psychology Review, 10*, 669–97.

Martin, M. A. and Metha, A. (1997). Recall of early childhood memories through musical mood induction. *The Arts in Psychotherapy, 24*, 447–54.

Matthews, B. R. et al. (2009). Pleasurable emotional response to music: a case of neurodegenerative generalized auditory agnosia. *Neurocase, 15*, 248–59.

Menon, V. and Levitin, D. J. (2005). The rewards of music listening: response and physiological connectivity of the mesolimbic system. *NeuroImage, 28*, 175–84.

Middleton, D. and Edwards, D. (1990). Conversational remembering: a social psychological approach. In: D. Middleton and D. Edwards (eds) *Collective Remembering.* London: Sage. pp. 23–45.

O'Rourke, N., Cappeliez, P., and Claxton, A. (2011). Functions of reminiscence and the psychological well-being of young-old and older adults over time. *Aging & Mental Health, 15*, 272–81.

Pignatiello, M. F., Camp, C. J., and Rasar, L. (1986). Musical mood induction: an alternative to the Velten technique. *Journal of Abnormal Psychology*, *95*, 295–7.

Platel, H. et al. (2003). Semantic and episodic memory of music are subserved by distinct neural networks. *NeuroImage*, *20*, 244–56.

Prickett, A. C. and Moore, R. S. (1991). The use of music to aid memory of Alzheimer's patients. *Journal of Music Therapy*, *28*, 101–10.

Rachman, S. (1981). The primacy of affect: some theoretical implications. *Behavior Research and Therapy*, *19*, 279–90.

Robottom, B. J., Shulman, L. M., and Weiner, W. J. (2010). Parkinson disease. In: W. J. Weiner, C. G. Goetz, R. K. Shin, and S. L. Lewis (eds) *Neurology for the Non-Neurologist*, 6th edition. New York: Lippincott Williams & Wilkins. pp. 222–40.

Rubin, D. C., Rahhal, T. A., and Poon, L. W. (1998). Things learned in early adulthood are remembered best. *Memory & Cognition*, *26*, 3–19.

Salmon, D. (1993). Music and emotion in palliative care. *Journal of Palliative Care*, *9*, 48–52.

Samson, S., Dellacherie, D., and Platel, H. (2009). Emotional power of music in patients with memory disorders: clinical implications of cognitive neuroscience. *Annals of the New York Academy of Sciences*, *1169*, 245–55.

Sarkamo, T. et al. (2008). Music listening enhances cognitive recovery and mood after middle cerebral artery stroke. *Brain*, *131*, 866–76.

Schacter, D. L. and Tulving, E. (1994). What are the memory systems of 1994? In: D. L. Schacter and E. Tulving (eds) *Memory Systems 1994*. Cambridge, MA: MIT Press. pp. 1–38.

Schenkenberg, T. and Miller, P. J. (2000). Issues in the clinical evaluation of suspected dementia. In: R. D. Hill, L. Bäckman, and A. S. Neely (eds) *Cognitive Rehabilitation in Old Age*. New York: Oxford University Press. pp. 207–23.

Schück, S. et al. (2002). Psychomotor and cognitive effects of piribedil, a dopamine agonist, in young healthy volunteers. *Fundamental & Clinical Pharmacology*, *16*, 57–65.

Schulkind, M. D., Hennis, L. K., and Rubin, D. C. (1999). Music, emotion, and autobiographical memory: they're playing your song. *Memory and Cognition*, *27*, 948–55.

Schwartz, B. L. (2011a). Episodic memory. In: *Memory: foundations and applications*. London: Sage. pp. 87–121.

Schwartz, B. L. (2011b). Memory disorders. In: *Memory: foundations and applications*. London: Sage. pp. 289–321.

Schwartz, B. L. (2011c). Memory in older adults. In: *Memory: foundations and applications*. London: Sage. pp. 351–75.

Soltys, F. G. (2007). Reminiscence, grief, loss, and end of life. In: J. A Kunz and F. G. Soltys (eds) *Transformational Reminiscence: life story work*. New York: Springer Publishing. pp. 197–214.

Stinson, C. K. (2009). Structured group reminiscence: an intervention for older adults. *Journal of Continuing Education in Nursing*, *40*, 521–8.

Suzuki, A. I. (1998). The effects of music therapy on mood and congruent memory of elderly adults with depressive symptoms. *Music Therapy Perspectives*, *16*, 75–80.

Sweatt, J. D. (2003). Aging-related memory disorders: Alzheimer's disease. In: *Mechanisms of Memory*. New York: Academic Press. pp. 337–65.

Thaut, M. H. (1999). Appendix: A session structure for music psychotherapy. In: W. B. Davis, K. E. Gfeller, and M. H. Thaut (eds) *An Introduction to Music Therapy: theory and practice*, 2nd edition. New York: McGraw-Hill Higher Education. pp. 339–41.

Thaut, M. H. (2002). Toward a cognition–affect model in neuropsychiatric music therapy. In: R. F. Unkefer and M. H. Thaut (eds) *Music Therapy in the Treatment of Adults with Mental Disorders: theoretical bases and clinical interventions*, 2nd edn. St Louis, MO: MMB Music, Inc. pp. 86–103.

Thaut, M. H. (2010). Neurologic music therapy in cognitive rehabilitation. *Music Perception, 27*, 281–5.

Thaut, M. H. and de l'Etoile, S. K. (1993). The effects of music on mood state-dependent recall. *Journal of Music Therapy, 30*, 70–80.

Thaut, M. H., Thaut, C., and LaGasse, B. (2008). Music therapy in neurologic rehabilitation. In: W. B. Davis, K. E. Gfeller, and M. H. Thaut (eds) *An Introduction to Music Therapy: theory and practice*, 3rd edn. Silver Spring, MD: American Music Therapy Association. pp. 261–304.

Thompson, P. M. et al. (2003). Dynamics of gray matter loss in Alzheimer's disease. *Journal of Neuroscience, 23*, 994–1005.

Walker, J. and Adamek, M. (2008). Music therapy in hospice and palliative care. In: W. B. Davis, K. E. Gfeller, and M. H. Thaut (eds) *An Introduction to Music Therapy: theory and practice*, 3rd edn. Silver Spring, MD: American Music Therapy Association. pp. 343–64.

Whittle, S., Allen, N. B., Lubman, D. I., and Yücel, M. (2006). The neurobiological basis of temperament: towards a better understanding of psychopathology. *Neuroscience and Biobehavioral Reviews, 30*, 511–25.

Chapter 27

Music in Psychosocial Training and Counseling (MPC)

Barbara L. Wheeler

27.1 Definition

MPC was originally called *music psychotherapy counseling*, and was described as employing;

> guided music listening, musical role playing, and expressive improvisation or composition exercises. It uses musical performance to address issues of mood control, affective expression, cognitive coherence, reality orientation, and appropriate social interaction to facilitate psychosocial functions. The techniques are based on models derived from affect modification, associative network theory of mood and memory, social learning theory, classical and operant conditioning, and mood vectoring based on iso principle techniques.
>
> (Thaut, 2005, p. 197)

More recently, the name was changed to *music in psychosocial training and counseling*, which is a better description of this NMT technique. This chapter details and expands upon ways in which MPC may be administered.

MPC focuses on psychosocial training, which is integral to NMT. When psychotherapy is involved, it may include techniques that have been described as activity or supportive, activities-oriented music therapy (Houghton et al., 2002; Wheeler, 1983), many of which may be appropriate for people whose cognitive and emotional functioning may be impaired by neurologic problems. It may also include techniques that are classified as insight music therapy with re-educative goals or re-educative, insight-, and process-oriented music therapy (Houghton et al., 2002; Wheeler, 1983), although the verbal aspects of this type of therapy may not be accessible to people with certain types of brain injuries or levels of impairment, and are not appropriate for those with cognitive deficits that impair insight-related functions such as self-monitoring, memory, ability to learn new material, or any combination of these. Certain types of brain damage, such as that involving frontal impairment, might contraindicate the use of insight-oriented therapies.

MPC can utilize any music-based method that can help people with neurologic problems to improve their psychosocial functioning. It uses "musical performance to address issues of mood control, affective expression, cognitive coherence, reality orientation, and appropriate social interaction to facilitate psychosocial functions" (Thaut, 2005, p. 197). Figure 27.1 illustrates the use of improvisation as part of an MPC session.

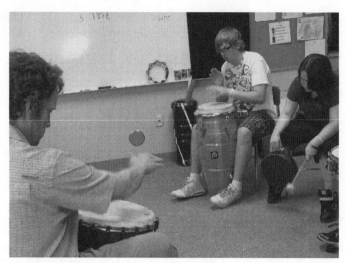

Fig. 27.1 Glen Helgeson, MEd, MT-BC, Neurologic Music Therapist, leads students at the MRVSEC Oasis program in Jordan, MN, in a group musical improvisation. MPC goals are to participate in a group improvisation, follow directions appropriately, listen to others, and take a risk by trying new instruments in front of their peers.

MPC may focus on psychosocial training, counseling, or a combination of both, depending upon the needs of the clients and on the training and skill of the therapist. While the training for neurologic music therapists includes MPC, it is not intended to develop skills for in-depth counseling. Some music therapists will have these skills and can therefore emphasize the counseling aspect of MPC, whereas others will not have enough training or experience to help clients to delve deeply into problems, and therefore should not attempt to work at this "deeper" level.

Prigatano (1999, pp. 219–20) offers practical considerations for the therapist when undertaking psychotherapy with a person who has had a brain injury. These are useful to keep in mind for MPC as well, and are listed (with some modifications) here:

1 Go slowly.

2 Present yourself as a consultant to the patient, not as a healer, boss, parent, etc.

3 Help the patient to sharpen their perspective on reality repeatedly.

4 Recognize the complexity of behavior and the role of conscious and unconscious factors that may motivate a given behavior. See behavior as an ongoing attempt to adapt to the present in the light of past experiences.

5 Focus on the present, but with an understanding of how the past may have contributed to the patient's behavior.

6 Help the patient to recognize the time limitations to rehabilitation, and that it must have a focused problem-solving approach. The intent is to help the patient to become independent of the therapist.

7 Deal with the patient's misperceptions, angry outbursts,[1] inappropriate behavior anxiety, and depression slowly, honestly, and empathetically.

8 Heed Jung's admonishment that if people think a certain way, they may feel considerably better.

9 Help the patient to establish a sense of meaning in the presence of, not despite, brain injury.

The primary goals of MPC can be loosely divided into affect identification and expression, mood control, and social competence and self-awareness. Information on these goal areas is presented in the remainder of this chapter.

27.2 **Target populations**

MPC is typically used with people with the following diagnoses and problems:

- ◆ autism and autism spectrum disorders (ASD)
- ◆ traumatic brain injury (TBI) or stroke, to enable them to adjust to their changed status and to deal with deficits
- ◆ other neurological problems (e.g. Parkinson's disease), to enable them to adjust to their changed status and to deal with deficits
- ◆ older adults and patients with dementia, to enable them to deal with decreased cognitive and physical skills, including emotional reactions to losses, and to maintain functioning for as long as possible
- ◆ depression secondary to TBI, stroke, or other problems; it is also applicable to those with depression as an independent psychiatric diagnosis.

MPC may be contraindicated for neurobehavioral populations with frontal impairments or with post-traumatic amnesia, as people with these problems often do not have the ability to benefit from insight-oriented therapies.

27.3 **Therapeutic mechanisms**

27.3.1 **Affect identification and expression**

The use of music and other methods that access emotions more directly than words do has been advocated for many years. Zwerling (1979) proposed that the arts, including music, have the unique ability to tap into the emotional component of behaviors, thoughts, and memories and elicit emotional reactions, making them powerful therapeutic stimuli to facilitate emotional processing in therapy. Emotional processing in therapy is needed when emotions, consciously or unconsciously attached to maladaptive behaviors, hinder the

---

[1] Patients with frontal impairments may have oversensitive triggers and therefore express behavior that is disinhibited. This does not mean that the anger is any less felt or inappropriate, but it might be disproportional to the trigger, difficult to modulate, and expressed very suddenly and more expressively, and is likely to be difficult to de-escalate.

development of more adaptive, healthy behaviors, or when emotional experiences such as fear, trauma, or loss arise and disrupt normal behaviors.

Applying this to music therapy, Thaut suggested that "methods and stimuli which have the unique qualities to evoke emotions and influence mood states" (Thaut, 1989a, pp. 55–6) could complement traditional verbal and behavioral interventions. Because music can access affective/motivational systems in the brain, it can influence and modify affective states and also access the totality of a patient's cognitions and perceptions, feeling states, and behavior organization (Thaut and Wheeler, 2010).

What mechanisms underlie the positive effect of music on affective change? Thaut (1989a, 2002) and Thaut and Wheeler (2010), in a model developed for psychiatric music therapy, have postulated that an "affective-evaluative response" comprised of three interacting response systems lies at the core of the emotional/mood reaction to music. This includes a primary affective response (Zajonc, 1984) or primary appraisal (Lazarus, 1984), cognitive elaborations on the primary response that determine the quality and meaning of the stimulus, and a differential neurophysiological arousal response. A therapeutic music experience involves three therapeutic effects: (1) music exercises designed for therapeutic leaving, (2) affective qualities inherent in the process of music perception that address relevant emotional materials in the therapeutic process directly, and (3) musical mood induction to access therapeutically desired associative memory networks, making mood-congruent cognitive information more accessible. Thus specific clinical music therapy techniques, including verbal processing, serve as training experiences in which music-induced affect modification drives cognitive, affective, and behavioral change related to therapeutic goals (Thaut and Wheeler, 2010).

27.3.2 Mood control

People with neurological problems may have problems with mood control in various aspects of their lives. Some may have depression, either related to their neurological problem or as an ongoing issue that may have preceded the neurological problem. Tension and anxiety may also be related to mood.

Cognitive reorientation (de l'Etoile, 1992; Thaut, 1989a) may help to control moods or deal with a mood disorder. A positive affective experience may help the individual to be amenable to cognitive change in therapy. Music may help to organize therapeutic experiences around their affective/motivational content and value for the individual, and may lead to rethinking personal problems, changing perceptions of others, learning new coping skills, processing significant life experiences, dealing with fears, and setting new goals (Gfeller, 2002).

One explanation for what occurs within cognitive reorientation is provided by the *associative network theory of mood and memory* (Bower, 1981), which suggests that when an event or information is stored in memory, connections are established with other elements of the event that occur at the same time and are then stored as nodes in memory and can be activated when a stimulus enters the memory.

A client may symbolically re-create a problematic life situation through imagery. Music may help to elicit images from memory, possibly based on associative memory network operations (Bower, 1981), and also helps to retrieve the mood/emotional quality of a particular life situation in the imaging process (Goldberg, 1992).

MPC can offer methods to alter or induce desired mood states that may directly influence feelings of depression, elation, anxiety, rest, relaxation, motivation, or levels of activation and energy. The ability of music to help to deal with depression may be useful as a person with neurologic injuries begins to come to grips with what has happened and its effect on their life.

27.3.3 Social competence and self-awareness

Sears (1968) and Zwerling (1979) have written of the social nature of the musical experience. Sears suggests that music provides "experience in relating to others" (Sears, 1968, p. 41), and Zwerling speaks of the "intrinsic social or reality-based character" (Zwerling, 1979, p. 844) of the creative arts therapies.

Bandura's social learning theory (Bandura, 1977) and social cognitive theory (Bandura, 1986) suggest that people learn by observing the behavior of others and the outcomes of those behaviors. The concept of self-efficacy, positing that people decide how to behave based largely on their belief in their own capabilities, is central to social cognitive theory and is critical for the ability of individuals to engage in the sort of self-regulation to which Bandura refers.

Thaut (2002) suggests that most psychiatric rehabilitation is concerned with the social aspects of behavior. Since many therapeutic music exercise methods offer opportunities for social learning, a neurologic music therapist can develop strategies to elicit social behaviors. Within the structure of an MPC session, participants can exhibit typical behaviors, some of which may be maladaptive, and then reflect upon and make plans to change them, as well as experimenting with more adaptive behaviors. Similar methods may be used with people with neurological problems, assuming that insight and learning are intact. In addition, because affect modification is seen as a prerequisite for certain types of behavior modification, establishing more direct therapy procedures for affect modification to facilitate behavior modification is suggested.

People with autism and autism spectrum disorder (ASD) have difficulty regulating their level of arousal (Bachevalier and Loveland, 2006; Gomez, 2005; National Autism Center, 2009, p. 39). MPC exercises can be used to help people to focus on the state of their bodies and use this awareness to help to change or regulate their level of arousal, bringing it to a more adaptive state.

27.4 Research summary

27.4.1 Affect identification and expression

Music's ability to evoke and alter emotional reactions has been documented. Hodges (1996) and Hodges and Sebald (2011) surveyed the literature on affective-mood responses to music and provided evidence that (1) music evokes emotional and mood reactions, including emotional peak experiences, (2) music can alter a listener's mood, (3) emotional and mood responses to music are accompanied by physiological changes, and (4) existing mood, musical preference, cultural expectations, and arousal needs also play a role in determining affective responses (Thaut, 2002).

Both cognitive and physiological responses are important for processing emotions, and there are numerous models of how they combine and are sequenced. One model is that of Mandler (1984), who suggested that an emotional reaction is preceded by biological arousal of the autonomic nervous system, caused by an interruption of expectancy patterns that are based on perceptual–motor schemata. When something unexpected happens, arousal is triggered as an alerting signal to search for an interpretation of the interruption, and an emotional experience of a particular quality is produced. The cognitive interpretation of the arousal-triggering circumstances defines the quality of the emotional experience. Another model is that of Huron (Hodges and Sebald, 2011; Huron, 2006), whose *ITPRA (Imagination–Tension–Prediction–Response–Appraisal) theory of expectation* includes two responses (imagination and tension) that occur prior to an event, and three responses (prediction, reaction, and appraisal) that occur after the event. (Appraisal assumes the ability to self-monitor and to learn new material for insight, and to integrate these, an ability that might be impaired in some individuals with brain injuries.)

Emotional processing of music occurs in both cortical structures (i.e. related to the cerebral cortex) and subcortical structures. Peretz (2010) points out that activity in cortical structures, including the orbitofrontal cortex, the superior temporal cortex, and the anterior cingulated cortex, is reported frequently in relation to musical emotions.

The limbic system, which is a subcortical structure, is important for processing music and emotion. Evidence of this includes findings from PET studies (Blood et al., 1999; Blood and Zatorre, 2001) that cerebral blood flow changes in subcortical neural structures as the intensity of physiological and psychological responses increases and as people experience musical "chills", as well as increased activation (in musicians) in the ventral striatum (containing the nucleus accumbens, which is involved in reward) and decreased activation in the amygdala (Peretz, 2010).

Many cortical and subcortical regions are also involved in emotional responses to music (see Damasio, 1994; LeDoux, 1996). Peretz (2010) has summarized research suggesting that emotional responses to music occur subcortically, and has reported activation of the nucleus accumbens in response to music (Brown et al., 2004; Koelsch et al., 2006; Menon and Levitin, 2005; Mitterschiffthaler et al., 2007). Since the nucleus accumbens is activated in response to highly rewarding or motivationally important stimuli, it appears that music can access subcortical structures associated with primary reinforcers. The amygdala can also be engaged by scary music (Gosselin et al., 2005, 2007), which suggests that music may be as effective as food, drugs, and facial expressions in eliciting subcortically mediated affective responses.

There is also evidence that the release of neurotransmitters may affect emotional responses to music. Menon and Levitin (2005) found correlations pointing to an association between dopamine release and response in two areas involved with reward—the nucleus accumbens and the ventral tegmental area—in response to pleasant music. Evers and Suhr (2000) found an increase in the release of serotonin (a neurotransmitter associated with feelings of satisfaction) when listening to unpleasant music. Hodges (2010, pp. 287–8) has provided an extensive table of research on biochemical responses to music.

Music can induce a variety of emotions. These can be specific emotions (Gabrielsson and Juslin, 1996; Krumhansl, 1997; Peretz, 2001) as well as emotional states (Gendolla and Krüsken, 2001; Gomez and Danuser, 2004; Khalfa et al., 2002).

Other aspects of music can also evoke emotional responses. Salimpoor et al. (2009) found a strong positive correlation between ratings of pleasure and emotional arousal, as well as indications that pleasure was necessary to experience emotional arousal. Kreutz et al. (2008) found instrumental music to be effective for the induction of basic emotions in adult listeners. Baumgartner et al. (2006) studied the influence of visual and musical stimuli on brain processing, and found that music could enhance the emotional experience evoked by affective pictures.

Juslin and Västfjäll (2008) have proposed six underlying mechanisms through which listening to music may induce emotions, and suggest that these may help to improve research in this area. These mechanisms are brainstem reflex, evaluative conditioning, emotional contagion, visual imagery, episodic memory, and musical expectancy.

Some studies suggest that individuals with autism can understand simple and complex emotions in music, although they have difficulty interpreting people's non-verbal, facial, and bodily expressions of emotion (Molnar-Szakacs and Heaton, 2012). This may make music useful for processing and expressing emotion.

27.4.2 **Mood control**

Music can affect cognition and related behaviors and can induce mood. It has been found that elated mood can help to remove intrusive, unwanted cognitions (Sutherland et al., 1982), depressed mood induced by music is associated with psychomotor retardation (Clark and Teasdale, 1985; Pignatiello et al., 1986; Teasdale and Spencer, 1984), mood influences the accessibility of positive and negative cognitions (Albersnagel, 1988; Clark and Teasdale, 1985), and induced mood states influence individuals' estimates of past and future success on a task (Teasdale and Spencer, 1984). Mood induction by music may support cognitive therapies of depression by helping the client to be more accessible to positive cognitions (Clark, 1983; Sutherland et al., 1982; Teasdale, 1983).

Music may elicit affective responses and influence therapeutically relevant behaviors. Studies document the efficacy of "happy" and "sad" music in inducing depressed and elated mood states in normal subjects. Albersnagel (1988), Clark (1983), Clark and Teasdale (1985), and Sutherland et al. (1982) reported that subjects reached predetermined mood change criteria and had stronger subjective mood ratings when music mood induction was used than with verbal methods (Velten, 1968).

Studies of the effects of music on depression provide initial evidence that music may have a positive influence on affective responses. A Cochrane review (Maratos et al., 2008) included four studies (Chen, 1992; Hanser and Thompson, 1994; Hendricks, 2001;

Radulovic et al., 1997) that found greater reductions in symptoms of depression among individuals randomized to music therapy, although one study (Zerhusen et al., 1995) found no such change.

Music has been found to decrease depression. Scheiby (1999) presented a case study of supportive music psychotherapy with four clients with dementia and depression and who had experienced neurological traumas. Nayak et al. (2000) found trends suggesting improved mood in people who had had strokes and TBI. Magee and Davidson (2002) found that music therapy, including short-term intervention, was helpful in improving mood states of people with a variety of neuro-disabilities. Eslinger et al. (1993) found a significant improvement in emotional empathy measures, as reported by family members and friends, in individuals who had had brain injuries. Purdie et al. (1997) found that long-term institutionalized patients who had had strokes showed signs of being less depressed and anxious after 12 weeks of music therapy than did those who had not received music therapy. Cross et al. (1984) found lower anxiety levels according to post-therapy emotional measures after the music therapy process had begun. Pacchetti et al. (1998, 2000) found improvements in emotional functioning in patients with Parkinson's disease. Participants in Sing for Joy (Magee, in press), a user-led investigation of the effects of communal singing for patients with Parkinson's disease and other chronic conditions and their carers, were found to show statistically significant improvements in feelings of energy and fear following the experience of communal singing.

Sarkamo et al. (2008) conducted a randomized controlled trial of 54 patients who had had strokes and who listened to self-selected music or audio books daily, or were part of a control group for 2 months, as well as receiving standard care. Verbal memory and focused attention domains improved significantly more in the music group than in the other two groups. The music group also experienced less depression and confusion than the control group. A follow-up study (Sarkamo et al., 2010) found positive results for people who listened to music or audio books.

Overviews of research on the use of music therapy in patients with neurological problems, including mood control, social competence, and self-awareness—the areas on which this chapter is focused—have been provided by Purdie (1997) and Gilbertson (2005). A Cochrane review (Bradt et al., 2010) was also undertaken, but no studies with these areas as a focus met the inclusion criteria. Findings from Eslinger et al. (1993) are pending.

27.4.3 Social competence and self-awareness

Research by Teasdale and Spencer (1984) indicated that depressed individuals made lower retrospective estimates of success on experimental tasks than did non-depressed controls. Studies manipulating the mood of normal subjects have consistently found decreased recall of positive memories and increased recall of negative memories in depressed compared with elated mood (Bower, 1981; Teasdale, 1983; Teasdale and Taylor, 1981). It is suggested that the activation of the negative network enhances and focuses respondents on negative content, thus perpetuating negative perceptions (Lyubomirsky and Nolen-Hoeksema, 1993; Nolen-Hoeksema, 1991).

Research supports the affective–social function of music in therapy. The structure of music activities can draw people together, due to requiring group participation and cooperation (Anshel and Kipper, 1988). Thaut (1989b) reported on the effect of music group therapy in promoting less hostile and more cooperative group-related behaviors in psychiatric prisoner-patients. Goldberg et al. (1988) found that music therapy groups produced more therapeutic interaction among and emotional responses from patients than verbal therapy. Henderson (1983) found a positive effect of music therapy on awareness of mood in music, group cohesion, and self-esteem among adolescent psychiatric clients. Some of these positive effects may occur in a group session, such as that shown in Figure 27.2, where students are participating in a musical improvisation. Music therapy is frequently acknowledged to be helpful in social aspects of rehabilitation from brain injuries, and in aiding self-awareness and improving self-concept. Case descriptions constitute much of the literature supporting these uses. A number of sources of interventions that include reference to identity, self-perception, and self-esteem are found in a German compilation of indications for music therapy (Baumann et al., 2007).

A limited amount of research also supports positive effects of music therapy on the social competence and self-awareness of people with brain injuries and other neurological problems. Barker and Brunk (1991) found that most participants in a 1-year group moved from a passive role to a leadership role. Nayak et al. (2000) found patients receiving music therapy to be significantly more involved in their rehabilitation programs and more socially interactive than those who did not receive music therapy. Magee (1999) found that individuals with multiple sclerosis used singing and playing instruments to monitor their illness and physical functioning. Shifting self-concepts and improved identity constructs relating to feelings of ability, control, independence, and skill emerged in participants' data.

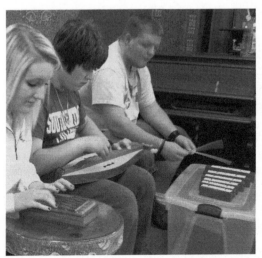

Fig. 27.2 Students at the MRVSEC Oasis program in Jordan, MN, participating in a group musical improvisation. MPC goals are to participate in a group improvisation, follow directions appropriately, listen to others, and take a risk by trying new instruments in front of peers. Glen Helgeson MEd, MT-BC, Neurologic Music Therapist, is facilitating the session.

27.5 **Clinical protocols**

The following protocols may elicit verbal material, insights, and behaviors that may be helpful for the person undergoing NMT. They can be powerful experiences, and the therapist should be cautious about the material that comes up, and not delve more deeply than the therapist's level of competence and the client's level of functioning allow. The levels of therapy that were discussed earlier (Houghton et al., 2002; Wheeler 1983) were developed for this purpose, to help music therapists to work at the level at which they are competent and that is appropriate for their clients.

It should also be emphasized that the relationship with the client and the way that the music is used within this relationship are of primary importance. The suggested techniques listed in this chapter should be understood within this context. They are not stand-alone ways to help people, but must be used within the context of a relationship and with care.

One additional point should be made about the interventions that are described in this chapter. The therapist must select and adapt them to meet the client's needs at the level at which the client is functioning. Considerations will include diagnosis, capacity to process, progress made from session to session, developmental age and chronological age, preferences, and culture. Most of the interventions that are presented here can be adapted for children or adults, and all of the techniques must be individualized.

27.5.1 **Affect and mood**

Active and receptive therapeutic music exercises can be used to facilitate the "feeling" experience of emotion, the identification of emotion, the expression of emotion, the understanding of emotional communication of others, and the synthesis, control, and modulation of one's own emotional behavior (Thaut and Wheeler, 2010).

27.5.1.1 Emotional continuum

Skill/area targeted: Recognition and expression of emotions.

Age group: Adults or adolescents; children at a simpler level.

Setting: Group.

Equipment needed: A range of simple percussion and melodic instruments.

Step-by-step procedure:

1 Form the group into a circle.

2 Each group member selects an instrument that they will use to represent an emotion.

3 The leader/therapist directs all of the participants to improvise in order to portray changes in emotional states (from 1 to 5), where 0 is very sad, 3 is neutral, and 5 is very happy.

4 Each individual plays a specific emotion and also practices playing and/or adjusting to others' emotional states, from 1 to 5.

5 The same activity is now performed in reverse (from 5 to 1) to demonstrate and practice emotional control.

6 Experiment with the form ABACAD, with each letter standing for a different emotion, alternating emotions.

Figure 27.3 shows a training session in the use of improvisation with MPC.

27.5.1.2 Continuum of arousal

This can be used to provide a different focus from emotional continuum.

Skill/area targeted: Awareness and expression of level of arousal.

Age group: Adults or adolescents; children at a simpler level.

Setting: Group.

Equipment needed: A range of simple percussive and melodic instruments.

Step-by-step procedure:

1 Form the group into a circle.

2 Each participant selects an instrument to use to represent a level of arousal.

3 The leader/therapist directs all of the participants to improvise in order to portray changes in level of arousal (from 1 to 5), where 1 is calm/serene, and 5 is restless.

4 Each individual plays a specific level and also practices playing and/or adjusting to others' level of arousal, from 1 to 5.

5 The same activity is now performed in reverse (from 5 to 1) to demonstrate and practice control of arousal.

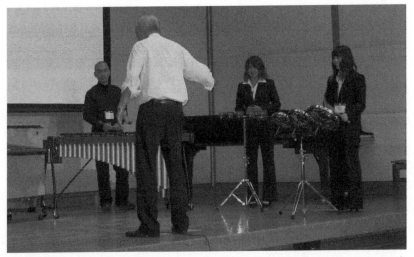

Fig. 27.3 Michael Thaut leads Japanese trainees through an improvisation based on a specific theme, demonstrating how to use the instruments and elements of the music to represent non-musical themes or context.

27.5.1.3 Modifying arousal

Skill/area targeted: Modification of over- or under-arousal, which is most likely to occur in people with autism and ASD.

Age group: All ages.

Setting: Group or individual.

Equipment needed: Hand drums or rhythm sticks.

Step-by-step procedure:

1 Form a circle (if a group setting is being used).

2 The individual or group member selects an instrument that they will use to represent their level of arousal.

3 The leader/therapist directs the individual or group members to improvise, portraying their current level of arousal.

4 The therapist and the individual or group members label their current state of arousal on a scale of 1 to 5, where 1 is under-aroused and 5 is over-aroused.

5 The individual or group member uses their instrument to heighten their awareness of their arousal level and to modify it (i.e. to decrease or increase their arousal level to a more functional state).

6 If the individual or group member is unable to self-regulate, the therapist facilitates the modification of their state of arousal by playing their rhythm and then gradually bringing it up or down to arrive at a more functional state of arousal.

7 The individual or group members can then discuss the experience if appropriate.

Additional information: In Magee et al. (2011), Case Vignette 6, familiar songs were sung live with guitar accompaniment to a man with post-traumatic amnesia. The goals were to reduce agitation and target increased orientation.

> Familiar music is thought to lead to optimal arousal rather than *maximal levels of arousal* (Baker, 2002, 2009; Soto et al., 2009), whereas non-preferred music may over-arouse patients. Imaging studies provide evidence of neural networks that are activated by preferred music related to arousal (Soto et al., 2009).

(Magee et al., p. 11)

27.5.1.4 Dealing with anger

Skill/area targeted: Anger management.

Age group: Adults or adolescents; children at a simpler level.

Setting: Group.

Equipment needed: Hand drums or rhythm sticks.

Step-by-step procedure:

1 Seat the group in a circle.

2 Each participant is given a hand drum, and the group then warms up by sharing a rhythm on the drums.

3 The group discusses how to express anger on a drum.

4 Each participant has opportunity to express an angry feeling on the drum.

5 The therapist sits facing the person who is expressing anger and helps him or her to deal with the anger as follows:

   a The participant is encouraged to express strong anger on the drum.

   b The therapist matches the angry expression on their own drum.

   c The therapist gradually makes their own drumming quiet and relaxed, influencing the participant to drum in a calm manner.

6 Each participant has the opportunity to pair up with another group member, express anger on the drum, and have their partner match the angry expression and bring it down to a calm feeling.

7 Each participant also has the opportunity to help another person come down from an angry feeling.

8 After everyone has had a chance to participate, the group discusses the exercise and its application to everyday experiences with anger.

27.5.1.5 Empathy through drumming

Skill/area targeted: Empathy.

Age group: Adults or adolescents; children at a simpler level.

Setting: Group.

Equipment needed: A variety of drums.

Step-by-step procedure:

1 Seat the group in a circle, allowing room for each person to play a drum.

2 Explain the purpose of the exercise.

3 Ask each group member to choose a musical instrument.

4 The group leader portrays an emotion to the rest of the group by playing a musical instrument. Facial expressions are kept to a minimum, so that the emotion comes through the music as much as possible.

5 Each group member is asked to state the emotion or experience that is being portrayed.

6 Each group member can express an emotion or experience to the rest of the group, and then ask the group to guess what was being portrayed.

27.5.1.6 Improvisation for mood change

Skill/area targeted: Mood for which change is desired.

Age group: Adults or children.

Setting: Individual or group.

Equipment needed: A range of simple rhythm and melodic instruments.

Step-by-step procedure:

1 Seat the participants in a circle (if a group setting is being used), with room to play their instruments.

2 Each participant selects an instrument to play to convey emotions.

3 The group members talk about their current mood(s) and how their mood(s) might change so that they would feel better.

4 All of the participants improvise with the goal of moving the mood(s) of the improvisation to a more positive place, in line with the discussion in Step 3.

5 Discussion of the participants' experience may occur after the improvisation.

27.5.1.7 Musical mood induction (guided music listening)

This can be used to access associative mood and memory networks to direct specific memory access and to gain access to positive networks of thoughts and emotions (e.g. in the treatment of depression).

Skill/area targeted: Depression, sadness.

Age group: Adults or adolescents; children at a simpler level; participants must have at least a minimal level of verbal understanding.

Setting: Individual or group.

Equipment needed: Recorded music conveying various moods; instruments for improvisation are optional.

Step-by-step procedure:

1 The therapist selects music that may help the client who is depressed to access more positive thoughts.

2 The therapist plays the music (live or recorded).

3 The therapist and client discuss the client's feelings in response to the music; according to the theory, these are likely to be more positive than previously.

4 After more positive thoughts have been accessed, music can be used to guide the client to topics of discussion that are deemed helpful and relevant (by the client or the therapist); this can be verbal or lead to additional selections of music or improvisation to process feelings.

This approach is called *cognitive reorientation through associative network theory* or *associative mood and memory training (AMMT)*.

27.5.1.8 Mood induction and vectoring (using the iso principle)

This is an adaptation of musical mood induction.

Skill/area targeted: Mood.

Age group: Adults or adolescents; children at a simpler level; participants must have at least a minimal level of verbal understanding.

Setting: Individual or group.

Equipment needed: Recorded music that conveys a range of moods.

Step-by-step procedure:

1 Match the music to the client's mood. This can be their self-identified mood or their mood as the therapist identifies it. The music can be live or recorded, pre-composed or improvised.

2 Gradually change the music, while remaining aware of the client's mood. The goal is to change the mood gradually toward a preferred or more adaptive mood by changing the music.

Adaptation: Participants can create their own music relaxation iPod playlists or CDs. This can be very helpful for clients with ASD who get stuck in emotional motor plans, and they can use it when they know that a situation is going to produce a particular negative and often explosive emotional reaction. It is also particularly effective when they have been stuck in a negative emotive state to help them to move from that state to a neutral response. For higher-functioning clients, creating their own playlists or CDs, listening to music, identifying their own physical responses to various music samples, and translating those responses into feeling words/labels is very important. This step is necessary due to different sensory processing in individuals with ASD and similar disorders in order to increase awareness of physical responses and then associate these with a particular emotive state. It is helpful for the therapist to verbally identify emotive states with lower-functioning or younger clients.

27.5.2 Social competence and self-awareness

Many therapy methods offer opportunities for social learning. Within the model of "affect modification", MPC exercises can offer two unique contributions to social experiences in therapy. First, they organize social behaviors around the affective/motivational experience of social interaction using affect-evoking materials (i.e. music-based experiences) (Zwerling, 1979). Secondly, they emphasize the practice and learning of social skills experientially through performance in a positive emotional context (Thaut, 2002). Individuals who have difficulties in social situations may be motivated through these activities to become interested in social settings.

27.5.2.1 Interaction and communication

Skill/area targeted: Interaction/communication.

Age group: Adults or adolescents; children at a simpler level.

Setting: Individual or group.

Equipment: A variety of percussion instruments.

Step-by-step procedure:

1 Form the group into a circle, with plenty of room for playing musical instruments.

2 Each participant chooses an instrument to express a non-verbal message.

3 Two group members face each other; one will initiate, the other will receive.

4 The initiator starts an instrumental conversation and the receiver responds, continuing until they are ready to end the conversation.

5 After they have finished, they discuss what occurred and how it felt.

6 Other members of the group may provide feedback.

7 They may repeat the instrumental interaction to make changes, when appropriate.

8 The procedure is then repeated with a different pair of participants.

27.5.2.2 Leading and following

Skill/area targeted: Group skills of leading and following.

Age group: Children or adults.

Setting: Group.

Equipment: A variety of simple rhythmic and melodic instruments.

Step-by-step procedure:

1 Form the group into a circle, with plenty of room for playing musical instruments.

2 Explain that they will be improvising under the leadership of one of the group members.

3 Each group member selects an instrument.

4 The therapist can model initial improvisation, taking the leadership role and providing non-verbal leadership.

5 One by one the group members take the leadership role, if they are capable of this; it may be too demanding or threatening for some, and they should not be required to lead.

6 Improvise to practice leading and following.

7 Sample improvisations include the following:

    a with changes of volume

    b with changes of tempo

    c modal, without harmonic grounding.

Figure 27.4 shows students participating in an improvisation led by a peer.

27.5.2.3 Music as a reinforcer

This is also called *musical incentive training for behavior modification*.

Skill/area targeted: Any specific behavior or skill can be targeted.

Age group: Children or adults.

Setting: Individual (can be adapted for a group).

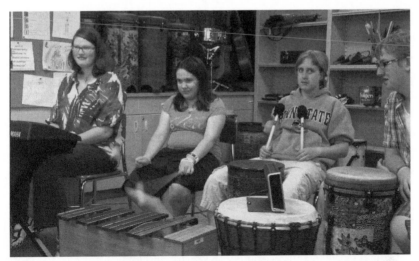

Fig. 27.4 Students in the MRVSEC Oasis program in Jordan, MN, waiting for their turn to participate in a musical improvisation led by a peer. MPC goals are to practice turn taking, build self-confidence, practice leadership skills, and create a meaningful therapeutic musical experience within the group setting. Glen Helgeson, MEd, MT-BC, Neurologic Music Therapist, is facilitating the session.

Equipment: Live or recorded music.

Step-by-step procedure:

1 Select the behavior to be targeted.

2 Determine the amount or number of occurrences of behavior that will be required to obtain reinforcement.

3 Determine the music to use for reinforcement (e.g. 3 minutes of listening to the chosen music, participation in 5 minutes of instrument playing).

4 Make the requirement and reinforcement clear to the participant.

5 After the behavior occurs, administer the reinforcement.

6 Keep track of the responses, and make adjustments as appropriate (e.g. decrease or increase the number of occurrences of the behavior that are needed for reinforcement).

Adaptations: This exercise can be used to target delayed gratification, anywhere from 5 seconds to 45 minutes. It can also be used to help the client to "buy into" or tolerate being in the therapy space and engaging in the music therapy session.

27.5.2.4 Musical performance for relationship training

Skill/area targeted: Relationships.

Age group: Children or adults.

Setting: Group or dyad.

Equipment: A variety of simple rhythmic and melodic instruments.

Step-by-step procedure:

1 One group member selects an instrument to use to make a connection with another participant, and an instrument with which the other can respond (they may either share an instrument or use separate instruments).

2 That group member goes to one person in the group, sits facing them, and plays the instrument to them.

3 The other person responds.

4 The two participants play together.

5 After they have played, the two participants discuss what has occurred.

6 Other members of the group share their observations; the group may discuss what has occurred.

7 The two participants may play again, possibly to change the way that an interaction occurred.

8 The discussion continues for as long as it is productive.

9 The process is repeated with a different pair.

27.5.2.5 Musical role playing

Skill/area targeted: Self-awareness.

Age group: Adults or adolescents; children at a simpler level.

Setting: Group.

Equipment: A variety of simple rhythmic and melodic instruments.

Step-by-step procedure:

1 If working in a group, form a circle, with room for the participants to play musical instruments.

2 Each of the participants chooses an instrument that expresses their presentation of self.

3 Each participant plays something on their instrument.

4 The other group members give verbal feedback on this expression.

5 The participant who has just played can then work on new ways of learning to express self during the session by playing something in a new way.

6 The others group members provide further verbal feedback.

Variation: The musical instrument and way of presenting self can be selected and identified by someone else.

27.5.2.6 Progressive relaxation with music

Skill/area targeted: Stress, tension, anxiety.

Age group: Adults; may be adapted for children.

Setting: Individual or group.

Equipment: CD player or iPod to provide background music, or live music provided by the therapist or their assistant.

Step-by-step procedure:

1 Position the client(s) comfortably in chairs or lying on the floor.

2 Provide cues for deep breathing for a period of time. Instruct the clients to continue deep breathing and to close their eyes if they are comfortable doing so.

3 Explain that you will be introducing a relaxation method that uses tensing of muscles and then releasing them, and that the contrast between the two helps the relaxation. Tell the client(s) to follow the therapist's cues, but that if anything does not feel comfortable, they should not do it, or they should do it to a lesser degree.

4 Beginning with the toes, say slowly "Tighten your toes . . . and relax. Tighten your toes again . . . and relax." (The therapist should do all steps of the procedure along with the client(s) to help pacing.)

   a Move up the body slowly, using these general body parts—heels, feet, calves, knees, thighs.

   b Then go up the body using the front body parts—stomach, chest, shoulders, upper arms, lower arms, hands, and fingers.

   c Then go up the entire arm—"Tense your arm"—then the shoulders, neck, head, back, buttocks, thighs, calves, and feet.

   d Periodically, throughout the exercise, focus on the breathing and remind the clients to continue deep breathing.

5 Relaxation procedures can be ended at this point by reminding everyone to continue deep breathing, then focusing on the feeling and sensations of the room around them, opening their eyes when they are ready, and gradually "coming back" to awareness of others and the room. Remind them that they can recreate this sequence on their own when they need to relax.

6 If desired, this can move into an imagery session that continues the relaxation, by suggesting to the clients that they imagine a place that is relaxing to them (leaving the specifics to each person's imagination, since different people have different places in which they feel relaxed). Suggest that they experience the feel of the air, what is under them, the smells, etc., while continuing to be relaxed. After a period of time, follow the procedures in Step 5 to bring everyone back to the reality of the place and time.

Note: There are numerous procedures for relaxation in addition to progressive muscle relaxation (Jacobson, 1938) as used here. The reader is referred to Justice (2007, pp. 36–9, cited in Crowe, 2007) for additional suggestions.

27.5.2.7 Social story songs

Skill/area targeted: Appropriate social interactions and behavior.

Age group: Children, adolescents, or adults.

Setting: Individual or group.

Equipment: None needed.

Step-by-step procedure:

1 Introduce the story using MMT (musical mnemonics training) to help the client to learn the information, using the song to help the client recall the *rules* of behavior.

   MPC occurs in the next two steps:

2 Discuss the targeted skill.

3 Practice the skill in created and generalized settings.

27.5.2.8 Song about grief

Skill/area targeted: Dealing with grief.

Age group: Adults or adolescents; children at a simpler level.

Setting: Individual or group.

Equipment: A wide enough range of recorded or live music to allow meaningful choices by the client(s).

Step-by-step procedure:

1 The client selects a song to convey feelings of grief.

2 The song is then played or performed by the client or therapist.

3 The client shares verbally how the song conveys feelings about grief (optional).

4 The therapist and/or the group provide feedback, and this facilitates discussion.

Variation: Song writing rather than recorded music can be used.

27.5.2.9 Song about self

Skill/area targeted: Self-awareness, self-concept.

Age group: Adults or adolescents; children at a simpler level.

Setting: Individual or group.

Equipment: A wide enough range of recorded or live music to allow meaningful choices by the client.

Step-by-step procedure:

1 The client selects a song to convey some aspect of him- or herself.

2 The song is played or performed by the client or the therapist.

3 The client shares verbally how he or she feels that the song conveys information about him- or herself.

4 The therapist and/or the group provide feedback, and this facilitates discussion.

27.5.2.10 Song about something needed

Skill/area targeted: Self-awareness.

Age group: Adults or adolescents; children at a simpler level.

Setting: Individual or group.

Equipment: A wide enough range of recorded or live music to allow meaningful choices by the client.

Step-by-step procedure:

1 If working in a group, form a circle.

2 The client selects a song to convey something about him- or herself that needs to be integrated into who he or she is.

3 The client plays and/or sings the song.

4 The client shares verbally how he or she feels about the information conveyed.

5 The therapist and/or the group provide feedback, and this facilitates discussion.

27.5.2.11 Song story

Skill/area targeted: Self-esteem.

Age group: Adults or adolescents; children at a simpler level.

Setting: Individual or group.

Equipment: A wide enough range of recorded or live music to allow meaningful choices by the client.

Step-by-step procedure:

1 If working in a group, form a circle.

2 The therapist and the client select a song that is meaningful to the client.

3 The song is made available to the client for him or her to listen to and interact with repeatedly.

4 The therapist helps the client to explore meaningful parts of the song over time.

27.5.2.12 Scripts

Skill/area targeted: Assertiveness.

Age group: Children or adults.

Setting: Individual or group.

Equipment: A variety of simple rhythmic and melodic instruments.

Step-by-step procedure:

1 If working in a group, form a circle, with room to use musical instruments.

2 Work with the clients to decide upon non-music scripts to role play in order to practice rejection/assertion of will (e.g. "Go with me to the park", "No", "Please, come on", "Maybe", "Come on, let's go", "OK").

3 The clients select instrument(s) with which to express themselves.

4 The clients each take it in turn to interact musically with the therapist to act out the script/situation.

5 The interaction is discussed.

6 Modifications to the interaction are suggested by other group members and the therapist.

7 The musical interaction is repeated with these modifications, and then discussed again.

Variations:

1 Another client can perform the answering role; this is more difficult than having the therapist do this.

2 An area other than assertiveness (e.g. relationship problems, expression of specific emotions) can be targeted.

27.5.2.13 Self-awareness: reality orientation

Age group: Children or adults.

Setting: Individual or group.

Equipment: Varies.

Step-by-step procedure: This is not a specific intervention but rather a general principle that can be utilized during other interventions. Material can be repeated verbally and through music in a way that may help a person to "take it in." For example, information about the materials that are being used can be stated each time they are brought out (e.g. "We are passing the drum from person to person," "Each person is contributing one word to our lyrics"), or musical procedures can be repeated (e.g. first one person, then the next, expresses their feelings on a percussion instrument). Each of these repetitions allows the reality to be repeated and increases the likelihood that the client will be oriented to reality.

27.5.2.14 Song discussion

Skill/area targeted: Emotional issues.

Age group: Adults; can be adapted for older children.

Setting: Individual or group.

Equipment: CD player or iPod to play recorded music; live music played by therapist or assistant or performed by clients.

Step-by-step procedure:

1 Ask the client(s) to select a song that is meaningful to them or that elicits emotional or cognitive issues.

2 Listen to the song one or more times.

3 The therapist facilitates discussion, which may begin by asking the client(s) to describe the emotions represented in the song. Cues that have been suggested to facilitate this (see Baker and Tamplin, 2006, pp. 207–8) include the following questions:

   a What events took place?

   b Who was the main character?

c What type of person was the main character?

d What was the overall message of the song?

e What feelings were expressed in the song, and did they change?

4 Encourage the client(s) to reflect upon how the themes from the song are similar or different to their own situation. Baker and Tamplin suggest the following questions (from Gardstrom, 2001):

a What thoughts and feelings ran through your mind as you listened to the song?

b Did you attempt to suppress or control any feelings?

c What images, memories, or associations did the song evoke? And did you try to repress any of these?

d How closely did the song match your own thoughts and feelings?

5 Other questions that may be appropriate near the end of the session (from Baker and Tamplin, 2006) include the following:

a What have you learned about yourself, your situation, or that of others through listening to the song and our discussion together?

b Is there anything you can take with you from the song or from our discussion about the song that will help you this week?

27.5.2.15 Songwriting: I

Skill/area targeted: Adjustment issues.

Age group: Children or adults.

Setting: Individual or group.

Equipment: A board or large sheet of paper on which to write song words; an accompanying instrument (optional).

Step-by-step procedure:

1 Generate a range of topics.

2 Select a topic for further exploration.

3 Brainstorm ideas related to this topic.

4 Identify the principal idea, thought, emotion, or concept within the topic (which will be the focus of the chorus).

5 Develop the ideas identified as central to the topic.

6 Group related points together.

7 Discard the irrelevant or least important points.

8 Construct an outline of the main theme.

9 Write the lyrics.

Techniques that may be used within the above framework (for details, see Baker and Tamplin, 2006; see also examples in Robb, 1996) include the following:

1 *Filling in the blank (word substitution).* Select a pre-composed familiar song and adapt the lyrics to reflect the issues discussed in therapy.

2 *Song parody.* Use the music of a pre-composed song, but completely replace the lyrics with lyrics generated by the participant(s).

3 *Song collage.* The clients look through music books or lyric sheets and select words or phrases from pre-composed songs that stand out or have personal significance; the therapist may suggest songs.

4 *Rhyme technique.* The clients create lists of words that rhyme; the therapist may provide cues or give suggestions.

5 *Therapeutic lyric creation.* Original lyrics and music are created.

Figure 27.5 shows the words developed by students in an MPC session that used songwriting.

27.5.2.16 Songwriting: II

Skill/area targeted: Self-concept after injury.

Age group: Children or adults.

Setting: Individual or group.

Equipment: A board or large sheet of paper on which to write song words; an accompanying instrument (optional).

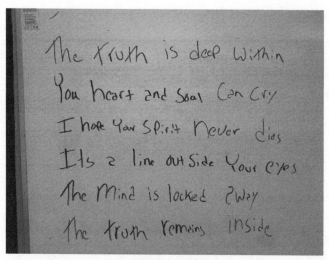

Fig. 27.5 Lyrics written by students in the MRVSEC Oasis program in Jordan, MN, to the song "A Beautiful Lie" by the band 30 Seconds To Mars. Students first listened to the original lyrics, and then participated in a group discussion of the question "What does the song mean to you?" The last step was to write their own verse to the song and sing the new lyrics, led by music therapist Glen Helgeson, MEd, MT-BC, Neurologic Music Therapist. The MPC goals were to explore feelings and express those feelings in a music therapy setting.

Step-by-step procedure (to be used in conjunction with the procedure from Songwriting: I):

1 Discuss details of the client's pre-injury self, including their goals and aspirations, likes, dislikes, personality, and characteristics.

2 Facilitate the client's discussion of their post-injury self, including the same areas as in Step 1.

3 Facilitate the client's brainstorming of strengths, in particular the similarities and differences between their pre- and post-injury self.

4 Use this material within the songwriting exercise to facilitate reflection, or use cognitive strategies (e.g. generating positive statements) and incorporate these into the song.

Acknowledgments

The author wishes to thank the following colleagues for feedback on and assistance with this chapter: Felicity Baker, Shannon de l'Etoile, Rachel (Firchau) Gonzalez, James Gardiner, Glen Helgesen, Donald Hodges, Ben Keim, Blythe LaGasse, Wendy Magee, Katrina McFerran, Suzanne Oliver, Edward Roth, Jeanette Tamplin, and Sabina Toomey. Some of the exercise examples presented in the Clinical Protocols section were developed by James Gardiner, Rachel (Firchau) Gonzalez, Glen Helgesen, Suzanne Oliver, and Michael Thaut, or adapted from Hiller (1989) or Prigatano (1991).

References

Albersnagel, F. A. (1988). Velten and musical mood induction procedures: a comparison with accessibility of thought associations. *Behavior Research and Therapy, 26*, 79–96.

Anshel, A. and Kipper, D. A. (1988). The influence of group singing on trust and cooperation. *Journal of Music Therapy, 25*, 145–55.

Bachevalier, J. and Loveland, K. A. (2006). The orbitofrontal-amygdala circuit and self-regulation of social-emotional behavior in autism. *Neuroscience and Biobehavioral Reviews, 30*, 97–117.

Baker, F. (2002). Rationale for the effects of familiar music on agitation and orientation levels of people experiencing posttraumatic amnesia. *Nordic Journal of Music Therapy, 10*, 31–41.

Baker, F. (2009). *Post Traumatic Amnesia and Music: managing behaviour through song*. Saarbrücken, Germany: VDM Verlag.

Baker, F. and Tamplin, J. (2006). *Music Therapy Methods in Neurorehabilitation: a clinician's manual*. London: Jessica Kingsley Publishers.

Bandura, A. (1977). *Social Learning Theory*. Englewood Cliffs, NJ: Prentice Hall.

Bandura, A. (1986). *Social Foundations of Thought and Action: a social cognitive theory*. Englewood Cliffs, NJ: Prentice-Hall.

Barker, V. L. and Brunk, B. (1991). The role of a creative arts group in the treatment of clients with traumatic brain injury. *Music Therapy Perspectives, 9*, 26–31.

Baumann, M. et al. (2007). *Beiträge zur Musiktherapie [Indications for Music Therapy in Neurological Rehabilitation]*. Berlin: Deutsche Gesellschaft für Musiktherapie.

Baumgartner, T., Esslen, M., and Jäncke, L. (2006). From emotion perception to emotion experience: emotions evoked by pictures and classical music. *International Journal of Psychophysiology, 60*, 34–43.

Blood, A. J. and Zatorre, R. J. (2001). Intensely pleasurable responses to music correlate with activity in brain regions implicated in reward and emotion. *Proceedings of the National Academy of Sciences of the USA*, *98*, 11818–23.

Blood, A. J., Zatorre, R. J., Bermudez, P., and Evans, A. C. (1999). Emotional responses to pleasant and unpleasant music correlate with activity in paralimbic brain regions. *Nature Neuroscience*, *2*, 382–7.

Bower, G. H. (1981). Mood and memory. *American Psychologist*, *36*, 129–48.

Bradt., J. et al. (2010). Music therapy for adults with acquired brain injury. *Cochrane Database of Systematic Reviews*, *Issue 7*, CD006787.

Brown, S., Martinez, M. J., and Parsons, L. M. (2004). Passive music listening spontaneously engages limbic and paralimbic systems. *NeuroReport*, *15*, 2033–7.

Chen, X. (1992). Active music therapy for senile depression. *Chinese Journal of Neurology and Psychiatry*, *25*, 208–10.

Clark, D. and Teasdale, J. (1985). Constraints of the effects of mood on memory. *Journal of Personality and Social Psychology*, *48*, 1595–608.

Clark, D. M. (1983). On the induction of depressed mood in the laboratory: evaluation of the Velten and musical procedures. *Advances in Behavior Research and Therapy*, *5*, 27–49.

Cross, P. et al. (1984). Observations on the use of music in rehabilitation of stroke patients. *Physiotherapy Canada*, *36*, 197–201.

Crowe, B. J. (2007). Supportive, activity-oriented music therapy: an overview. In: B. J. Crowe and C. Colwell (eds) *Music Therapy for Children, Adolescents, and Adults with Mental Disorders*. Silver Spring, MD: American Music Therapy Association. pp. 31–40.

Damasio, A. (1994). *Descartes' Error*. New York: Penguin.

de l'Etoile, S. K. (1992). *The effectiveness of music therapy in group psychotherapy for adults with mental illness*. Master's thesis. Fort Collins, CO: Colorado State University.

Eslinger, P., Stauffer, J. W., Rohrbacher, M., and Grattan, L. M. (1993). Music therapy and brain injury. *Report to the Office of Alternative Medicine at the NIH*. Bethesda, MD: National Institutes of Health.

Evers, S. and Suhr, B. (2000). Changes of the neurotransmitter serotonin but not of hormones during short time music perception. *European Archives of Psychiatry and Clinical Neuroscience*, *250*, 144–7.

Gabrielsson, A. and Juslin, P. N. (1996). Emotional expression in music performance: between the performer's intention and the listener's experience. *Psychology of Music*, *24*, 68–91.

Gardstrom, S. (2001). Practical techniques for the development of complementary skills in musical improvisation. *Music Therapy Perspectives*, *19*, 82–7.

Gendolla, G. H. E. and Křusken, J. (2001). Mood state and cardiovascular response in active coping with an affect-regulative challenge. *International Journal of Psychophysiology*, *41*, 169–80.

Gfeller, K. (2002). Music as therapeutic agent: historical and sociocultural perspectives. In: R. F. Unkefer and M. H. Thaut (eds) *Music Therapy in the Treatment of Adults with Mental Disorders*. Gilsum, NH: Barcelona Publishers. pp. 60–67.

Gilbertson, S. K. (2005). Music therapy in neurorehabilitation after traumatic brain injury: a literature review. In: D. Aldridge (ed.) *Music Therapy and Neurological Rehabilitation: performing health*. London: Jessica Kingsley Publishers. pp. 83–137.

Goldberg, F., McNiel, D., and Binder, R. (1988). Therapeutic factors in two forms of inpatient group psychotherapy: music therapy and verbal therapy. *Group*, *12*, 145–56.

Goldberg, F. S. (1992). Images of emotion: the role of emotion in guided imagery and music. *Journal of the Association for Music and Imagery*, *1*, 5–17.

Gomez, C. R. (2005). Identifying early indicators for autism in self-regulation difficulties. *Focus on Autism and Other Developmental Disabilities*, *20*, 106–16.

Gomez, P. and Danuser, B. (2004). Relationships between musical structure and psychophysiological measures of emotion. *Emotion, 7*, 377–87.

Gosselin, N. et al. (2005). Impaired recognition of scary music following unilateral temporal lobe excision. *Brain, 128*, 628–40.

Gosselin, N., Peretz, I., Johnson, E., and Adolphs, R. (2007). Amygdala damage impairs emotion recognition from music. *Neuropsychologia, 45*, 236–44.

Hanser, S. B. and Thompson, L. W. (1994). Effects of a music therapy strategy on depressed older adults. *Journal of Gerontology, 49*, 265–9.

Henderson, S. M. (1983). Effects of music therapy program upon awareness of mood in music, group cohesion, and self-esteem among hospitalized adolescent patients. *Journal of Music Therapy, 20*, 14–20.

Hendricks, C. B. (2001). A study of the use of music therapy techniques in a group for the treatment of adolescent depression. *Dissertation Abstracts International, 62*(2-A), 472.

Hiller, P. U. (1989). Song story: a potent tool for cognitive and affective relearning in head injury. *Cognitive Rehabilitation, 7*, 20–23.

Hodges, D. A. (ed.) (1996). *Handbook of Music Psychology*, 2nd edition. San Antonio, TX: IMR Press.

Hodges, D. (2010). Psychophysiological measures. In: P. Juslin and J. Sloboda (eds) *Handbook of Music and Emotion*. Oxford: Oxford University Press. pp. 279–312.

Hodges, D. and Sebald, D. (2011). *Music in the Human Experience: an introduction to music psychology*. New York: Routledge.

Houghton, B. A. et al. (2002). Taxonomy of clinical music therapy programs and techniques. In: R. F. Unkefer and M. H. Thaut (eds) *Music Therapy in the Treatment of Adults with Mental Disorders*. Gilsum, NH: Barcelona Publishers. pp. 181–206.

Huron, D. (2006). *Sweet Anticipation: music and the psychology of expectation*. Cambridge, MA: MIT Press.

Jacobson, E. (1938). *Progressive Relaxation*. Chicago: University of Chicago Press.

Juslin, P. N. and Västfjäll, D. (2008). Emotional responses to music: the need to consider underlying mechanisms. *Behavioral and Brain Sciences, 31*, 559–75.

Khalfa, S., Peretz, I., Blondin, J.-P. and Manon, R. (2002). Event-related skin conductance responses to musical emotions in humans. *Neuroscience Letters, 328*, 145–9.

Koelsch, S. et al. (2006). Investigating emotion with music: an fMRI study. *Human Brain Mapping, 27*, 239–50.

Kreutz, G. et al. (2008). Using music to induce emotions: influences of musical preference and absorption. *Psychology of Music, 36*, 101–26.

Krumhansl, C. L. (1997). An exploratory study of musical emotions and psychophysiology. *Canadian Journal of Experimental Psychology, 51*, 336–52.

Lazarus, R. S. (1984). On the primacy of cognition. *American Psychologist, 39*, 124–9.

LeDoux, J. E. (1996). *The Emotional Brain*. New York: Simon & Schuster.

Lyubomirsky, S. and Nolen-Hoeksema, S. (1993). Self-perpetuating properties of dysphoric rumination. *Journal of Personality and Social Psychology, 65*, 339–49.

Magee, W. (1999). 'Singing my life, playing my self': music therapy in the treatment of chronic neurological illness. In: T. Wigram and J. De Backer (eds) *Clinical Applications of Music Therapy in Developmental Disability, Paediatrics and Neurology*. London: Jessica Kingsley Publishers. pp. 201–23.

Magee, W. L. (in press). Music-making in therapeutic contexts: reframing identity following disruptions to health. In: R. MacDonald, D. Miell, and D. Hargreaves (eds) *The Oxford Handbook of Musical Identities*. Oxford: Oxford University Press.

Magee, W. L. and Davidson, J. W. (2002). The effect of music therapy on mood states in neurological patients: a pilot study. *Journal of Music Therapy*, *39*, 20–29.

Magee, W. L. et al. (2011). Music therapy methods with children, adolescents and adults with severe neurobehavioural disorders. *Music Therapy Perspectives*, *29*, 5–13.

Mandler, G. (1984). *Mind and Body*. New York: Norton.

Maratos, A. S., Gold, C., Wang, X., and Crawford, M. J. (2008). Music therapy for depression. *Cochrane Database of Systematic Reviews*, Issue *1*, CD004517.

Menon, V. and Levitin, D. J. (2005). The rewards of music listening: response and physiological connectivity of the mesolimbic system. *NeuroImage*, *28*, 175–84.

Mitterschiffthaler, M. T. et al. (2007). A functional MRI study of happy and sad affective states induced by classical music. *Human Brain Mapping*, *28*, 1150–62.

Molnar-Szakacs, I. and Heaton, P. (2012). Music: a unique window into the world of autism. *Annals of the New York Academy of Sciences*, *1252*, 318–24.

National Autism Center (2009). *National Standards Report*. Randolph, MA: National Autism Center.

Nayak, S., Wheeler, B. L., Shiflett, S. C. and Agostinelli, S. (2000). The effect of music therapy on mood and social interaction among individuals with acute traumatic brain injury and stroke. *Rehabilitation Psychology*, *45*, 274–83.

Nolen-Hoeksema, S. (1991). Responses to depression and their effects on the duration of depressive episodes. *Journal of Abnormal Psychology*, *100*, 560–682.

Pacchetti, C. et al. (1998). Active music therapy in Parkinson's disease: methods. *Functional Neurology*, *13*, 57–67.

Pacchetti, C. et al. (2000). Active music therapy in Parkinson's disease: an integrative method for motor and emotional rehabilitation. *Psychosomatic Medicine*, *62*, 386–93.

Peretz, I. (2001). Listen to the brain: the biological perspective on musical emotions. In: P. Juslin and J. Sloboda (eds) *Music and Emotion: theory and research*. Oxford: Oxford University Press. pp. 105–34.

Peretz, I. (2010). Towards a neurobiology of musical emotions. In: P. N. Juslin and J. A. Sloboda (eds) *Handbook of Music and Emotion: theory, research, applications*. New York: Oxford University Press. pp. 99–126.

Pignatiello, M. F., Camp, C. J., and Rasar, L. (1986). Musical mood induction: an alternative to the Velten technique. *Journal of Abnormal Psychology*, *95*, 295–7.

Prigatano, G. P. (1991). Disordered mind, wounded soul: the emerging role of psychotherapy in rehabilitation after brain injury. *Journal of Head Trauma Rehabilitation*, *6*, 1–10.

Prigatano, G. P. (1999). *Principles of Neuropsychological Rehabilitation*. New York: Oxford University Press.

Purdie, H. (1997). Music therapy in neurorehabilitation: recent developments and new challenges. *Critical Reviews in Physical and Rehabilitation Medicine*, *9*, 205–17.

Purdie, H., Hamilton, S., and Baldwin, S. (1997). Music therapy: facilitating behavioural and psychological change in people with stroke—a pilot study. *International Journal of Rehabilitation Research*, *20*, 325–7.

Radulovic, R., Cvetkovic, M., and Pejovic, M. (1997). *Complementary musical therapy and medicamentous therapy in treatment of depressive disorders*. Paper presented at the World Psychiatric Association (WPA) Thematic Conference, Jerusalem, Israel, November 1997.

Robb, S. L. (1996). Techniques in song writing: restoring emotional and physical well being in adolescents who have been traumatically injured. *Music Therapy Perspectives*, *14*, 30–37.

Salimpoor, V. N. et al. (2009) The rewarding aspects of music listening are related to degree of emotional arousal. *PLoS ONE*, *4*, e7487.

Sarkamo, T. et al. (2008). Music listening enhances cognitive recovery and mood after middle cerebral artery stroke. *Brain*, *131*, 866–76.

Sarkamo, T. et al. (2010). Music and speech listening enhance the recovery of early sensory processing after stroke. *Journal of Cognitive Neuroscience*, *22*, 2716–27.

Scheiby, B. B. (1999). Music as symbolic expression: analytical music therapy. In: D. J. Wiener (ed.) *Beyond Talk Therapy: using movement and expressive techniques in clinical practice*. Washington, DC: American Psychological Association. pp. 263–85.

Sears, W. (1968). Processes in music therapy. In: E. T. Gaston (ed.) *Music in Therapy*. New York: Macmillan. pp. 30–44.

Soto, D. et al. (2009). Pleasant music overcomes the loss of awareness in patients with visual neglect. *Proceedings of the National Academy of Sciences of the USA*, *106*, 6011–16.

Sutherland, G., Newman, B., and Rachman, S. (1982). Experimental investigations of the relations between mood and intrusive, unwanted cognitions. *British Journal of Medical Psychology*, *55*, 127–38.

Teasdale, J. (1983). Negative thinking in depression: cause, effect, or reciprocal relationship? *Advances in Behaviour Research and Therapy*, *5*, 3–25.

Teasdale, J. and Taylor, R. (1981). Induced mood and accessibility of memories: an effect of mood state or of induction procedure? *British Journal of Clinical Psychology*, *20*, 39–48.

Teasdale, J. D. and Spencer, P. (1984). Induced mood and estimates of past success. *British Journal of Clinical Psychology*, *23*, 149–50.

Thaut, M. H. (1989a). Music therapy, affect modification, and therapeutic change: towards an integrative model. *Music Therapy Perspectives*, *7*, 55–62.

Thaut, M. H. (1989b). The influence of music therapy interventions on self-rated changes in relaxation, affect and thought in psychiatric prisoner-patients. *Journal of Music Therapy*, *26*, 155–66.

Thaut, M. H. (2002). Toward a cognition–affect model in neuropsychiatric music therapy. In: R. F. Unkefer and M. H. Thaut (eds) *Music Therapy in the Treatment of Adults with Mental Disorders*. Gilsum, NH: Barcelona Publishers. pp. 86–116.

Thaut, M. H. (2005). *Rhythm, Music, and the Brain: scientific foundations and clinical applications*. New York: Routledge.

Thaut, M. H. and Wheeler, B. L. (2010). Music therapy. In: P. Juslin and J. Sloboda (eds) *Handbook of Music and Emotion*. Oxford: Oxford University Press. pp. 819–48.

Velten, E. (1968). A laboratory task for induction of mood states. *Behavioral Research and Therapy*, *6*, 607–17.

Wheeler, B. L. (1983). A psychotherapeutic classification of music therapy practices: a continuum of procedures. *Music Therapy Perspectives*, *1*, 8–12.

Zajonc, R. (1984). Feeling and thinking: preferences need no inferences. *American Psychologist*, *35*, 151–75.

Zerhusen, J. D., Boyle, K., and Wilson, W. (1995). Out of the darkness: group cognitive therapy for depressed elderly. *Journal of Military Nursing Research*, *1*, 28–32.

Zwerling, I. (1979). The creative arts therapies as "real therapies." *Hospital and Community Psychiatry*, *30*, 841–4.

Author Index

Subject Index

M

MalletKat 17
massed practice 48
mediating models 4, 5
melodic intonation therapy (MIT) 140–3
  aphasia 140, 187
  children 142
  clinical protocols 142–3
  definition 140
  error correction 143
  patient selection criteria 140
  research summary 141
  shortened version 142–3
  target populations 140
  therapeutic mechanisms 141–2
melodica 170, 171
melody 85
  auditory perception training 244–5
  memory improvement 297
  speech production 199–200
memory
  external aids 296
  temporal processing 5
  types of 294–5
  see also associative mood and memory training;
    musical echoic memory training; musical
    mnemonics training
mental flexibility 281
meta-analysis 8
meter
  improvisation 26
  patterned sensory enhancement 111
  rhythmic speech cueing 150, 156, 158
mid stance 99
mid swing 99
MIDI interface 14
mirror neurons 222
mixed dysarthria 152, 153, 159
mnemonics 294
modeling 201, 204
modes, improvisation 29–30
mood
  arousal and 223
  cognitive reorientation 334, 344
  induction 317–18, 344–5
  memory and 316
  music and 39, 85, 337–8
  music in psychosocial training and counseling
    44–5, 334–5, 337–8, 340–5
  state-dependent memory 316–17, 318
  tempo 26
motivation
  motor learning 9
  musical executive function training 284
  therapeutical instrumental music performance 120
Motor Activity Log (MAL) 50–1
motor impairment classification 116–17
motor learning
  constraint-induced therapy 48
  elementary rules 9–10
  musical instrument playing 121

rhythm 5, 118
motor performance, attention and 57
motor scales 66
movement sensors 17–18
multiple sclerosis
  associative mood and memory training 315
  musical attention control training 258
  musical executive function training 280
  musical mnemonics training 295, 297
  rhythmic auditory stimulation 95, 104
  self-awareness 339
  therapeutic singing 186
  vocal exercises 180
multisystem atrophy 189–90
Munich Intelligibility Profile 154
muscle activity
  patterned sensory enhancement 112–13
  priming 96
  rhythmic entrainment 120
  tempo 26
  timbre 37
muscular dystrophy 162–3, 169
music in psychosocial training and counseling
    (MPC) 6, 331–55
  affect 333–4, 335–7, 340–5
  anger management 342–3
  arousal 335, 336, 341–2
  clinical protocols 340–55
  communication 345–6
  definition 331–3
  emotional continuum 340–1
  empathy 343
  improvisation 39, 44–5, 343–4
  interaction 345–6
  iPod/iPad 18–19
  Kaossilator 19
  keyboards 15
  leading and following 346
  mood induction and vectoring 44–5, 334–5,
    337–8, 340–5
  reality orientation 352
  reinforcement (behavior modification) 346–7
  relationship training 347–8
  relaxation 348–9
  research summary 335–9
  role playing 348
  scripts 351–2
  self-awareness 335, 338–9, 345–55
  social competence training 39, 44, 335, 338–9,
    345–55
  songs 349–51, 352–5
  Soundbeam 18
  target populations 333
  therapeutic mechanisms 333–5
  writing songs 353–5
music technology 12–22
  brain–music interface system 21
  digital hand-held devices 18–19
  hardware 14–19
  instruments and triggers 14–17
  movement sensors 17–18